Vascular Access for Hemodialysis—IV

Vascular Access for Hemodialysis—IV

MITCHELL L. HENRY, M.D.
RONALD M. FERGUSON, M.D., Ph.D.

W.L. Gore & Associates, Inc.
Precept Press

Library of Congress Cataloging-in-Publication Data
Vascular access for hemodialysis—IV / [edited by] Mitchell L. Henry.
Ronald M. Ferguson.
p. cm.
Includes bibliographical references and index.
ISBN 0-944496-45-8 (cloth)
1. Hemodialysis. 2. Blood-vessels-Surgery. I. Henry Mitchell L. II. Ferguson, Ronald M.
[DNLM: 1. Vascular Surgery—methods. 2. Kidney Failure, Chronic—therapy. 3. Hemodialysis. 4. Arteriovenous Shunt, Surgical. 5. Catheters, Indwelling.
WG 170 V32755 1995]
RC901.7.H45V37 1995
617.4'61059—dc20
DNLM/DLC
for Library of Congress 95-16238
CIP

99 98 97 96 95 5 4 3 2 1

CONTENTS

ACKNOWLEDGMENTS

Drs. Mitchell L. Henry and Ronald M. Ferguson wish to thank the Medical Products Division of W.L. Gore and Associates, Inc., for their substantial support and help in organizing the ongoing series of two-day symposia on hemodialysis access. Their support has been essential to make possible this unique gathering of individuals interested in vascular access. W.L. Gore also made a substantial contribution toward underwriting the publication cost of this book, which is a direct result of the Fourth Symposium of Dialysis Access. The authors would also like to thank Cindy Narcross and Joni Ashcraft for their time and effort in organizing the conference and transcript preparation. A special thanks to the many efforts of Joni Ashcraft in final preparation and editing of the manuscripts for this book.

PREFACE

In our previous book, *Vascular Access for Hemodialysis-III*, it was demonstrated that vascular access related morbidity was, by a wide margin, the most common cause for hospital admission in a large population of patients with end-stage renal disease. In this same patient population, hospital days due to vascular access problems nearly doubled from the beginning of 1989 to the end of 1990. These data continue to remind us of the significance of these problems to the physicians caring for the patients, the resources allocated to correct the problems, and, most important, to the patients themselves.

This book is the direct result of the Fourth Symposium on Dialysis Access. Presentations at the symposium included many of the standard issues in vascular access, but also touched on newer technologies as they are applied to these same problems. The presenters, authors, and participants really made this a valuable experience and in this book we hoped to capture these and share them with others.

We hope to continue to gather together regularly to ponder, consider, and debate these issues in order to have a positive impact on the morbidity of vascular access. We may then be able to improve the delivery of care of end-stage renal disease patients.

SECTION I

1

INCIDENCE AND CAUSES OF ACCESS FAILURE

Richard Dickerman, M.D., James Robison, M.D., and Jeffrey Seigel, M.D.

THE APPROACH TO THE NONFUNCTIONING DIALYSIS GRAFT continues to be a frustrating and challenging procedure for the vascular access surgeon. The number of patients on chronic dialysis continues to increase as nephrologists accept older candidates, patients live longer, and loss of transplanted kidneys return people to dialysis and renew the need for dependable access.[1] Long-term function of these grafts has been shown to be dependent upon the surgeon's or radiologist's ability to salvage graft failure.[2] As with any vascular graft, the basic requirements of adequate inflow and outflow are tantamount. In addition, the conduit that is placed will, to some degree, have an effect on long-term function.

Study Methods

Methodist Medical Center, Dallas, serves as a referral center for approximately 600 of the 1,100 patients on chronic hemodialysis in the city. A retrospective study was done on 225 patients who underwent 930 procedures between 1989 and 1993 for failed grafts. Patients who were undergoing placement of new grafts or those undergoing revision of functioning grafts on an elective basis were not included in this study.

The mechanism of failure of the graft was divided into venous thrombosis, which included diseases of the venous outflow tract (as well as peridialysis hypotension) and four other causes of failure. These mechanisms and the number and percentage of patients affected by each are shown in table 1-1. The operative procedures included embolectomy and dilation, interposition grafting, and patch angioplasty. New grafts were placed in 10% of the patients. Embolectomy with

Table 1-1. Dialysis Access Failure Mechanisms, 1989-1994 (930 Procedures in 225 Patients)

Failure mechanism	No.	%
Venous thromboses (peridialysis hypotension)	573	67
Arterial inflow	46	5
Conduit disease	101	12
Infection	53	6
Aneurysm	74	9

Table 1-2. Operative Procedure

Interposition grafting	36%
Embolectomy and dilation	36%
Patch angioplasty	18%
New graft	10%
Embolectomy and angiography	14%

Table 1-3. Number of Procedures

1	18%
2–4	36%
5–7	29%
8–10	11%
>10	6%

arteriography alone where no local anatomical problem was detected was seen in 14% of the patients within the operating room (table 1-2). Also included was an attempt to divide the patients according to the number of procedures performed for each (table 1-3). Additional data revealed an average hemoglobin of 9.3 g and a hematocrit of 28 volumes/percent. We identified 12 patients who had subclavian vein thrombosis, eight of whom were found to be bilateral.

Surgery Versus Radiology

Whether the approach to the failed graft is surgical or radiological, the knowledge of how the pathological processes involve the graft will determine the long-term outcome. The question of whether to approach the failed graft by radiological thrombolysis or surgical exploration will vary at each center. Relative contraindications of recent surgery, gastrointestinal bleeding, or hypotension may deter some radiologists, while others, believing that the systemic effect of urokinase (UK) used with graft salvage is minimal, will proceed. At our center, we have found certain clinical settings that one may term curable, others that are helpful, and finally those that are doomed to failure. The best setting appears to be that of graft thrombosis that has been documented with hypotension. There is a definite dialysis population that because of their disease process, i.e., diabetes, or because of attempts that remove of large volumes of fluid, will experience a drop in their

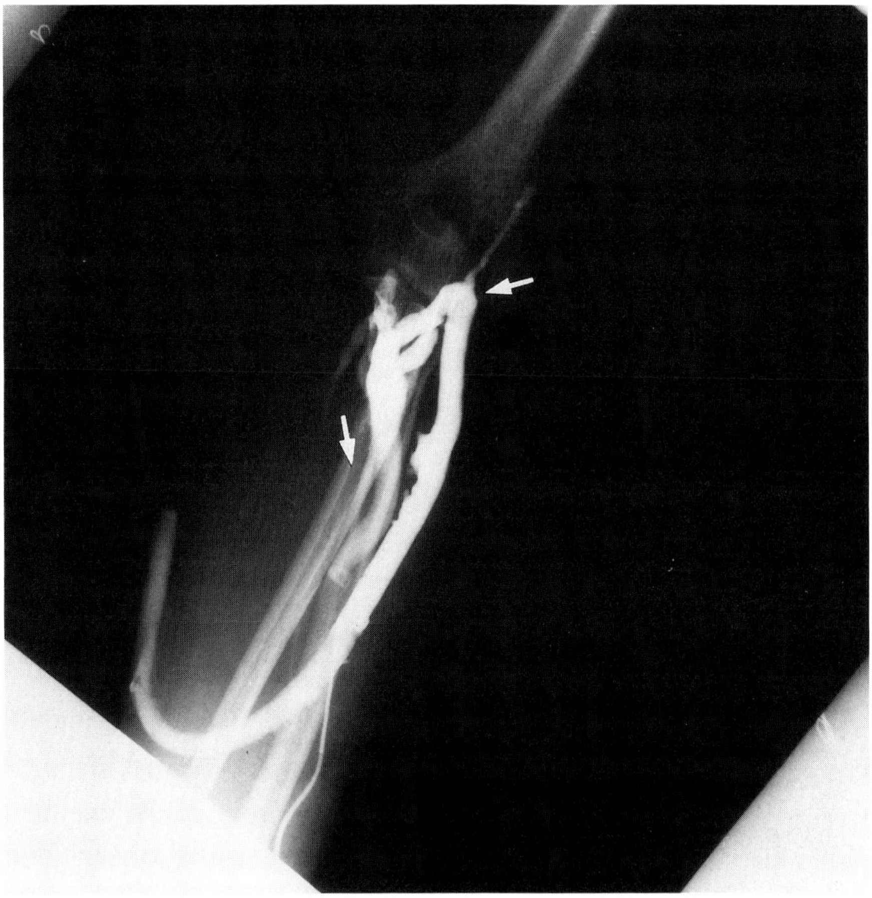

Figure 1-1. Venous outflow of forearm graft.

systolic pressure after dialysis. In our hands, this group is the best for UK thrombolysis. Other patients who may sustain cardiac arrhythmias or cardiac arrests are good candidates following stabilization. Finally, the small population of patients who do have a hypocoagulable state or in whom no anatomical or rheological abnormalities have been detected have had excellent outcomes.

Patients who have thrombosed grafts that have been functional for long periods will have only a fair long-term result in the radiologist's hands. The reason for this is obvious to most surgeons who deal with these patients routinely. The venous outflow obstruction that is detected as the culprit is so dense that rethrombosis is frequent (figure 1-1). The recent addition of balloon angioplasty with stent placement has increased the immediate patency results; however, the long-term patency may not be as encouraging.[3,4] An important fact to remember is that even if the graft re-thromboses early following thrombolysis, the experienced radiologist will be able to provide a study that will act as a "road map" for the surgeon to define the exact level of obstruction and the number of sites involved (figure 1-2). For this reason, we have not discouraged our radiologists from performing these procedures.

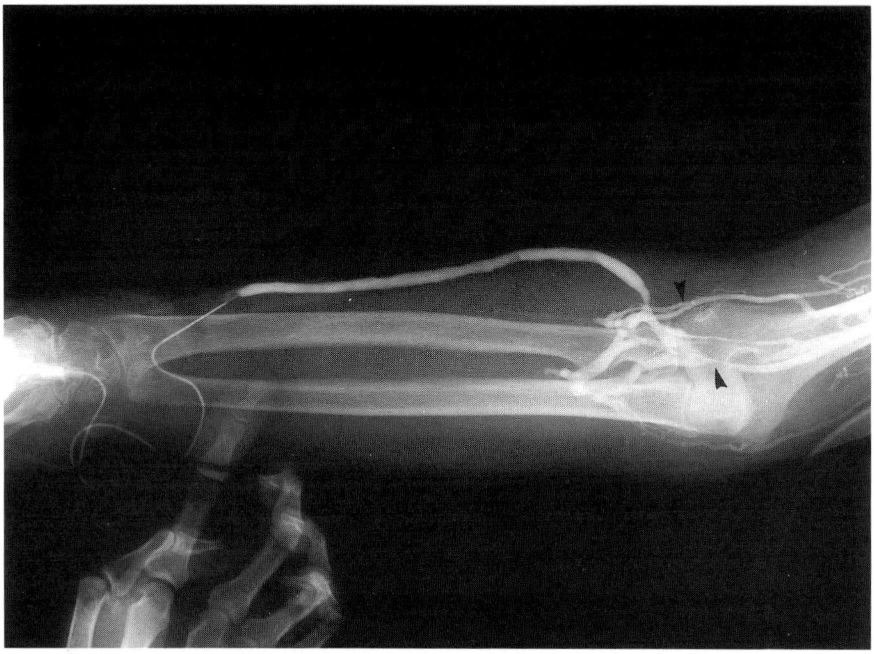

Figure 1-2. Angiogram demonstrating abnormalities of direct surgical consideration.

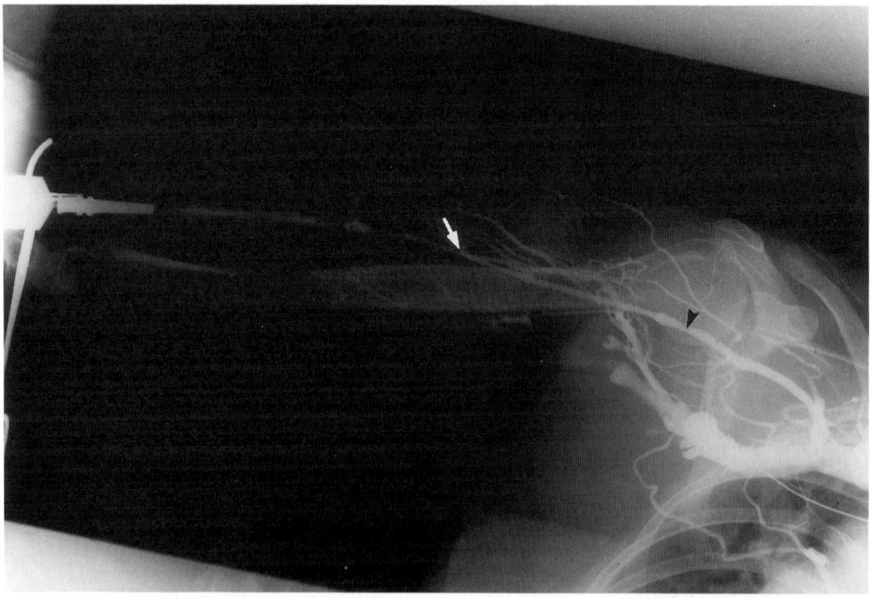

Figure 1-3. Angiogram demonstrating inadequate venous caliber precluding graft placement.

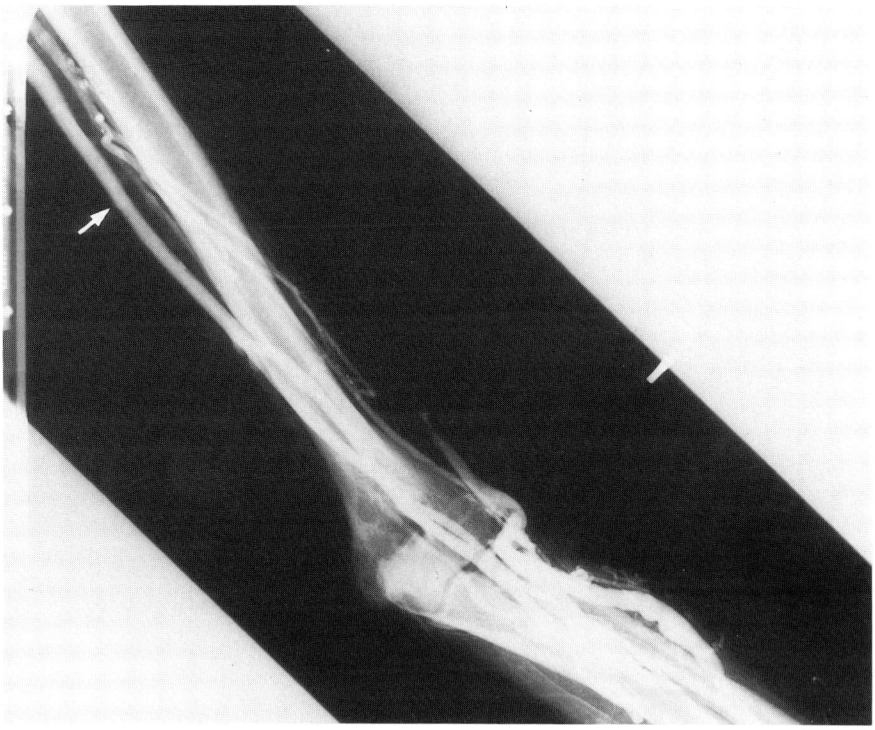

Figure 1-4. Angiogram demonstrating large basilic vein that can readily be used for outflow tract.

The group of patients in which we have virtually abandoned thrombolysis is made up of those who have had recent graft placement and thromboses within one to three months. The reason for this is that if there is no hypotension or trauma to the graft, the grafts in this group invariably will have poor outflow secondary to vein caliber size and will need exploration for an alternate site of venous outflow (figure 1-3).

Surgical Approaches

The decision to approach the failed graft in the operating room should be done with a logical approach based on the disease process involved. After almost 15 years at our institution, which deals with more than 900 dialysis patients, we continue to use inflow, outflow, and conduit as our guideline for approach and treatment.

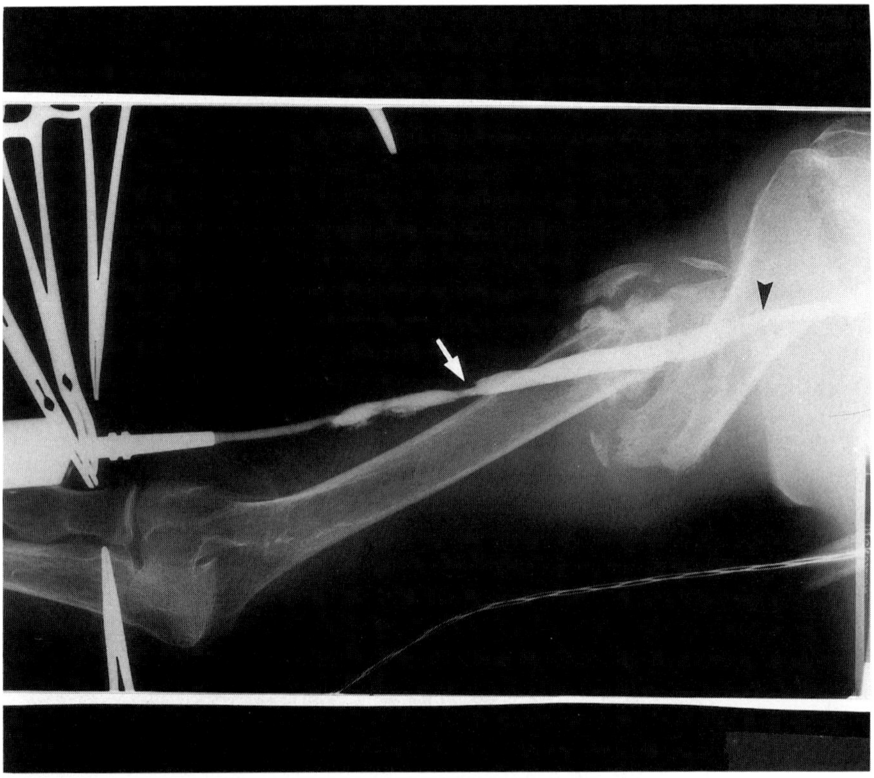

Figure 1-5. Segmental stenotic lesions.

The venous outflow of the graft continues to be the most common site for graft failure. The point of anastomosis at the graft to the vein elicits a fibroplastic reaction that has been extensively described.[5,6] This area of injury, which can vary from gelatinous to fibrotic, should be the first area approached surgically. Repair of this area can be accomplished by several methods. Almost exclusively, we now use interposition grafting of small segments of new graft to vein just above the affected site or to new outflow system if the original one is too involved with fibrosis or clot. The use of patch angioplasty with polytetrafluoroethylene (PTFE) or autogenous tissue has been used and will fare well with short segmental areas of stenosis. An important secondary outflow system to remember is that of the basilic vein, which lies just above the olecranon process medially (figure 1-4). On occasion, when the graft has been placed from the brachial artery to the axillary vein, and the area of fibrosis is at the anastomotic site, the distal end of the graft can be excised, mobilized, and re-anastomosed to a segment of vein without the use of a new segment.

The experienced access surgeon should remember that the venous outflow system does not stop at the point of vein-to-graft anastomosis. This important corollary can be the single most common reason for failure to salvage a thrombosed graft. One must find a reason for the graft failure in the operating room if thrombosis is not secondary to hypotension or technical problems surrounding needle punctures. If no significant fibrodysplasia is found at the vein-to-anastomotic site, then the venous system needs to be investigated from the arm to the heart by intraoperative

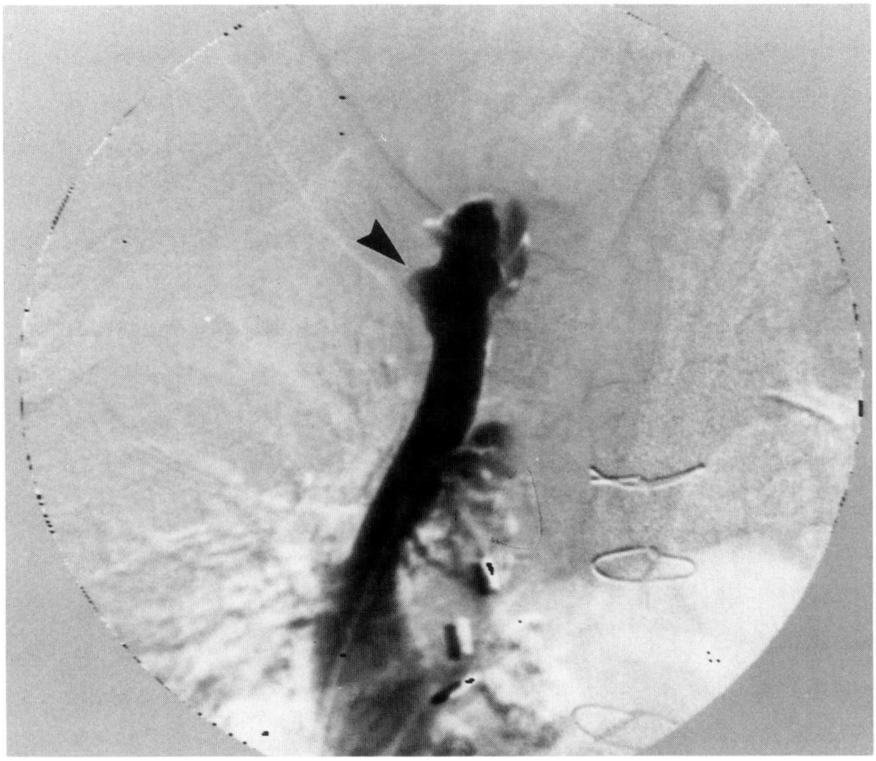

Figure 1-6. Subclavian vein occlusion.

angiography and vessel exploration. A significant number of our patients have continued to present with segmental stenotic lesions or thrombosis of cephalic or basilic venous systems well into the axillary and subclavian veins (figure 1-5).

The literature currently contains increasingly frequent descriptions of incidences of subclavian vein thrombosis, most probably secondary to long-term cannulation with temporary dialysis catheters.[7] When no technical reason can be found at the venous outflow and a good pulsatile inflow is returned to the graft following thrombectomy, the surgeon should expect underlying subclavian vein thrombosis if the area of stenosis cannot be found in the outflow of the arm (figure 1-6). If intraoperative angiography is done on the outflow system in the normal arm, an attempt should be made to obtain films near the thoracic inlet. Even if one cannot demonstrate the actual occlusion, the course of the dye going up into the neck will be indicative of a central thrombosis and alert the surgeon to the presence of subclavian vein thrombosis (figure 1-7). The surgeon should be alerted to the presence of this condition if the patient has multiple collaterals in the arm or a history of significant swelling of the arm prior to the thrombosis. Exploration of the venous outflow tract with dilators and Fogarty catheter is helpful in detecting stenotic areas that are closer to the anastomotic site and may be found in tandem with disease at a more proximal level. These areas may be treated by dilation itself or can be approached by intraoperative balloon angioplasty. It has been an extremely productive relationship to have the radiologist present in the operating room with the surgeon who is

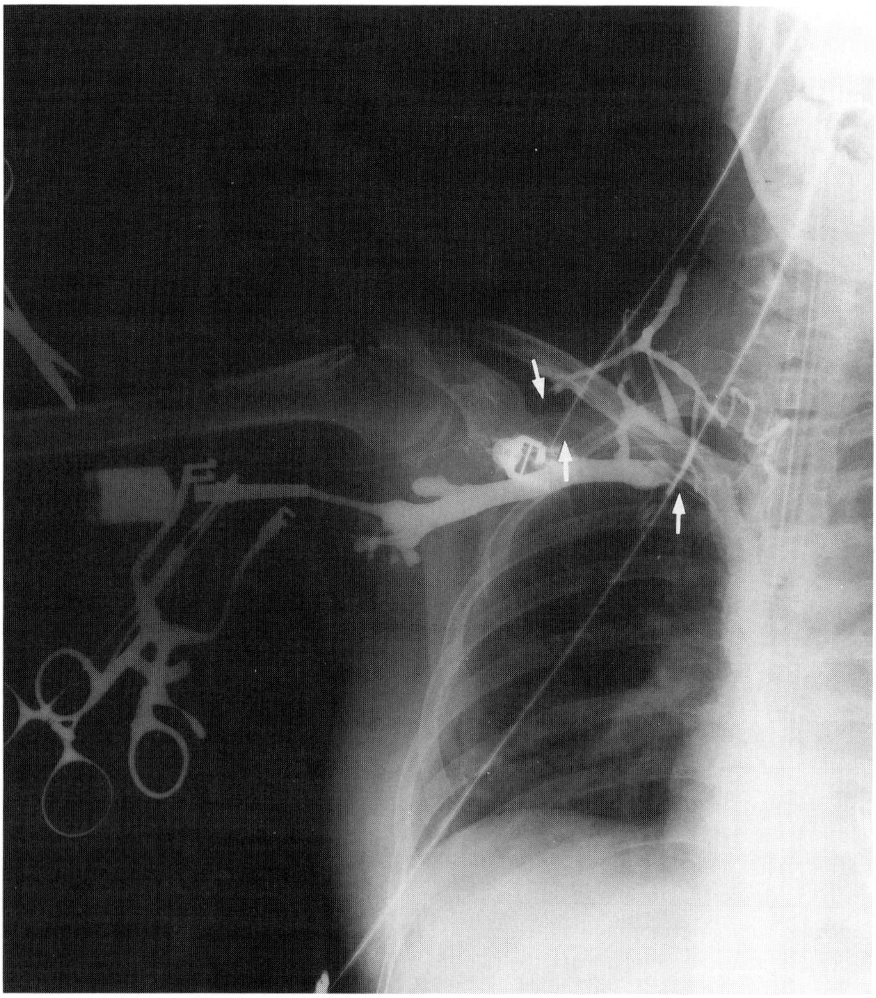

Figure 1-7. Multiple collateral vessels indicating subclavian vein occlusion.

uniformly inexperienced with the different types of balloon catheters and the newer atherectomy devices and stents. When used properly, these tools can be valuable in the operating room as well as in the angiography suite.

The outflow system of primary arteriovenous systems is unique in that the conduit and outflow are of an autogenous nature. The areas of needle puncture sites and aneurysmal disease appear to be the main source of thrombosis. Although these autogenous veins undergo repeated needle punctures, the longevity is remarkable, and they continue to be the first choice for access. Most problems with fistula thrombosis are relative to aneurysm formation in locally stenotic areas. These areas are easily detected in the operating room and can be repaired by local excision with primary re-anastomosis or short segment interposition grafts. Once again, disease at the site of the artery-to-vein anastomosis is common and should still be explored when the fistula presents thrombosed. If the source of thrombosis is a stricture or aneurysm following thrombectomy, the pulse will stop at the point of obstruction and can be detected and repaired as described above.

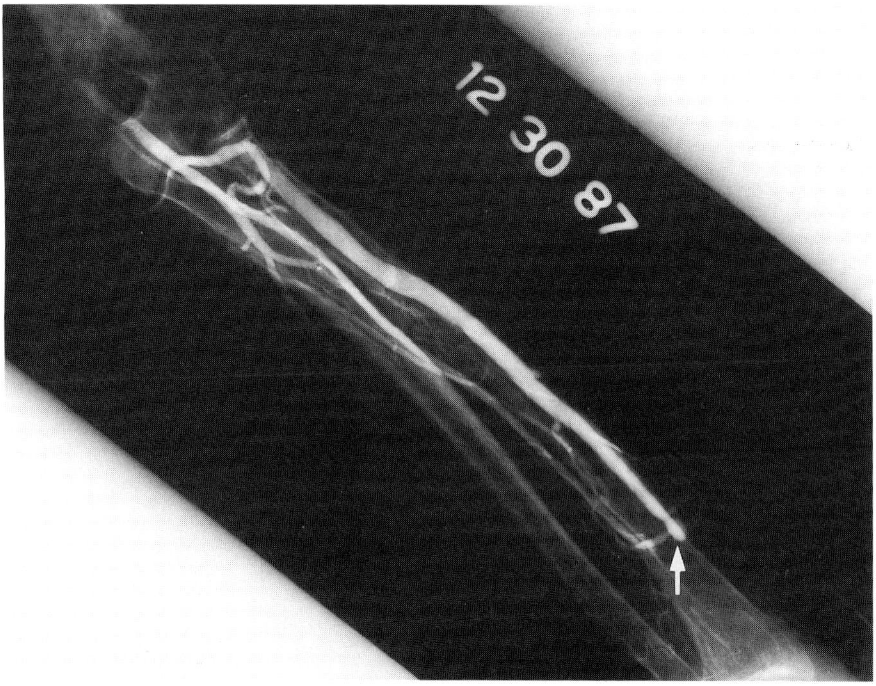

Figure 1-8. Poor flow at arterial anastomosis documented by angiogram.

Evaluation of the inflow system can be helped by a careful history as well as findings within the operating room. Graft failure in diabetic and older patients is not statistically more prevalent, but careful attention must be paid in these individuals to the caliber and quality of the arterial inflow. The history of poor flow through the arterial site of the graft, as well as a poor thrill and "soft graft," may be helpful to identify prior to approaching this type of failed graft in the operating room (figure 1-8). In our review, only about 5% of grafts failed because of poor inflow. The findings in the operating room are relatively simple to evaluate when the balloon catheter cannot pass at the arterial anastomosis or the flow restored initially stops. We will commonly obtain an angiogram through the shunt retrograde into the arterial system, which will reflux proximally and distally in the arterial tree to delineate the anatomy (figure 1-9). If this is the cause of failure of the graft, then parallel grafting from an alternative arterial inflow is the procedure of choice.

Graft Disease as Cause of Failure

Disease of the graft itself is another common cause of failure. The two most common problems are stricture secondary to repeated needle puncture sites and aneurysmal disease (figure 1-10). The first problem can be remedied by continued patient and technician education. These areas are usually easy to detect in the operating room by palpation and by the inability of the balloon catheter to navigate the

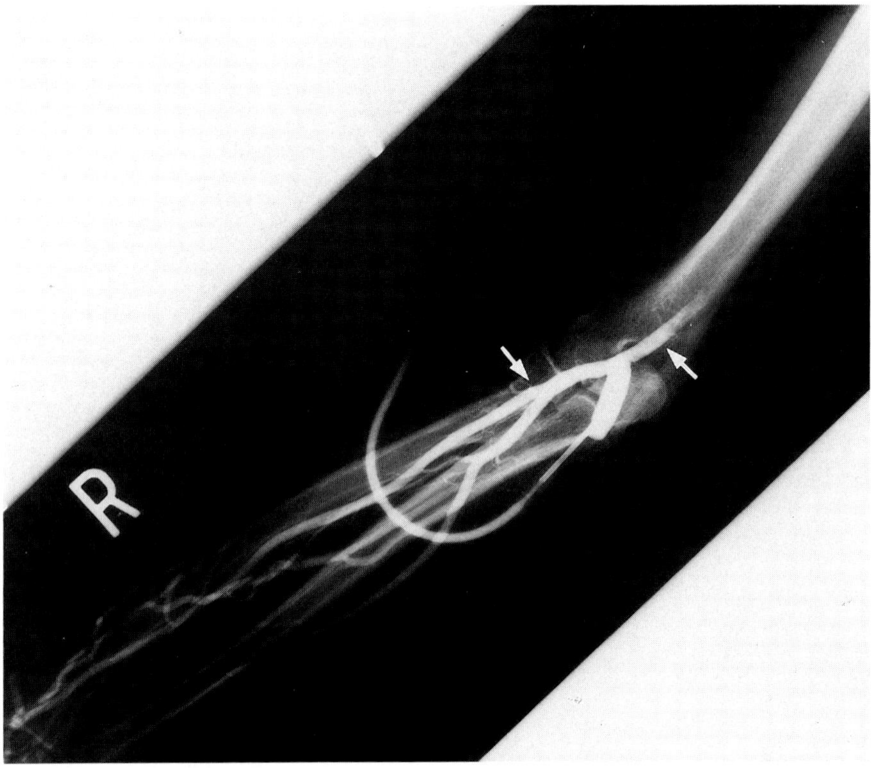

Figure 1-9. Retrograde angiogram to delineate arterial anatomy.

site during embolectomy. We have been successful at dilating these areas with 6-mm common duct dilators. These can help to dislodge the fibroplastic plug, which can then be easily removed. Curettage and metal brushes have also been employed, but they have the potential of damaging the graft itself. If these areas cannot be dilated, then parallel grafting appears to be the procedure of choice with most success in our hands.

Aneurysmal disease of the graft will continue to be problematic until conduits that are lined with true intimal cells can be developed. Until then, and for as long as dialysis technicians continue to use poor technique, aneurysmal disease will be a cause of graft failure. Most centers have extensive experience with bovine heterograft and PTFE grafts, and although reports indicate that bovine grafts do well and have only a slightly higher incidence of aneurysmal disease, PTFE grafts continue to be the most common choice of graft material.[9-11] When graft failure is either caused by or associated with aneurysmal disease, more extensive surgery may be required to replace segments of the graft. A local approach to an aneurysmal segment of the graft is possible with repair of the defect in the graft by patch angioplasty; however, the area needed for control and exposure may significantly cut down on the available area needed for needle puncture site in the future.

Although infection can be problematic in dialysis access, few grafts will present as actual thrombosis as a result of an infected needle puncture site or aneurysm. We found that only 6% of the grafts we operated on for salvage presented with

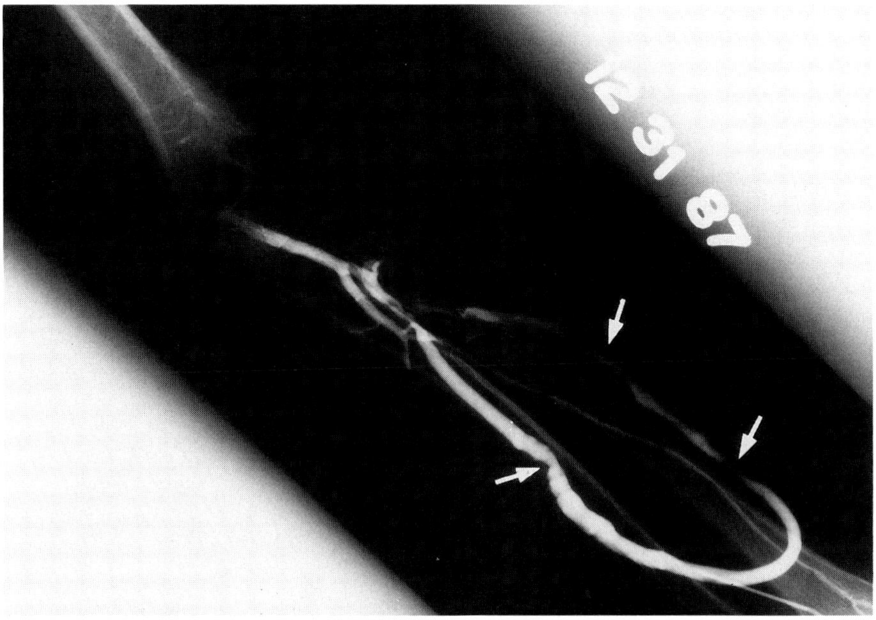

Figure 1-10. Multiple structure secondary to repeated needle puncture sites.

significant infection from rupturing graft or infected pseudoaneurysms. About half of these grafts are salvaged by excision and bypass of the infected segment, but others require ligation of the graft because of significant edema and cellulitis of the involved extremity. The remaining causes of graft failure make up a small group of patients with peridialysis hypotension, trauma from needle puncture sites, and the very occasional hypercoagulable state.

Conclusion

Our data reflected that there were 225 patients reviewed over a five-year period who underwent 930 procedures. The subpopulation of conduit failure included 16 procedures that were related to significant laceration of the graft, needle punctures that caused large perigraft hematomas and eventual thrombosis. Our belief differs greatly from that of the group advocating early PTFE puncture.[12,13] Also included in the 573 procedures in which venous thrombosis was listed as the cause were 34 procedures in 12 patients where continued hypotension was documented as the cause of graft failure. Most of these patients were eventually placed on permanent Silastic catheters for dialysis.

Another small group of patients that needs to be identified is the extremely small group presenting with a hypercoagulable state.[14] We found only an additional three patients over that five-year period that we could identify with abnormal clotting studies, two of whom had lupus and one who was HIV-positive. When a hypercoagulable state is suspected, a battery of tests should be given that includes the

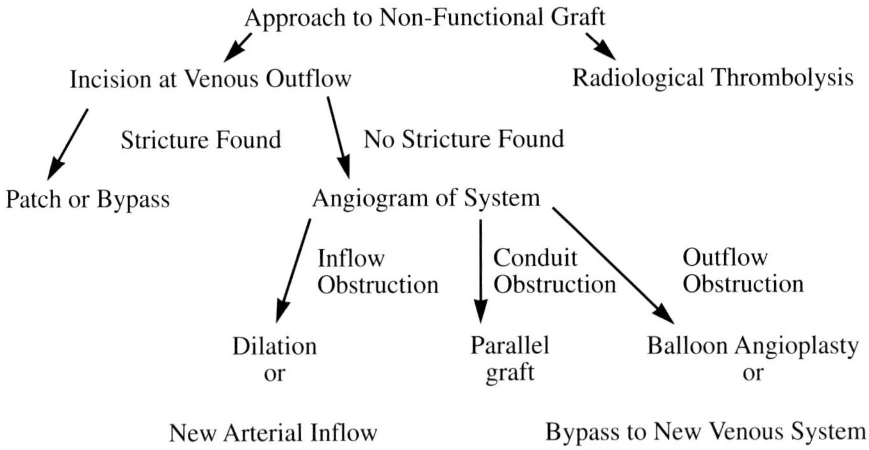

Figure 1–11. Flow chart of approaches to treatment of clotted grafts.

detection of antithrombin III deficiency and protein C and S deficiency. Disorders of the fibrinolytic system, including hypoplasminogenemia, abnormal plasminogen, and plasminogen activator factor, dysfibrinogenemia, factor 12 deficiency, and lupus anticoagulant should also be identified. One factor that was suspected as a cause of a higher incidence of graft failure compared to our initial experience was the use of recombinant erythropoietin. The average hematocrit of our patients was 28 volumes/percent, whereas eight years before, in a similar group of patients with graft thrombosis, hematocrit averaged 22 volumes/percent. However, no direct effect on graft thrombosis could be identified.

The above discussion grew out of many years of experience with graft failure. The knowledge acquired from these patients has now led us to approach the clotted grafts as shown in figure 1-11. Once the decision to proceed with operative therapy has been reached, we always approach the graft at the venous anastomosis first unless the graft is infected and hemorrhaging. If obvious pathology is found, we approach this with either interposition grafting or patch angioplasty to suitable venous outflow. If no stricture is found at the venous anastomosis, then we proceed with investigation of more distal venous outflow. If this move is again not productive, the inflow and conduit are evaluated by the techniques described in this paper. The treatment of pathology found is based on good angiographic and surgical findings as summarized in the algorithm. One should remember that although the goal is salvage of the failed access, the surgeon should not pursue a totally diseased outflow system or a graft that is decimated by strictures when the placement of a totally new graft will take less time in the operating room and cause less discomfort for the patient. If these logical steps are followed and good surgical technique is applied, the difficult problem of graft failure can be made somewhat more tolerable in this difficult patient population.

References

1. Byre C, Vernon P, Cohen JJ. Effect of age and diagnosis on survival of older patients beginning chronic dialysis. JAMA 1994; 271(1)34-41.
2. Leapman SB, Pescovitz MD, Thomalla JV, Milgrom M, Filo RS. Salvage surgery for arteriovenous conduits: Does it make sense? In: Henry ML, Ferguson RM, eds. Vascular access for hemodialysis—III. Chicago: W.L. Gore & Associates, Inc., and Precept Press, 1993; 169-174.
3. Voeqwek D, Gunther RW, Bohndorf K, Kistler D, Gladziwa U, Sieberth HG. Follow-up results after stent placement in failing arteriovenous shunts: A three-year experience. Cardiovasc Intervent Radiol 1991; 14(5):285-289.
4. Zollikofer CL, Antonucci F, Stuckmann G, Mattias P, Bruhlmann WF, Slomonowitz EK. Cardiovasc Intervent Radiol 1992; 15(5):334-341.
5. Swedberg SH, Brown BG, Sigley R, et al. Intimal fibromuscular hyperplasia at the venous anastomosis of PTFE grafts in hemodialysis patients: Clinical, immunohistochemical, light and electron microscopic assessment. Circulation 1989; 80:1726-1736.
6. Fillinger MF, Kerns DB. Biologic mediators of intimal hyperplasia. In: Henry ML, Ferguson RM, eds. Vascular access for hemodialysis—III. Chicago: W.L. Gore & Associates, Inc., and Precept Press, 1993; 14-40.
7. Surratt RS, Picus D, Hicks ME, Darcy MD, Kleinhoffer M, Jendrisak M. The importance of preoperative evaluation of the subclavian vein in dialysis access planning. Am J Roentgenol 1991; 156(3):623-625.
8. Puckett JW, Lindsay SF. Graft curettage. In: Henry ML, Ferguson RM, eds. Vascular access for hemodialysis—III. Chicago: W.L. Gore & Associates, Inc., and Precept Press, 1993; 186-195.
9. Hurt AV, Batello-Cruz MB, Skipper BJ, et al. Bovine carotid artery heterografts versus polytetrafluoroethylene grafts. Am J Surg 1983; 146:844-847.
10. Tellis VA, Kohlberg WI, Bhat DJ, et al. Expanded polytetrafluoroethylene graft fistulae for chronic hemodialysis. Ann Surg 1980; 189:101-105.
11. Burbridge GE, Bigger JA, Remmers AR, et al. Late complications and results of bovine xenografts. Trans Am Soc Artif Intern Organs 1976; 22:377-379.
12. Haag BW, Paramesh V, Roberts T, Taber T. Early use of polytetrafluoroethylene grafts for hemodialysis access. In: Henry ML, Ferguson RM, eds. Vascular access for hemodialysis—III. Chicago: W.L. Gore & Associates, Inc., and Precept Press, 1993; 173-178.
13. Taucher LA. Immediate, safe hemodialysis into arteriovenous fistulae created with a new tunneler. Am J Surg 1985; 150:212-215.
14. Schafer AI. The hypercoagulable states. Ann Intern Med 1985; 102:814-828.

2

IMPACT OF ERYTHROPOIETIN THERAPY ON DIALYSIS PATENCY

Ralph H. Didlake, M.D.

THE EFFICACY OF RECOMBINANT HUMAN ERYTHROPOIETIN (EPO) in the treatment of chronic anemia in end-stage renal disease (ESRD) patients has made EPO therapy routine in the care of hemodialysis patients. The beneficial effects of hematocrit elevation in these patients, including reduction of transfusion requirements, increased exercise capacity, and improved quality of life, have been well documented.[1-5] A concern was raised in the initial clinical trials of this therapy that normalization of the hematocrit levels in these heretofore anemic patients would result in a higher rate of vascular access thrombosis.[6] The relationship between vascular access thrombosis and EPO therapy remains a subject of debate and is a question with great relevance for the ESRD population.

An efficient vascular access is a critical component of modern hemodialysis therapy. Dialysis prescriptions based on kinetic modeling assume that a hemo-access device with sufficient flow volume and minimal recirculation is present. This assumption is essential in the case of conventional hemodialysis and is critical in the case of high-flux hemodialysis. Any factors that have an impact on the flow dynamics of an access device, whether of patient or of graft origin, can significantly alter the adequacy of the patient's dialysis. Dependable vascular access is also a major determinant of rehabilitation for the ESRD patient. The rehabilitation potential of a hemodialysis patient—and certainly his or her degree of meaningful employability—are directly related to the patient's ability to establish and maintain a schedule for dialysis therapy. The most common cause of disruption of such schedules is dialysis access dysfunction.

All currently available technologies for the construction of access shunts, including autogenous vein, expanded polytetrafluoroethylene (ePTFE), human umbilical vein, and bovine carotid artery, are vulnerable to the complications of infection, pseudoaneurysm formation, and thrombosis. Of these, thrombosis is the most common cause of hemo-access failure and was the operative indication for 65% of patients receiving surgical procedures on already established PTFE access grafts.[7] It is critical, therefore, to assess carefully any change in the care of hemodialysis patients that may have a negative impact on access patency.

The goals of this chapter are (1) to provide an overview of anemia in the ESRD patient, (2) to review the physiology of EPO, (3) to review the rheological principles relevant to blood flow in an access graft, (4) to outline the theoretical impact of elevated hematocrit on blood flow, and (5) to review published data on the impact of EPO therapy on access patency.

Anemia

Anemia is a central clinical feature of the patient with chronic renal failure. This anemia is characterized as normochromic and macrocytic and is usually associated with a reticulocyte count that is inappropriately low for the level of the anemia. Other marrow-dependent elements, specifically the leukocyte and platelet, are generally spared. The etiology of this anemia is erythroid-specific marrow failure owing to the inability of the end-stage kidney to produce adequate amounts of the hematopoietic hormone erythropoietin. Although the uremic state itself inhibits erythropoiesis and shortens red blood cell survival, these factors are only minor contributors to the anemia seen in the chronic dialysis patient. The central factor is the absence of EPO stimulation of the erythroid progenitor cell line in the bone marrow. The morbidity associated with anemia in the ESRD patient is significant. In addition to the constitutional symptoms of fatigue, dyspnea, exercise intolerance, and angina, the need for repeated red cell transfusion carries the risks of viral infection and iron overload. Repeated transfusion can also result in sensitization of the patient to HLA antigens, which potentially limits the success of renal allografting. After renal failure patients are stabilized on dialysis, some mild improvement in hematocrit levels may be seen, but anemia remains a substantial management issue.

Physiology of EPO

The prominent role of the kidney as an endocrine organ has been recognized for almost 100 years. Tigerstedt and Bergman isolated renin from kidney extracts and demonstrated its pressor activity in 1898.[8] More recently, renal metabolism of 1,25 vitamin D[9] and renal prostaglandin production[10] were described. The existence of a hematopoietic hormone of renal origin was suggested by Carnot and Deflandre early in this century and was ultimately identified as erythropoietin.[11] Biochemically, EPO is a peptide hormone consisting of 163 amino acids with a molecular weight of 18,399 daltons.

Although EPO is produced in both the kidney and liver, hepatic synthesis contributes only 10% of the total production, and the liver is unable to maintain normal EPO levels in the anephric individual. The kidneys, therefore, are essential for maintenance of normal hematocrit levels. The exact cell or cells responsible for renal EPO synthesis in man have not been positively identified, but are likely tubular or peritubular cells.[12] The major stimuli for renal EPO synthesis are increased oxygen demand or reduced oxygen delivery.

Although thyroxine and growth hormone increase EPO production in experimental models and in man, these stimuli are minor compared to the response of the hypoxic kidney. Reduced oxygen delivery due to anemia or increased hemoglobin-oxygen affinity and hypoxia due to high altitude or cardiopulmonary pathology directly stimulate renal production of EPO and its release into the circulation. A closed feedback loop decreases renal EPO production when the increased red cell mass returns oxygen delivery to normal. The cellular and biochemical pathways for the oxygen-sensing, EPO-producing feedback loop in the kidneys are not well defined. When EPO is secreted by the kidney, the site of action is the erythroid progenitor cell line of the bone marrow.

Successful production of human recombinant EPO was achieved in 1985 by Lin,[13] and the hormone became available for clinical trial in 1986. In 1989, Eschbach et al. reported the results of a phase 3 multicenter clinical trial and described the efficacy of recombinant EPO as a therapeutic agent.[1] Hematocrit values responded favorably in 97.4% of patients within 12 weeks of therapy, and most patients receiving the agent were noted to have decreased functional impairment and improved energy level. Subsequent reports have confirmed the efficacy as well as the safety profile of EPO in the treatment of anemia in the hemodialysis patient. Some early reports, however, suggested that the incidence of vascular access thrombosis and other thrombotic events was increased in patients receiving EPO.[6] It was postulated that increased blood viscosity associated with higher hematocrits following EPO administration was responsible for these thrombotic episodes.[14,15]

Rheology of Human Blood

The relationship between blood viscosity and hematocrit is well known. Blood viscosity increases dramatically when hematocrits exceed 40; below that point, this relationship is essentially linear and is quite linear over the range of hematocrit values seen in most hemodialysis patients. The linearity of this relationship over the range of hematocrit values seen in such patients (20-34) is confirmed by plotting the experimental values obtained by Pirofsky for blood viscosity at various hematocrits.[16] A regression plot with 95% confidence intervals for this clinically relevant hematocrit range is shown in figure 2-1.

The dynamics of blood flow in a vascular access graft can be conceptualized as flow in a semirigid tube. Fluid flow in such a system can be mathematically modeled using the standard form of the Poiseuille equation where Q is total flow volume in ml/sec, R is the radius of the tube through which the fluid flows, P_2-P_1 is the pressure gradient across the tube in dynes per cm^2, μ is the fluid viscosity in poises, and L is the length of the tube in cm. The appropriateness and limitations of

$$Q = \frac{\pi R^4 (P_2 - P_1)}{8 \mu L}$$

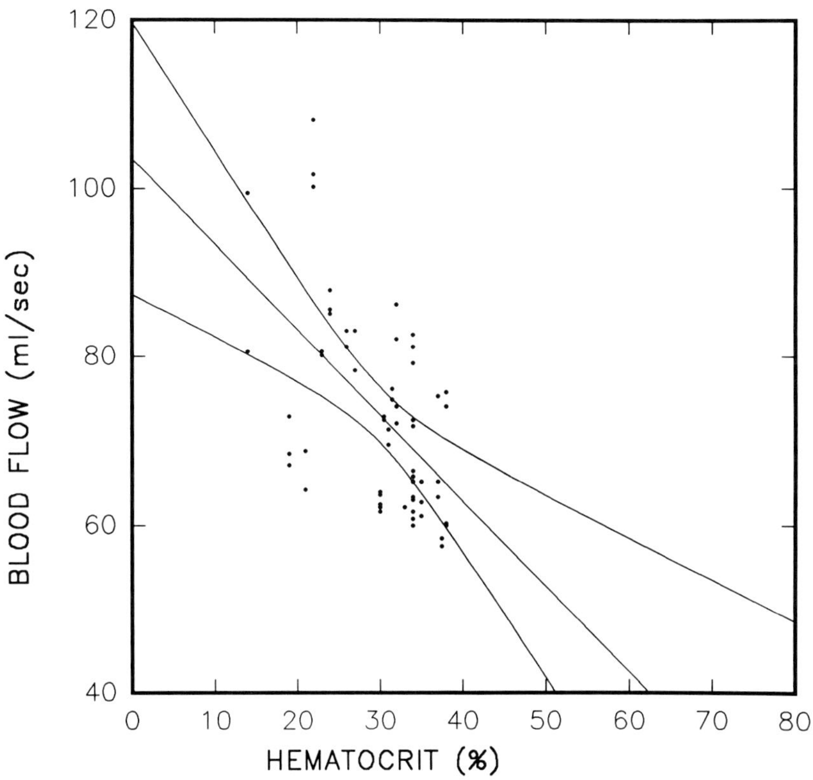

Figure 2–1. Linear relationships of viscosity and hematocrit value less than 40. Derived from data of Pirofsky.[16]

using this equation to describe flow in the human vascular system are based on certain assumptions. These assumptions, which have been thoroughly reviewed by Nichols and O'Rouke,[17] include accepting that blood is a homogenous fluid and that its viscosity does not change appreciably with flow velocity, that this velocity of flow is relatively steady, that flow is laminar with a parabolic flow velocity profile, and that the diameter of the conduit is constant. These assumptions are clearly inappropriate for the analysis of some aspects of the human circulation, but have great utility in the study of flow in prosthetic arteriovenous (A-V) vascular access grafts. Examination of the Poiseuille equation shows that flow is inversely related to flow viscosity.

Impact of Hematocrit on Blood Flow

The impact of hematocrit (i.e., viscosity) on blood flow in a theoretical vascular access conduit is demonstrated in figure 2-2. This curve was derived using the Poiseuille equation for a 6-mm diameter conduit 30 cm long flowing under a pressure gradient of 100 mm Hg. Examination of the resulting curve shows that increas-

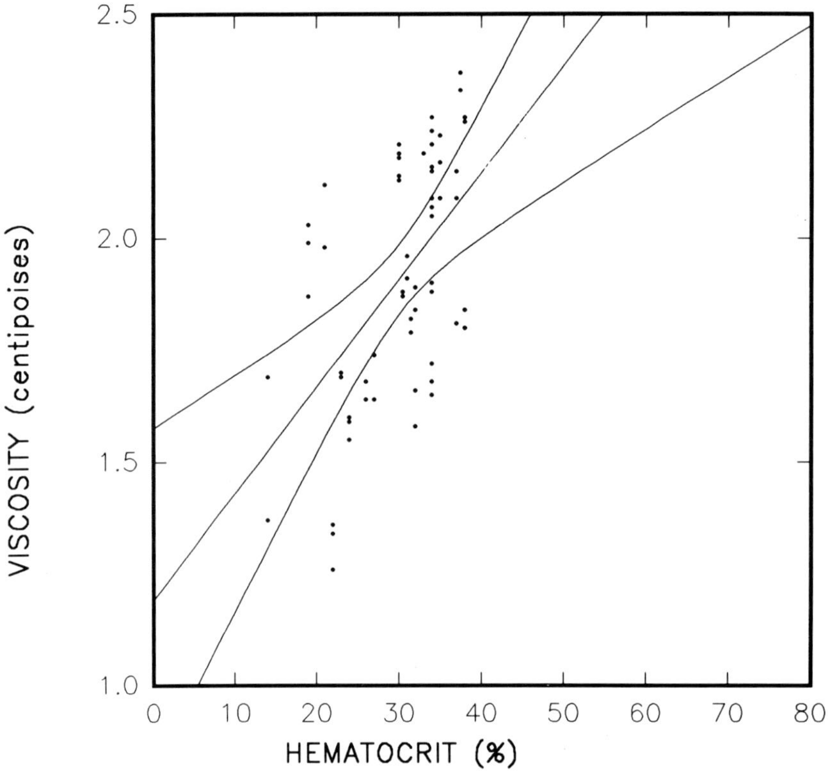

Figure 2-2. Relationship of blood flow to hematocrit in a theoretical 6-mm conduit.

ing the hematocrit by 50% (from 20 to 30) decreases blood flow from 81.25 ml/sec to 71.30 ml/sec. This drop in flow volume would appear to be modest in an adequately functioning access graft and is probably not of clinical significance unless other factors that compromise flow are also present. A more definitive answer to this question must await our ability to model, with mathematical confidence, the effects of inflow and outflow geometry, an irregular pseudointimal lining, and pulsatile blood flow.

The most common failure mode of vascular access grafts is thrombosis associated with pseudointimal hyperplasia in the region of the venous anastomosis. This response of intimal and vascular smooth muscle cells is thought to be related to hyperphysiologic flow dynamics, but a specific flow parameter responsible for hyperplasia has not been identified with certainty. It is, however, useful to examine the current theories relating flow dynamics to pseudointimal hyperplasia and how blood viscosity may be related.

The excellent work of Glagov relates wall shear stress and mural tensile stress to intimal thickenings in arterial and venous systems.[18] The dependence of wall shear (**Υ**) stress on flow dynamics is given by the function

$$\Upsilon = \frac{4\mu Q}{\pi r^3}$$

where μ is viscosity and Q is flow. If, as the Glagov hypothesis suggests, intimal hyperplastic reactions are related to regions of low shear, then increasing blood viscosity (i.e., hematocrit) may actually reduce the hyperplastic response. Other investigators have proposed that intimal and medial thickening occurs in areas of high shear stress, in which case increasing blood viscosity may have a detrimental effect.[19]

Fillinger et al. have made substantial contributions to the understanding of flow turbulence in vascular access grafts and its relationship to pseudointimal hyperplasia.[20,21] Turbulence is quantitated by the Reynold's number defined by the relationship

$$Re = \frac{\overline{DVp}}{\mu}$$

where D is the diameter of the conduit in question, V is the mean velocity of flow, p is fluid density, and μ is viscosity. Based on this relationship, one may expect decreased turbulence of flow with increasing hematocrit.

Kinetic energy loss across the venous anastomosis of vascular access grafts has also been implicated in the genesis of pseudointimal hyperplasia by both experimental work and clinical observation.[22,23] Total pulse wave energy Σ in ergs/cm is defined by

$$\Sigma = P + pgh = \tfrac{1}{2}\, pV^2$$

where P is the average pulse pressure in dynes/cm^2, p is the fluid density in grams/cm^3 , g is a gravitational constant, h is the height of the fluid column in cm and V is velocity in cm/sec. For our purpose, the potential energy due to gravitation (pgh) can be ignored and Σ can be considered to be a function of pressure and velocity. Fluid viscosity does not enter into the calculation of total fluid energy.

These three hypotheses of the relationship between flow dynamics and pseudointimal hyperplasia remain unproven, but this overview suggests that the increase in blood viscosity seen in EPO-treated patients would not play a major role.

Mechanisms other than increasing blood viscosity by elevating hematocrit have been proposed for any impact that EPO may have on access thrombosis. Anemia alone is known to prolong bleeding time. This prolongation returns to normal with correction of the anemia.[24] In this manner, bleeding time may be improved in dialysis patients on EPO therapy. Protein C and protein S are potent anticoagulants, the levels of which decrease with EPO administration.[25] Platelet count has also been noted to rise transiently during EPO therapy, but an improvement in platelet function appears to be sustained.[26,27]

Literature Review

Tang et al. analyzed vascular access thrombosis in a population of 63 patients receiving EPO therapy and found that those who experienced a thrombotic episode were significantly older, more likely to be diabetic, and more likely to have a PTFE access than an autogenous vein fistula.[28] Hematologic responses to EPO were not different between the patients who experienced thrombosis and those who did not. The period over which this mixed population of access types were followed was 23 months. The authors concluded that access thrombosis was unrelated to hematocrit, but no control data were provided.

Standage et al. divided a group of 64 patients into three EPO dosage groups and recorded the number of thrombotic events that occurred during an eight-month follow-up period.[29] No difference in the rate of access thrombosis was noted between the groups. An untreated control was not provided, but the authors concluded that EPO treatment does not increase the incidence of vascular access clotting.

The experience of Casati et al. with 14 hemodialysis patients treated with EPO led them to note "a tendency to vascular thrombosis."[30] An indepth analysis of these thromboses in the small patient cohort was not given. A group of 37 patients on EPO therapy reported by Duff et al. was found to exhibit no increase in access thrombosis when a three-month pretherapy and a six-month posttherapy interval were compared.[31] The type of access grafts used by these patients was not described. The authors did state that intradialytic heparinization was increased 25% at the onset of EPO treatment.

Vascular access thrombosis before and after EPO therapy was also studied by Dy et al.[32] This group found a significantly higher incidence of graft thrombosis in a group of 46 patients with PTFE grafts during 12 months of EPO as compared to the 12-month period before EPO was started.

The significant article by Powe et al. is a review of the Medicare claims database in which the causes of hospital admission for ESRD patients were studied.[33] A population of 23,806 patients on EPO therapy was compared to an untreated control cohort of 22,720 patients over an 18-month period. Hospital admission for vascular access morbidity was 11% more likely in the EPO group. A similar study was conducted by Lazarus, who retrospectively reviewed a five-year period of the National Medical Care, Inc., database.[34] This analysis noted an increase in vascular access morbidity that appeared to coincide with the clinical introduction of EPO, but no statistical relationship could be shown.

The results of the phase 3 clinical trial of EPO administration are reported in the widely quoted paper by Eschbach et al.[1] These investigators found that vascular access thrombosis occurred at a rate of 0.3 events per patient year in a population of 333 patients followed for 10 months after EPO treatment began. The types of access devices used by these patients and the age and status of the devices at the beginning of the study were not discussed. Eschbach et al. concluded that the incidence of access thrombosis was no greater than that observed in 1,111 dialysis patients who were not on EPO therapy. This "control" group was offered parenthetically as an unpublished observation without further analysis. Eschbach later reported data on 13 dialysis patients with normal hematocrits who were not receiving EPO therapy, concluding that the incidence of PTFE and bovine access thrombosis was not higher than that reported by others for anemic patients with similar graft types.[35]

Several of the reports examining the effect of EPO therapy contrasted vascular access thrombosis in a pretherapy control period to that in a posttherapy period and statistically compared the rate of thrombosis in each. Of the studies using this design, that of Besarab et al. provides the longest observation period and the largest patient population.[36] Forty percent of the patient population had autogenous vein A-V fistulas; its membership did not remain constant over the course of the study, with 49 patients leaving and 71 patients joining the population during the pretreatment period. Finding a decrease in the monthly rate of thrombotic events from 0.06 to 0.03 per patient month over the 32 months of the study, these investigators concluded that EPO therapy does not increase vascular access clotting.

The study by Klinkmann, based on the European multicenter study, used a semi-crossover design in which 362 patients were equally divided between an EPO treatment group and an untreated control group.[37] After one year, the control group was also started on EPO and the entire group was followed for an additional year. The number of vascular access thromboses was not different between the two groups. The author concluded that hematocrit levels of 30-35 do not have a significant impact on blood viscosity and rheology.

The findings of the Canadian Erythropoietin Study Group were reported in the *British Medical Journal* in 1990.[6] This is the only EPO study reported to employ a double-blind placebo control. The 118 patients were randomized to one of two EPO dosage groups and to the placebo control group. During the six months of the study, four patients in the low-dose EPO group and seven patients in the high-dose EPO group experienced clotting of a vascular access device, as compared to one patient in the placebo group. Statistical analysis led this study group to conclude that a positive association existed between EPO treatment and the incidence of vascular access thrombosis.

The study by Muirhead presented data for 128 patients with significant comorbid disease and a mixture of access devices.[38] Although this is one of the few reports to provide actuarial analysis of access patency during EPO therapy, no control data were provided to which these survival curves could be compared. The authors describe thrombotic events as "common" during EPO therapy but draw no other conclusions.

The frequently cited report by Paganini et al. reviewed 58 patients on EPO therapy who were followed for one year.[39] The types of access devices in this population were mixed. Clotting was described in 13 PTFE grafts, but no further analysis was offered. Of interest in this study is the assessment of fistula flow using noninvasively-determined cardiac parameters before and after fistula occlusion. The validity of such parameters in evaluating the flow dynamics, functional integrity, or long-term patency of vascular access grafts is not established.

A critical flaw shared by all of these reported series is that although they are longitudinal studies of EPO therapy, they are cross-sectional in their study of access patency. In each report, the patients were entered into the study at the beginning of EPO treatment and followed for various periods of time. This is an appropriate longitudinal design for the study of hematologic response to the therapy in question. However, the access grafts of these patients were of various ages at the time EPO therapy began. This results in a cross-sectional analysis of access graft patency during EPO therapy that compares newly placed access grafts and aging, multiply thrombectomized or revised grafts with equal weight. This is a standard of analysis that one would not accept in evaluating a new graft material or a new graft placement technique, and it is inappropriate to accept this standard in evaluating a factor that may have an adverse impact on access graft patency.

Unfortunately, the opportunity to perform a well-controlled study may have passed now that EPO administration is routine in dialysis patients and development of an untreated control group may not be possible. The issue of appropriate study design was recognized in a recent study by Churchill et al. in which graft thrombosis was compared between patients started on EPO either before or within three months of the first use of a permanent vascular access device and a matched cohort of patients who did not receive EPO.[40] Stratification of these patients by type of access showed no difference between treated and untreated patients in the rate of autogenous fistula thrombosis, but a significantly higher rate of prosthetic access thrombosis was noted in patients receiving EPO. Although the EPO–treated group had more cardiovascular disease than the control patients, the results of this well-designed study are compelling.

Conclusion

Based on the data available at this time, it appears that EPO therapy may have a subtle negative effect on vascular access patency. A definitive understanding of the relationship between EPO administration, hematocrit level, and vascular access patency and function would require a study that would be longitudinal both for vascular access life and for EPO therapy. Such a study must be of sufficient sample size and include appropriate control groups in order for statistical analysis to be meaningful. From a purely pragmatic viewpoint, one may question the need for such a study in that normalized hematocrit levels are the environment in which vascular access surgeons must now work. However, intelligent improvements in graft design and elucidation of the mechanisms of pseudointimal hyperplasia are dependent upon a more complete understanding of all factors that influence flow dynamics in a vascular access.

References

1. Eschbach JW, Abdulhadi MH, Browne JK, et al. Recombinant human erythropoietin in anemic patients with end-stage renal disease: Results of a Phase III multicenter clinical trial. Ann Intern Med 1989; 111:992-1000.
2. Evans RW, Rader B, Manninen DL. The quality of life of hemodialysis recipients treated with recombinant human erythropoietin. JAMA 1990; 263:825-830.
3. Robertson HT, Haley R, Guthrie M, Cardenas D, Eschbach JW, Adamson JW. Recombinant human erythropoietin improves exercise capacity in anemic hemodialysis patients. Am J Kidney Dis 1990; 15:325-332.
4. Mayer G, Thum J, Cada EM, Stummvoll HK, Graf H. Working capacity is increased following recombinant human erythropoietin treatment. Kidney Int 1988; 34:525-528.
5. Bommer J, Kugel M, Schwobel B, Ritz E, Barth HP, Seelig R. Improved sexual function during recombinant erythropoietin therapy. Nephrol Dial Transplant 1990; 5:204-207.
6. Canadian Erythropoietin Study Group. Association between recombinant human erythropoietin and quality of life and exercise capacity of patients receiving hemodialysis. Br Med J 1990; 300:573-578.
7. Didlake R, Curry E, Rigdon E, Raju S, Bower J. Outpatient vascular access surgery: impact of a dialysis unit–based surgical facility. Am J Kidney Dis 1992; 15:39-44.

8. Tigerstedt R, Bergman PG. Niere und Kreislauf. Skand Arch Physiol 1898; 8:223.
9. Fraser DR, Kodicek E. Unique biosynthesis by kidney of a biologically active vitamin D metabolite. Nature (London) 1970; 228:764.
10. Zins GR. Renal prostaglandins. Am J Med 1975; 58:14-24.
11. Carnot P, Deflandre C. Sur l'activité hemopoiétique de sérum au cours de le régenération du sang. CR: Acad Sci 1906; 143:384-386.
12. Stevens JM, Kurtz A, Eckardt K-U, Winearls CG. Anaemia in chronic renal failure. In: Cameron S, Davison AM, Grunfeld J-P, Kerr D, Ritz E, eds. Oxford textbook of clinical nephrology. vol. 2. Oxford: Oxford University Press, 1992; 1344-1360.
13. Lin F-K, Suggs S, Lin C-H, et al. Cloning and expression of the human erythropoietin gene. Proc Natl Acad Sci 1985; 82:7580-7589.
14. Bommer J, Barth HP, Zeier M, et al. Efficacy comparison of intravenous and subcutaneous recombinant human erythropoietin administration in hemodialysis patients. Contrib Nephrol 1991; 88:136-43.
15. Deniston OL, Luscombe FA, Buesching OP, Richner RE, Spinowitz BS. Effect of long-term epoetin beta therapy on the quality of life of hemodialysis patients. ASAIO Trans 1990; 36:M157-60.
16. Pirofsky B. The determination of blood viscosity in man by a method based on Poiseuille's law. J Clin Invest 1953; 32:292-298.
17. Nichols WW, O'Rourke MF. McDonald's blood flow in arteries. 3rd ed. Philadelphia: Lea & Febiger, 1990: 20-21.
18. Glagov S, Giddens DP, Bassiouny H, White S, Zarins CK. Hemodynamic effects and tissue reactions at graft to vein anastomosis for vascular access. In: Summer BG, Henry ML, eds. Vascular access for hemodialysis—III. Chicago: W.L. Gore & Associates, Inc., and Precept Press, 1991; 3-20.
19. Fry DL. Acute vascular endothelial changes associated with increased blood velocity gradients. Circ Res 1967; 22:165-197.
20. Fillinger MF, Reintz ER, Schwartz RA, Resetarits DE, Paskanik AM, Bredenberg CE. Beneficial effects of banding on venous intimal-medial hyperplasia in arteriovenous loop grafts. Am J Surg 1989; 158:87-94.
21. Fillinger MF, Reinitz ER, Schwartz RA, et al. Graft geometry and venous intimal-medial hyperplasia in arteriovenous loop grafts. J Vasc Surg 1990; 11:556-566.
22. Imperato AM, Bracco A, Kim GE, Zeff R. Intimal and neointimal fibrous proliferation causing failure of arterial reconstructions. Surgery 1972; 72:1007-1014.
23. Didlake R, Curry E, Bower J. Composite dialysis access grafts. J Am Coll Surg 1994; 178:24-28.
24. Anand A, Feffer SE. Hematocrit and bleeding time: an update. South Med J 1994; 87:299-301.
25. MacDougall IC, Davies ME, Hallett I, et al. Coagulation studies and fistula blood flow during erythropoietin therapy in haemodialysis patients. Nephrol Dial Transplant 1991; 6:862-867.
26. Azikawa T, Kinugasa E, Kitacka T, Koshikawa S. Effects of recombinant human erythropoietin and correction of anemia on platelet function in hemodialysis patient. Nephron 1996; 58:400-406.
27. Cases A, Escolar G, Reverter JC, et al. Recombinant human erythropoietin treatment improves platelet function in uremic patients. Kidney Int 1992; 42:668-672.
28. Tang IY, Vrahnos D, Valaitis D, Lau AH. Vascular access thrombosis during recombinant human erythropoietin therapy. ASAIO J 1992; 38:M528-M531.
29. Standage BA, Schuman ES, Ackerman D, Gross GF, Ragsdale JW. Does the use of erythropoietin in hemodialysis patients increase dialysis graft thrombosis rates? Am J Surg 1993; 165:650-654.

30. Casati S, Passerini P, Campise MR, et al. Benefits and risks of protracted treatment with human recombinant erythropoietin in patients having haemodialysis. Br Med J 1987; 295:1017-1020.
31. Duff DR, Golper TA, Sloan RS, Brier ME, Aronoff GR. Low-dose recombinant human erythropoietin therapy in chronic hemodialysis patients. Am J Kidney Dis 1991; 18:60-64.
32. Dy GR, Bloom EJ, Ijelu GK, Merritts GW, Kramer MS, Raja RM. Effect of recombinant human erythropoietin on vascular access. ASAIO Trans 1991; 37:M274-275.
33. Powe NR, Griffiths RI, Watson AJ, et al. Effect of recombinant erythropoietin on hospital admissions, readmissions, length of stay, and costs of dialysis patients. J Am Soc Nephrol 1994; 4:1455-1465.
34. Lazarus JM, Huang WH, Lew HL, Lowrie EG. Contribution of vascular access-related disease to morbidity of hemodialysis patients. In: Henry ML, Ferguson RM, eds. Vascular access for hemodialysis—III. Chicago: W.L. Gore & Associates, Inc., and Precept Press, 1993; 3-13.
35. Eschbach JW. Does treatment with erythropoietin cause vascular access thrombosis? Erythropoietin is not a cause of access thrombosis. Semin Dial 1993; 6:180-184.
36. Besarab A, Medina F, Musial E, Picanello N, Michael H. Recombinant human erythropoietin does not increase clotting in vascular accesses. ASAIO Trans 1990; 36:M749-M753.
37. Klinkmann H, Wirczorek L, Seigalla P. Adverse events of subcutaneous recombinant human erythropoietin therapy: Results of a controlled multicenter European study. Artif Organs 1993; 17:219-225.
38. Muirhead N. Does treatment with erythropoietin cause vascular access thrombosis? Erythropoietin is a cause of access thrombosis. Semin Dial 1993; 6:184-188.
39. Paganini EP, Latham D, Abdulhadi M. Practical considerations of recombinant human erythropoietin therapy. Am J Kidney Dis 1989; XIV (suppl 1):19-25.
40. Churchill DN, Muirhead N, Goldstein M, et al. Probability of thrombosis of vascular access among hemodialysis patients treated with recombinant human erythropoietin. J Am Soc Nephrol 1994; 4:1809-1813.

3

HEMODIALYSIS VASCULAR ACCESS: EFFECT ON HIGH-FLUX HEMODIALYSIS

David W. Butterly, M.D., and Steve J. Schwab, M.D.

THERE IS SUBSTANTIAL EVIDENCE that inadequacies in the delivery of the appropriate dose of dialysis contribute to the morbidity and mortality seen in end-stage renal disease (ESRD).[1] The results of the National Cooperative Dialysis Study showed a correlation between quantity of dialysis delivered and patient morbidity.[2] Gotch and Sargeant's mechanistic analysis that followed expressed the quantity of delivered dialysis mathematically as Kt/V and introduced the concept of urea kinetic modeling as a means of measuring the amount of delivered dialysis.[3] Unfortunately, however, many of our patients do not reach the desired or prescribed urea clearance. A recent article showed that only one-half of hemodialysis patients in a large metropolitan area reached a Kt/V of 1.0.[4] This occurs for a variety of reasons, but often vascular access dysfunction is a significant contributor. The rate-limiting step in the delivery of high-flux and high-efficiency hemodialysis is often the performance of the vascular access.

The effective delivery of dialysis requires repeated reliable access to the circulation. This access to the circulation continues to be the "Achilles' heel" in the delivery of long-term hemodialysis therapy. In addition, high-flux and high-efficiency dialysis require faster extracorporeal blood flows, thereby placing even greater demands on vascular access.

Vascular access complications remain the greatest cause of morbidity and account for about one-fourth of all admissions and hospitalization days in the hemodialysis population.[5,6] In addition, from a financial standpoint, as much as $500 million annually is spent on placement and maintenance of vascular access.[7] Thrombosis causes most access failures and is generally associated with venous stenosis.[8,9] In addition to causing thrombosis, these anatomic lesions lead to graft dysfunction by limiting dialyzer blood flow and promoting recirculation. Prospective identification and correction of stenoses not only prevents thrombosis but also improves graft function and dialysis efficiency.[9]

Fistula Blood Flow

Vascular access must provide adequate blood flow to support the extracorporeal circuit, since insufficient flow will lead to recirculation. The higher blood flows required for high-efficiency dialysis (400-500 ml/min) exacerbate this problem, as recirculation increases with increasing dialyzer pump speed. Studies using velocity flow probes and Doppler ultrasound have demonstrated that many native and synthetic fistulas achieve blood flows in excess of 800-1,000 ml/min, easily exceeding the demands of high-efficiency dialysis.[10,11] Blood flow in native arteriovenous (A-V) fistulas measured by intraoperative velocity flow probe is initially 200-300 ml/min but progressively increases with dilation of the venous runoff system.[10] In contrast, blood flow in synthetic grafts is initially much higher but tends to progressively decrease, presumably secondary to neointimal hyperplasia and subsequent venous stenosis.[8,10-12]

The location of the fistula may also affect blood flow. In general, grafts constructed from more proximal brachial arteries tend to have higher blood flows than radial artery grafts.[11,12] These differences probably relate to the size of the vessel used to construct the fistula. Even with these lower blood flows, there is no difference in upper-arm versus forearm graft survival. However, because of lower blood flows there may be increased recirculation in forearm grafts, which can negatively affect the urea clearance. For instance, at blood flows of 400 ml/min, Collins demonstrated that the mean recirculation rate in radial fistulas was higher than that seen in upper-arm grafts.[13] Despite these observations, it is clear that vascular access sites must be preserved to assure long-term hemodialysis. Thus, the dictum of "as distal as possible for as long as possible" in the placement of vascular access continues to apply even if dialysis durations need to be extended to meet hemodialysis goals.

Prospective Identification and Correction of Stenoses

Prospective identification of patients with vascular access stenoses followed by correction of these lesions can have a dramatic impact on fistula thromboses, significantly prolonging the life of the vascular graft.[13-16] We have shown that correction of venous and arterial stenoses prior to thromboses by using a combination of transluminal angioplasty and surgical revision dramatically improves thrombosis rates.[14] Fistula thromboses were decreased threefold when a rigorous program of preventive monitoring was employed and combined with proactive correction of anatomic stenoses.[14] Studies from our institution have shown that >80% of fistula thromboses are associated with anatomic stenoses.[8,9] We and others have also shown that correction of these stenoses improves the efficiency of hemodialysis.[13,17] The location of most stenoses is in the venous circuit, with a minority in the arterial inflow. Table 3-1 documents the location of stenotic lesions identified in patients from Duke University following prospective screening or in follow-up after thrombectomy. Table 3-2 shows the most commonly

Table 3-1. Location of Fistula Stenoses

Vein-graft anastomosis	58%
Proximal vein	22%
Central vein	14%
Artery-graft anastomosis	02%
Intrafistula	04%

Table 3-2. Techniques for Monitoring Fistulas

Physical exam
Arm edema
Manual compression test
Venous dialysis pressure
Urea recirculation
Urea kinetic parameters
Doppler ultrasound

used techniques for monitoring vascular access for patency and function. The monitoring techniques discussed below have been previously summarized.[7-9,16]

Physical Examination

Careful examination of the fistula is an important, inexpensive, and often overlooked screening tool for detecting venous stenosis and fistula dysfunction. Inspection and auscultation of the graft, combined with a few simple bedside maneuvers, can aid in detection of anatomic stenosis. Edema in the arm is common after graft placement. However, when edema fails to resolve or appears *de novo*, this may be indicative of central venous stenosis, particularly in a patient with previous ipsilateral cannulation of the subclavian vein.[15] Often, these patients may have no other clinical indication of stenosis, including normal clearances and venous dialysis pressures. Akmal et al. recently reported on five patients in whom limb edema was the only manifestation of subclavian stenosis proximal to the fistula.[18] Auscultation along the entire length of the graft can also be of value. Generally, the pitch of the bruit over the graft should gradually diminish from the arterial to the venous anastomosis. Because the velocity of blood flow increases through an area of stenosis, a localized increase in the pitch of the bruit may be indicative of an area of graft stenosis.[19]

Digital compression of the graft between the arterial and venous needles during dialysis, which can effectively short-circuit recirculation through the graft, is simple to perform and can be of assistance in identifying the patient with recirculation. In the case of high fistula recirculation, manual compression between the arterial and venous needles will effectively eliminate the recirculation pathway, causing a drop in arterial pressure and an increase in venous pressure. A recent report showed that an increase in a venous dialysis pressure(VDP) of >40 mm Hg had a sensitivity of 77% for detecting venous stenosis.[20]

Table 3-3. VDP Monitoring Protocol

1. Cannulate fistula with 15- or 16-gauge needles
2. Measuring VDP at QB 200 ml/min during first five minutes of dialysis
3. If VDP >150 mm Hg on three consecutive treatments, proceed to fistulogram (Gambro machine)

Urea Kinetic Modeling

In addition to measuring effective solute clearance and the dose of dialysis delivered, urea kinetic modeling can also be used as a tool to identify access dysfunction.[20] Recirculation can be detected directly from the results of urea kinetic modeling. The difference between the actual and predicted Kt/V is an indicator of the recirculation rate, assuming that no other errors in the model have occurred. Mathematical models estimating recirculation based on these differences are available.[20]

Venous Dialysis Pressures

Venous stenosis can be detected by measurement of the pressure in the venous return line of the dialyzer circuit. This measured pressure, or VDP, represents the clinically relevant intra-access pressure along with irrelevant hydrostatic pressure gradients between the needle and measuring site and the pressure gradient through the external venous tubing and return needle.[5,13,16] Measured VDP increases with increased blood flow. Thus, dialyzer blood flow, needle size and position, and blood viscosity and hematocrit all affect measured VDP.[8,21] Venous obstruction leads to elevations of intrafistula pressure, which subsequently elevates VDP. Elevations in VDP occurs both in stenosis involving the venous anastomosis as well as the more proximal central veins.[12,13,16] However, Sullivan et al. showed that in patients with high-grade stenosis, those with central venous stenosis had the lowest VDP.[22] This was felt to be secondary to the capacity of the veins to form collateral circulation around the stenosis. Venous dialysis pressures can be falsely low in the presence of stenosis when significant recirculation is occurring.[19] It is therefore important to combine VDP with urea recirculation measurements.

We try to minimize the potentially confounding variables affecting VDP by using the established protocol shown in table 3-3. Only 15–16-gauge needles are used to cannulate the fistula, and VDP is measured at the beginning of the treatment with blood flow (QB) 200 before increasing to maximum flows. As blood flow rates are increased beyond 225 ml/min, VDP increases, and there is poor correlation between pressures and anatomic lesions.[7,8,13] In our dialysis units, VDP is measured and recorded with each treatment. Patients with VDP of >150 mm Hg on three consecutive treatments are routinely referred for venography. We have previously demonstrated that at blood flows of 200 ml/min, VDP can accurately predict the presence of functionally significant anatomic lesions. We referred patients with VDP of >150 mm Hg on three consecutive treatments for fistulogram. Using this protocol, 50/58 patients (86%) referred for fistulogram were found to have venous stenosis. When the stenoses were corrected, thrombosis rates in this patient population declined dramatically.[14]

Recirculation

Hemodialysis recirculation occurs whenever dialyzed blood from the venous needle reenters the extracorporeal circuit without first passing through the systemic circulation.[23] This occurs whenever dialyzer blood flow exceeds fistula blood flow. This is usually caused by stenosis proximal to the venous needle, which forces blood flow retrograde into the arterial dialyzer circuit. Much less commonly, an arterial lesion limiting arterial inflow can be present, necessitating blood flow retrograde to meet the flow demands of the blood pump. Other factors that decrease fistula blood flow, e.g., low cardiac output, intravascular volume depletion, and hypotension, along with improper needle position, can also increase recirculation.[19,23] Because recirculation decreases the solute concentration entering the dialyzer circuit, it decreases the efficiency of the dialysis procedure. Thus, for any given dialysis prescription, effective urea clearance decreases with increasing recirculation. Recirculation rate is calculated by the following formula:

$$\text{recirculation} = \text{P-A/P-V} \times 100$$

$$\text{P} = \text{peripheral urea}$$

$$\text{A} = \text{arterial (dialyzer inflow) urea}$$

$$\text{V} = \text{venous (dialyzer outflow) urea}$$

A detailed review of recirculation is beyond the scope of this article (see reference 23 for a more detailed discussion). The higher blood flows required for high-efficiency dialysis lead to increased recirculation, particularly if an anatomic stenosis is present.[13,23] Occasionally, recirculation can increase to the point that it negates the improvement in urea clearance gained with increased blood flow.

Several authors have demonstrated that monitoring recirculation can identify patients with anatomic stenoses, and that correction of these stenoses prevents fistula thromboses.[13,17] When anatomic lesions are corrected, urea recirculation returns to normal, in most instances dramatically improving dialysis efficiency. Monitoring fistula urea recirculation monthly or quarterly is our recommendation.

Ultrasound

Duplex Doppler color flow studies are newer techniques that may provide additional information on fistula flow and function. These techniques have not been rigorously tested, but may ultimately prove useful in identifying venous stenoses and

Table 3-4. Indications for Fistulogram

Clinical
Thrombosis
Prolonged bleeding
Fistula arm edema
Monitoring indicators
Elevated venous dialysis pressure
Elevated fistula recirculation
Unexplained decrease in urea kinetics

fistula dysfunction. Duplex Doppler can accurately measure fistula blood flow, and when used serially can predict graft stenosis and imminent graft failure. Shackelton et al. demonstrated that a Doppler flow of <450 ml had a sensitivity of 83% and a specificity of 75% for the development of graft thrombosis within six weeks.[24] Similarly, Rittgers et al. reported that a significant drop in fistula blood flow predicted thrombosis.[12] The usefulness of this technique, however, is currently limited by high cost and operator variability. In comparison, VDP and urea recirculation are both physiologic measurements that can be performed repetitively and at a minimum cost. Stenoses that are detected still require angiography prior to correction.

Angiography

Although fistulograms cannot give detailed assessment of actual fistula function, they are the "gold standard" for identifying anatomic lesions in the fistula circuit. By providing detailed visualization of the fistula lumen, the arterial and venous anastomosis, and proximal venous runoff, fistulography allows the clinician to identify anatomic lesions at any site.[7] These studies are not used as a routine screening tool for fistula evaluation because of high cost and low prevalence of stenosis in the general dialysis population.

We use the clinical and monitoring parameters as indications for fistulogram, as outlined in table 3-4. Patients with elevated VDP on three consecutive treatments or elevated recirculation rates (checked monthly) are referred for elective fistulogram. Because venous stenosis is the most common cause of thrombosis, patients who experience graft thrombosis are referred for fistulogram even if VDP and recirculation are normal. Once detected, stenoses are corrected by either angioplasty or surgical revision.

Treatment of Stenosis

Once an anatomic lesion causing graft dysfunction has been identified, this may be corrected with either surgical revision or angioplasty. Surgical revision has the advantage of low recurrence rates, but often requires extension of the graft more proximally, thereby eliminating future potential access sites. Angioplasty has the advantage that it can be done on an outpatient basis at the time of fistulogram. It also can be performed on single or multiple lesions and can be used in central venous lesions, which are difficult to correct surgically.[9]

The major drawback to angioplasty is re-stenosis, which varies from 30-80% at one year. In our experience, the initial technical success of angioplasty is 85% for anastomotic, 85% for peripheral venous, and 95% for central venous lesions, with stenosis rates of 20%, 33%, and 50%, respectively, at one year.[25] Beathard reported an initial success rate of 94%, with 38.7% six-month and 61.8% one-year re-stenosis rates.[16] However, most re-stenoses can be opened with repeat angioplasty. Our approach is to attempt angioplasty in all approachable lesions. We reserve surgical revision for patients with technical failures, nonangioplastiable anatomy, and repeated re-stenosis after the procedure. We and others have performed clinical trials with endovascular stents in an attempt to minimize recurrence of venous stenoses following angioplasty.[26,27] Results from these trials showed that stents are of limited value in preventing recurrence because of exuberant endothelial hyperplasia. Only the subset of elastic lesions responded favorably to stent placement.[26]

It has been shown previously that prospective identification and treatment has profound effects on graft patency and long-term graft survival.[14] In addition, addressing these lesions can improve fistula function and dialysis efficiency. Collins et al. and Windus et al. reported that correction with either surgery or angioplasty led to an improvement in recirculation rates and improvements in dialysis efficiency.[13,17] Therefore, prospective identification of venous stenoses and correction by surgery or angioplasty reduces recirculation and improves the dialysis procedure by increasing solute clearance.

References

1. Hakim RA, Depner TA, Parker TF. Adequacy of hemodialysis. Am J Kidney Dis 1992; 20:107-123.
2. Lowrie EG, Laird NM, Parker TF, Sargeant JA. Effect of hemodialysis prescription on patient morbidity. N Engl J Med 1981; 305:1176-1181.
3. Gotch FA, Sargeant JA. A mechanistic analysis of the National Cooperative Dialysis Study. Kidney Int 1985; 28:526-534.
4. Delmez JA, Windus DA, for St. Louis Nephrology Study Group. Hemodialysis prescription and delivery in a metropolitan community. Kidney Int 1992; 41:1023-1028.
5. Besarab A, Dorrell S, Moritz M, Sullivan K, Michael H. What can be done to preserve vascular access for dialysis? Semin Dial 1991; 4:155-156.
6. Carlson DM, Duncan DA, Naessens JM, Johnson WJ. Hospitalization in dialysis patients. Mayo Clinic Proc 1984; 59:769-775.
7. Windus DW. Permanent vascular access: a nephrologist's view. Am J Kidney Dis 1993; 21:457-471.
8. Fan PY, Schwab SJ. Vascular access: concepts for the 1990's. J Am Soc Nephrol 1992; 3:1-11.
9. Butterly D, Schwab SJ. Hemodialysis vascular access: effect on urea kinetics and dialysis prescription. Am J Nephrol (in press).
10. Anderson CB, Etheredge EE, Harter HR, Codd JE, Graff, Newton WT. Blood flow measurements in arteriovenous dialysis fistulas. Surgery 1977; 81:459-461.
11. Burdick ZJF, Scott W, Cosimi AB. Experience with Dacron graft arteriovenous fistulas for dialysis access. Ann Surg 1978; 187:262-266.
12. Rittgers SE, Garcia-Valdez C, McCormick JT, Posner MP. Noninvasive blood flow measure-

ments in expanded polytetraflouroethylene grafts for hemodialysis access. J Vasc Surg 1986; 3:635-642.

13. Collins DM, Lambert MB, Middleton JP, Proctor R, Davidson CJ, Newman GE, Schwab SJ. Fistula dysfunction: Effect on rapid hemodialysis. Kidney Int 1992; 41:1292-1296.
14. Schwab SJ, Raymond JR, Saeed M, Newman GE, Dennis P, Bollinger RR. Prevention of hemodialysis fistula thrombosis. Early detection of venous stenosis. Kidney Int 1989; 36:707-711.
15. Schwab S, Quarles D, Middleton JP, Cohan RH, Saeed M, Dennis VW. Hemodialysis associated subclavian vein stenosis. Kidney Int 1988; 33:1156-1159.
16. Beathard GA. Percutaneous transvenous angioplasty in the treatment of vascular access stenosis. Kidney Int 1992; 42:1390-1397.
17. Windus D, Audrain J, Vanderson R, Jendrisak MD, Picus D, Delmez JA. Optimization of high-efficiency hemodialysis by detection and correction of fistula function. Kidney Int 1990; 38:337-341.
18. Akmal M, Hanks SE, Katz MD, Kapstein EM. Limb edema as a complication of venous catheterization and arteriovenous access creation for hemodialysis. J Am Soc Nephrol 1993; 4:330A.
19. Depner TA. Techniques for prospective detection of venous stenosis. In: SJ Schwab, ed. Advances in renal replacement therapy (in press).
20. Daniels ID, Hoffer EK, George-Cipriani JA, Friedman EA, Lundin AP. Clinical tests detect hemodialysis stenosis. J Am Soc Nephrol 1993; 4:102A.
21. Michael H, Dorrell S, Besarab A, Moritz M. Vascular dialysis accesses. Determinants of measured venous dialysis pressures and relationship to intra-access venous pressure. J Am Soc Nephrol 1990; 1:369A.
22. Sullivan KL, Besarab A, Bonn J, Shapiro MJ, Gardiner GA, Moritz MJ. Hemodynamics of failing dialysis grafts. Radiology 1993; 186:867-872.
23. Sherman RA. The measurement of dialysis access recirculation. Am J Kidney Dis 1993; 22:616-621.
24. Shackelton CR, Taylor DC, Buckley AR, Rowley VA, Cooperberg PL, Fry PD. Predicting failure in polytetrafluoroethylene vascular access grafts for hemodialysis. Can J Surg 1987; 30:442-444.
25. Newman GE, Davidson CJ, McCann RL, Schwab SJ. Functional restenosis rate after hemodialysis graft angioplasty. J Am Soc Nephrol 1991; 2:341A.
26. Kovalik E, Newman G, Suhocki P, Schwab SJ. Treatment of central vein stenoses: role of angioplasty and endovascular Wallstents. Kidney Int 1994; 45:1177-1181.
27. Beathard G. Gianturco self expanding stents in the treatment of stenoses in hemodialysis grafts. Kidney Int 1993; 43:872-877.

DISCUSSION

Moderator:
Mitchell L. Henry, M.D.
Panelists:
Richard Dickerman, M.D.
Ralph H. Didlake, M.D.
Phillip Held, M.D.
Steve Schwab, M.D.

Discussant: Dr. Schwab, could you comment on the use of venous pressures to screen vascular access for future failure? My understanding from Dr. Besarab's papers is that this is not terribly effective.

Dr. Schwab: I think you are right. Dr. Besarab has pointed out that at least in primary arteriovenous fistulas, he finds venous dialysis pressures to be less predictive. To a certain extent, that is also our observation. Because we do not have a large number of A-V fistulas and they clot less often, it is more difficult to reach statistical significance. However, we certainly do detect stenoses in primary A-V fistulas and we correct them. The truth of the matter is that the stenoses occur much less frequently, for reasons that I do not understand.

Discussant: Dr. Schwab, a procedural question. You are talking about doing venous pressures in the first 10 minutes at the low blood flow rates. Is there some magic to the first 10 minutes and to keeping the blood flow down for that long? Is there any reason you could not do it midway through the dialysis over a two-minute period?

Dr. Schwab: A subset of patients will develop venous spasm after needle insertion, and we would like for the venous spasm to resolve itself prior to measuring venous dialysis pressure. We chose 10 minutes because Beathard made that work. Originally, we liked to wait 15 to 20 minutes, but in his 1992 paper, Beathard showed that he could get reliable measurements in 10 minutes. Ten minutes resulted because people want to run blood flows of 400–450 cc/min to deliver a good hemodialysis treatment and do not want to wait much longer. The reason that we wait 10 minutes is it is probably the soonest you can still get reproducible measurements. The third question is, Can you measure it at any time in the treatment? Can you do that in the treatment when they are coming off of the machine? The answer is that you may well be able to do so. We have routinely not done it then because at the beginning of the treatment the patient usually is stable, with a stable blood pressure, and I believe the measurements will be more consistent. Hypotension tends to occur toward the end of the ultrafiltration period. The cardiac output falls toward the end of the treatment. I believe that at the beginning of the treatment it is just more reproducible.

Discussant: Two questions for Dr. Schwab. One may be more logistical with your surgeons. Why do you keep your revisions in house 24 hours? I think many folks do it as an outpatient without much trouble. Second, when you look at all of the studies of thrombosis that occurs, it is clear that there is a small number of patients who require a repeated number of procedures and become a thorn in the side of most of us here in this room. Did you look at that group of patients, those with reduced thrombosis and revision rates, and is that group positively affected by screening?

Dr. Schwab: Why do we put revisions in house for 24 hours? We admit patients undergoing revision for 24 hours because although our vascular access surgeons do thrombectomies as an outpatient procedure, they believe that new PTFE, with its antecedent swelling, should be observed for 24 hours. The answer to the second question is yes, I believe you have a subset of patients who tend to repetitively clot. I believe those patients repetitively clot because you did not solve the problem in the first place. What we have seen is that these patients do better once their stenoses are fixed.

Dr. Henry: Dr. Dickerman, do you think that everybody needs to be admitted overnight after the placement of access or revisions?

Dr. Dickerman: We do about 60 procedures per month, all on outpatients. The only reason we admit them is if they are hyperkalemic or if they are volume overloaded. Again, these are patients with failed access, not patients with new grafts.

Dr. Henry: Dr. Didlake, would you want to comment now?

Dr. Didlake: I will comment just briefly now. We do not feel that patients with revisions need to be admitted a priori. There are some specific indications for admissions, but we do about 80% of all of our access surgery on an outpatient basis.

Discussant: I have a question for the people who are constantly thrombosing their grafts. In our institution, we are having a lot of heparin antibodies discovered. I do not know whether that is pertinent or not, but what are your thoughts on heparin antibodies and clotting of access?

Dr. Schwab: We do not necessarily look for antiplatelet or antiheparin antibodies unless we come up with a problem. Because we have low-molecular-weight heparin and heparinoids available on investigational protocol, those patients who develop heparin-associated thrombocytopenia are those whom we believe to have thrombosis-related heparin antibodies. We will initially conduct a trial on experimental protocol of one of the two or three available heparinoids. The disadvantage of the heparinoids is there is some crossover, about 30%, of patients who will still maintain antibody positivity. The other disadvantage is that the low-molecular-weight heparins are expensive. When they are on protocol, I can use them, but when I have to pay for them I am not sure I will be able to.

Discussant: I have a question for Dr. Dickerman and the rest of the panel as well. Let's say the Health Care Financing Administration capitated the end-stage renal disease program. Would your algorithm of how you handle a clotted access change? You are using a lot of interventions such as thrombolysis and percutaneous angioplasty. Would it change, and if so, how?

Dr. Dickerman: I think it absolutely would. I still think taking the patient to the operating room for treatment is still the least expensive procedure. Whether or not that is the patient or the nephrology preference, it is hard to say. I understand the point you are making and I still think in 90% of the cases, taking the patient to the operating room is the quickest and most cost-effective mode of treatment.

Dr. Didlake: I agree completely. Taking the patient to the operating room electively is probably the most cost-effective way we have currently. In the future, I think it depends on our ability to have a cheap and reliable screening method. A quick and clean method that the nurses can perform at the bedside at each dialysis session.

Dr. Schwab: We are in the process right now of trying to examine what aggressive intervention costs. That is difficult because we do not have a positive control group. If we were capitated, I think we would maintain the concept of prospective intervention.

Discussant: Do you use Coumadin following stent placement?

Panelist: No.

Discussant: Do you do on-table angiograms with your revisions or primary grafts?

Panelist: No.

Discussant: You talk a lot about strictures or stenoses. If these patients are given angiograms after the graft has been used for a while, they all show narrowing in the body of the graft or at the venous end. How do you know which stenoses are significant? Do you measure pressure gradients? How do you decide what is important to deal with?

Dr. Schwab: I think you reviewed a couple of my papers. I think that is an excellent question, but if you look at the study design, we did not take stenoses that did not have a physiologic variable. Patients in our group who went on to intervention either thrombosed their fistula, had an elevated urea recirculation (which is a physiologic proof of an upstream stenosis), or met our protocol for elevated venous dialysis pressure. All of these are a physiologic, although indirect, flow variable. In the report on our study, I did not mention where we used intravascular ultrasound. We actually mapped a cross-sectional diameter and did pullback pressures. And in roughly 70% of the stenoses, there was a positive pressure gradient across the lesion. But I think your point is well taken. What you are asking is, if we did not use a physiologic screen such as venous dialysis pressure or urea recirculation, and if we just looked at the images, how would we know that the intervention helped or did not help? The only way you would know would be to randomize the groups and then follow them to see if the intervention made a difference. I would argue that in an unplanned and imperfect way, we did that. I can say if you have a physiologic variable—elevated urea recirculation, for example—and you leave it alone, it clots. I can tell you that if you correct the stenoses, urea recirculation and venous pressure return to near normal.

Discussant: What about failure as it involves the body of the graft, the conduit?

Dr. Henry: I am going to talk more about that later, but measuring flow in the graft with color flow Doppler can help determine whether that graft is going to fail in the future.

Discussant: I agree with that, because you and I have both shown data that flow correlates, with clotting, rather than stenosis. You can predict which stenotic lesions are going to clot using Doppler. I want to make a comment about cost data. We presented at ASIO a paper comparing thrombolytic therapy for acutely occluded PTFE grafts to the use of surgery. We showed a cost difference of about $6,000 between groups favoring surgery. I wondered if you all have had that same experience and whether you have looked at that?

Dr. Henry: I will comment briefly on the cost issue. A lot of cost studies have been cross-sectional rather than logitudinal views of costs. If you do not look at re-thrombosis or re-stenosis rates over time, all costs may not be addressed. In multicenter trials, the major problem from institution to institution is that the protocols may be quite different. For a patient with a patent graft, an overnight hospitalization for a thrombectomy and patch angioplasty surgically probably is going to cost more than a percutaneous transluminal angioplasty in a stable outpatient setting. Those differences need to be taken into close consideration when examining cost data.

Dr. Held: I would like to make a quick comment on the question about what a capitation scheme would mean. I think it gets to the heart of a really tremendous change that would likely occur if such a scheme were put in place. A lot of work was done a long time ago on the design of a capitation plan and it was not well received at that time. But the point made in the question is a very good one. We know in general that putting decision making and resource control at the local level and letting a person who is making the choices care for the full patient is a good thing. We saw, for example, that when capitation came in for transplantation, a kidney transplant length of stay was cut in half. My guess is that most people would think that is not a bad thing. But a real problem with capitation, one that should be of tremendous concern for everybody, is that capitation often brings with it terrible quality and incentive problems. The incentive is to spend as little as you can get by with. I am not saying everybody does that, but that is what the question is.

I was recently put on the spot at the National Renal Administrators meeting when asked if I would I support a motion to put the cost of erythropoietin into the composite rate, that is to make a pot of money. My response was that I thought placing the decision making for this at the local level, thus leaving that choice to the physician, was a good idea. Then I went around the room and asked them a similar question. I said, "Let's put it another way. If your child had kidney failure, would you rather have EPO as a separate charge or combined?" I was stunned that every administrator in the room said that if it were their child, they would rather have a separate charge. So to get back to the question, I would like to ask this group today, If the patient were your child, would you elect to do the procedure, on an outpatient basis?

Dr. Dickerman: We deal with a patient population that is largely undereducated and has limited resources. In that population, we have found that outpatient management of most access-related problems is entirely safe. I believe that I would be comfortable taking care of my child on an outpatient basis.

Dr. Didlake: I would agree with that. We have done more than 1,000 of these procedures in the past several years on an outpatient basis and we have had not had a single mortality. We have had several of them come back during the night with problems, but we have not had a mortality. I would continue to push for these to be done on an outpatient basis.

Discussant: We are finding that we are using more and more low-dose Coumadin in patients in whom we cannot identify anatomic causes. Does this make sense to you?

Dr. Schwab: There was a recent paper in *Kidney International* that looked at the use of antiplatelet agents and gave us some very confusing guidance. This paper said that aspirin does not work. This paper said that in certain doses, Persantine works in patients who have not had a thrombosis, but does not work in patients who have had a thrombosis. So I would tell you that the use of antiplatelet agents has to be questionable at best. I have not used low-dose Coumadin, despite its proven benefit in total parenteral nutrition catheters because I am afraid of low-dose Coumadin. I think my patients who have been anticoagulated for heart valves have had disastrous morbidity and mortality compared with those patients who get porcine valves and are not anticoagulated. I have learned to fear anticoagulation in patients with either a PTFE graft or hemodialysis fistula.

Dr. Dickerman: The key is low-dose Coumadin. We have found it to be extremely helpful in some problem patients. I think the problem is when you get too much Coumadin on board. We are starting to use more and more low-dose Coumadin, and I would encourage you to do the same in that problem population with re-thrombosis.

Dr. Didlake: We also have a very small population of patients who are recurrent clotters with no apparent anatomic problem, and we have put them on a relatively homeopathic dose of Coumadin. I am greatly concerned about the side effects of Coumadin and about antiplatelet therapy generally. First is the question of which agent do you use. All of the antiplatelet drugs have their own set of complications. It is an issue that we need to look into very carefully because it may have direct biochemical and cellular effects on pseudointimal hyperplasia. I believe that this area needs a lot more research.

SECTION II

4

STENTS IN HEMODIALYSIS ACCESS

Scott O. Trerotola, M.D.

VENOUS STENOSIS COMPLICATING VASCULAR ACCESS is a chronic and recurrent problem in patients undergoing hemodialysis, contributing significantly to morbidity, hospitalization, and cost. Stenosis of outflow veins of native fistulas and synthetic grafts results in access malfunction and ultimately thrombosis, while central venous stenosis ipsilateral to a functioning vascular access can lead to debilitating arm swelling as well as access failure. Although prevention of these stenoses would be ideal, to date this goal has not been achieved. Instead, numerous approaches to the treatment of venous stenosis in hemodialysis access have been developed, all with less than optimal results.[1-4] Percutaneous transluminal angioplasty (PTA) and atherectomy, although they are associated with relatively good initial results, suffer from early re-stenosis, and surgical revision can deplete future access sites. Vascular endoprostheses, or stents, have been introduced during the past decade and are used in the treatment of failed angioplasty in the arterial system, primarily the iliac arteries. Because of the excellent results achieved with metallic stents in the arterial system, they have been considered for use in the treatment of hemodialysis-related venous stenosis. The purpose of this review is to describe these prostheses, their current role in hemodialysis access, and potential future uses for them.

Stent Designs

Different types of metallic stent have been tried in hemodialysis access, but only three are currently available in the United States. None of these are FDA-approved for venous use; all are approved for biliary use, and one, the Palmaz stent (Johnson and Johnson Interventional Systems, Warren, New Jersey), is approved for iliac arterial use. Use of metallic stents in this country, therefore, is limited to compassionate "off-label" use or clinical trials.

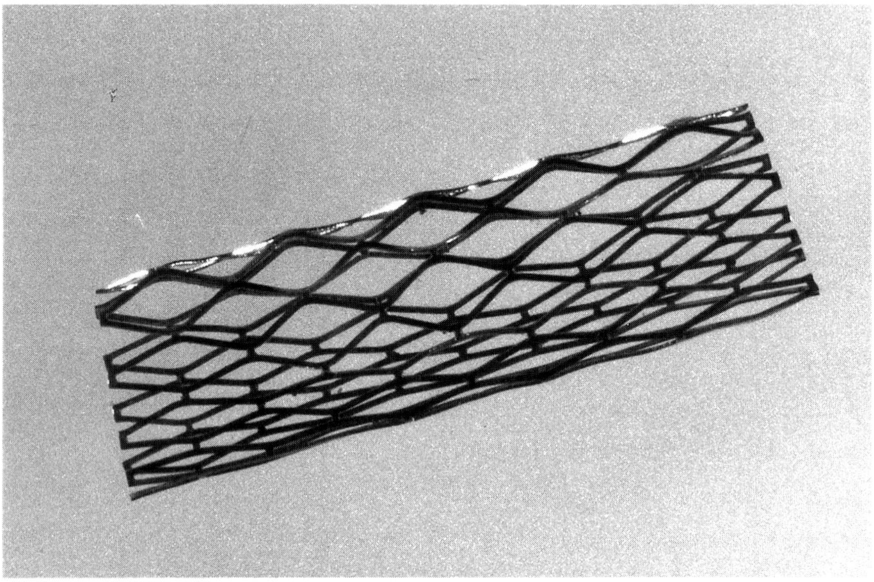

Figure 4-1. Palmaz balloon expandable stent.

The Palmaz stent (figure 4-1) is a stainless steel, balloon-expandable endoprosthesis. This device is delivered through a 7-9 Fr sheath and expanded to 4-12 mm using a balloon, depending upon the specific stent size. Once expanded, the stent may collapse if exposed to extrinsic crushing force, making it unsuitable for use in hemodialysis access. The role of this stent in central venous stenosis is discussed below. The advantages of this stent are availability, radiopacity, and ease of use. The stent is rigid and therefore poorly suited for use in curved vessels.

The Gianturco Z stent (Cook Inc., Bloomington, Indiana) may be configured several ways. The basic building block of the stent is a zigzag stainless steel wire barrel, hence the name Z stent. The barrel segments may be held together by metallic struts (Wallace modification, figure 4-2) or by suture (Roesch modification), or the stent may consist of a single spiral zigzag wire held together with suture (spiral Z stent).[5] These stents are self-expanding; therefore, if they are exposed to extrinsic crushing force they will resume their shape once the force is removed. Their design allows for some vessel curvature. Depending upon the size of stent used, the delivery sheath size may range from 8.5 to 16 Fr or more. The only commercially available Z stent is the Roesch modified stent, used almost exclusively in the biliary tree. However, the simple stent design has allowed investigators to make their own stents, which have been used clinically.[6,7] One of the significant potential advantages of this stent design over other stents is the low amount of metallic surface area, which may offer some advantage in patency.[8]

The Wallstent (Schneider, Minneapolis, Minnesota,) (figure 4-3) is a stainless steel alloy woven stent that is also self-expanding. This stent is available in 8–12-mm size ranges in this country and in much larger diameters in Europe. The 8–12-mm size stents are delivered through a 7 Fr sheath. The stent is very flexible, allowing its use in curved vessels and tortuous access. The metallic surface area is significantly higher than the previously described stent designs. Due to availability, flexibility and self-expansion, this stent has been the preferred stent for venous stenoses in hemodialysis patients among most investigators.

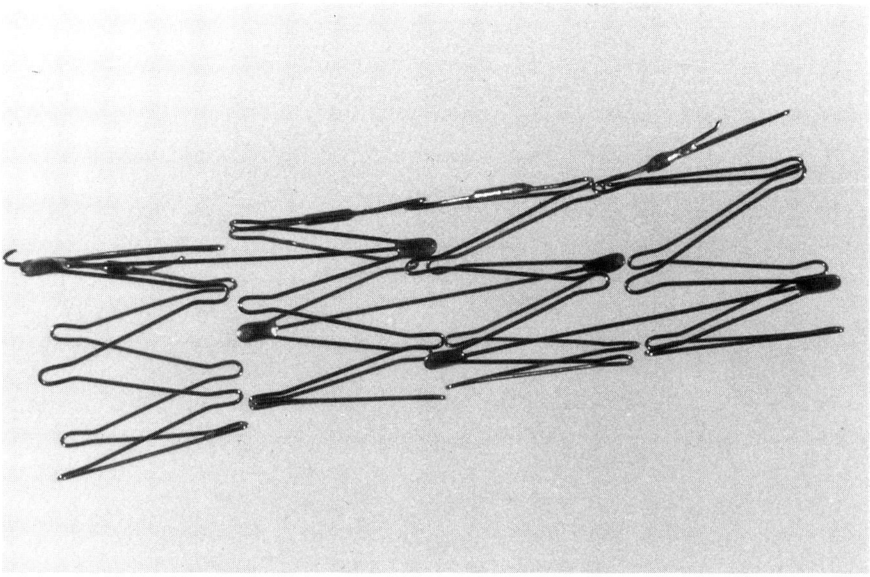

Figure 4-2. Wallace modified Gianturco Z stent. This stent is self-expanding.

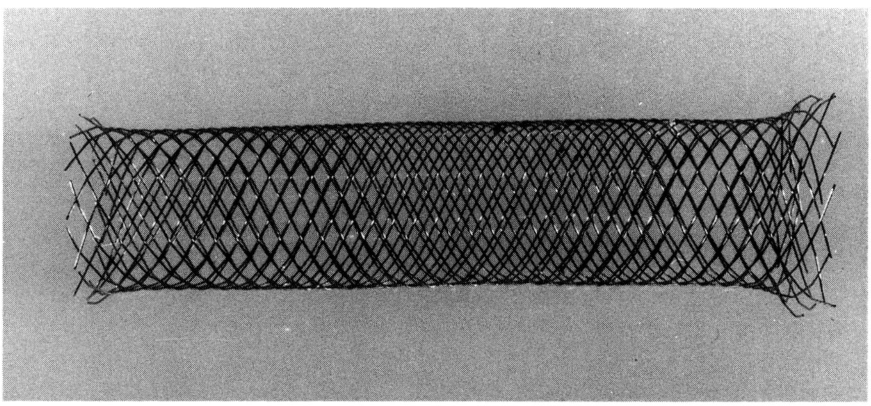

Figure 4-3. Wallstent. Note the braided design of this self-expanding stent.

Peripheral Stenoses

The first clinical application of metallic endoprostheses in hemodialysis access is generally attributed to Maass et al.[9], who used a spiral support in bovine heterografts to prolong the life of these grafts. The first application of percutaneously placed metallic stents was reported by Zollikofer et al in 1988,[10] and since then multiple reports and small series have been published describing the use of stents in hemodialysis access.[11-17]

Investigators have not used stents until all other percutaneous means of access salvage had been exhausted (e.g., PTA, atherectomy). The stents most commonly used have been Wallstents, although Gianturco[6,7] and Strecker (not available in the United States) stents[15] have also been used. In general, Palmaz stents have not been used in peripheral lesions due to their nonself-expandingnature. Technical success in stent placement has been excellent, with success rates in excess of 90%, but stents in peripheral venous lesions have been plagued by problems with re-stenosis. Vorwerk et al., in a series of 18 patients with Wallstents used to treat venous outflow stenoses, described multiple events of re-thrombosis and re-stenosis following stent placement with only 27% patency at 18 months.[12] With aggressive reintervention, however, 77% cumulative patency was achieved. Beathard, using Gianturco stents in 28 patients, showed no difference in patency between stented grafts and a control group treated with PTA alone, demonstrating one-year patency of 17% (although only primary patency was evaluated).[7] Quinn et al., in a study combining central and peripheral stents, reported two-year primary patency of 25%, secondary patency of 34%, and tertiary patency of 42%.[6] Other investigators have reported similar results.

Re-stenosis within stents has been treated with thrombolysis, and if necessary, PTA, new stents, and the Simpson atherectomy device as needed, with the ability to significantly prolong access life with these aggressive interventions. However, given the satisfactory results of surgical revision, there are several reasons that this approach will likely remain the mainstay of therapy in most patients after failure of PTA/atherectomy. First, the cost of stents (nearly $1,000 per device) may be prohibitive, erasing any potential advantages of the percutaneous approach. Second, stents may not be punctured with needles, thus in Brescia-Cimino fistulas their presence could impede hemodialysis. Third, if stents are not judiciously placed to minimize coverage of normal vein, they may deplete access "real estate."

What, then, is the role of stents in peripheral stenoses in hemodialysis access? We have reserved use of stents for failures of PTA (usually two procedures within a three-month period, whereas some investigators use a six-month period)[17] in patients in whom surgical revision is either not an option or is undesirable for some reason. Figures 4-4A and 4-4B illustrate this type of situation. In patients in whom no other access is available, stents can prolong the life of the existing access almost indefinitely, provided aggressive treatment of re-stenosis is performed. This type of approach has been reported by one group to yield 71% cumulative patency at 3 years.[17]

Central Venous Stenosis

Whereas widespread use of stents in peripheral venous lesions awaits control of re-stenosis, stents have found an important role in the treatment of hemodialysis-related central venous stenosis. The reasons for this paradox are several: They include the lack of viable surgical options in central venous stenosis and the fact that re-stenosis, while present, may be less significant in these larger stents. All stents, arterial and venous, are subject to some amount of re-stenosis as the stent is incorporated into the vessel wall and healing occurs.[18] The larger the initial lumen of the stent, the less significant the intimal hyperplasia will be. This is not to say that re-stenosis

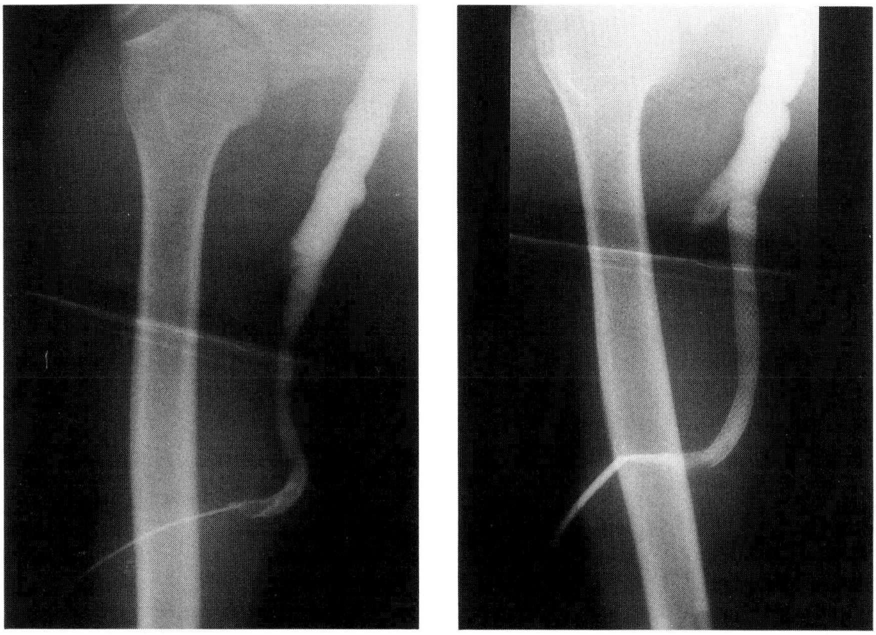

Figure 4-4A. (Above left) Stenosis in venous outflow of upper-arm PTFE dialysis graft. After several angioplasties over a six-month period, lesion became unresponsive to PTA. Residual stenosis seen here after PTA. had significant pressure gradient across it. The patient had no other available access sites, thus stent placement was considered.

Figure 4-4B. (Above right) After placement of 42-mm long by 10-mm diameter Wallstent, angiographic result is excellent. Note that very little normal vein has been covered, an important principle in preserving access sites.

in central venous stents is not a problem; it is just that it takes longer to become a problem in a 10–12-mm or larger stent than in a 6-mm stent. Unfortunately, unlike stents used to treat arterial and nonhemodialysis-related venous stenoses (where intimal hyperplasia peaks after a few months, then may actually regress), intimal hyperplasia in the hemodialysis population is a relentless, progressive process.

Despite problems with re-stenosis, stents in hemodialysis-related central venous stenosis can offer substantial prolongation of patency once PTA has failed. Similar to peripheral lesions, stents should be reserved until PTA is no longer successful. Unfortunately, the results of PTA in central lesions are even worse than peripheral lesions, with 10-35% one-year patency.[3,19] Despite these results, PTA is less costly, does not involve the implantation of a permanent device, can be repeated easily, and can offer long-term benefit in a subset of patients. Thus, it should be used as the primary treatment modality. Unlike peripheral lesions, however, when PTA fails, the surgical options are limited to bypasses that generally offer poor patency or abandonment of access in the affected limb. Thus, stents offer a viable intermediate option and can stave off loss of access in the affected

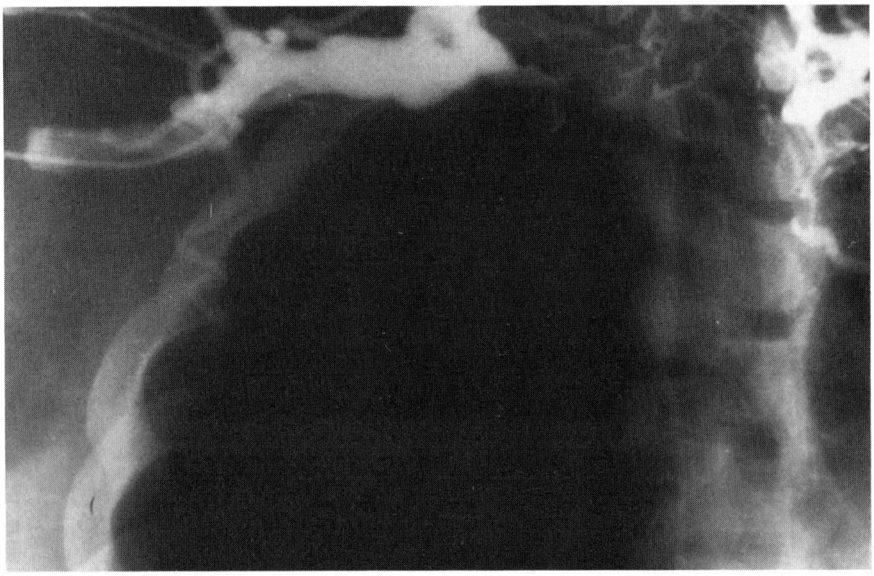

Figure 4-5A. Central venous stenosis/occlusion in patient with ipsilateral PTFE access graft. Catheter was inserted via graft; contrast injection shows complete occlusion of right subclavian vein with multiple collaterals. Patient had disabling arm swelling.

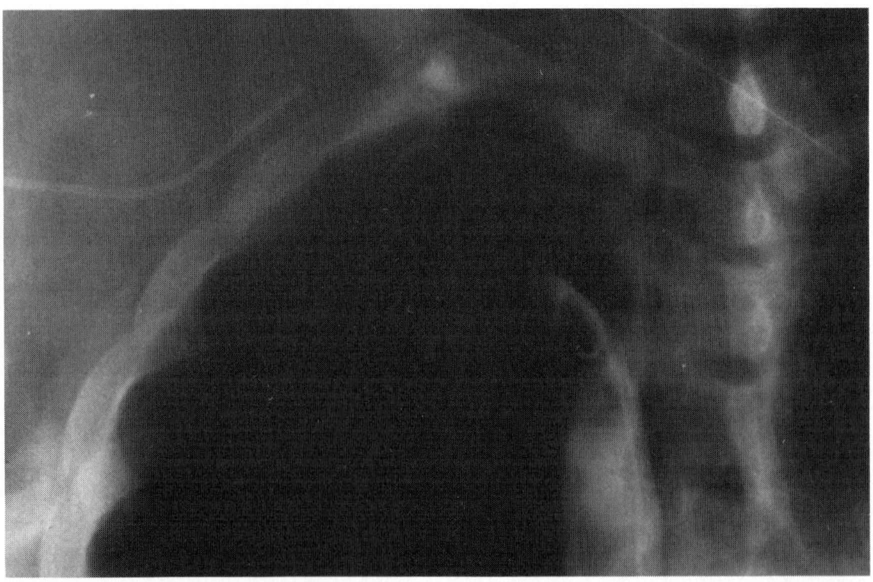

Figure 4-5B. Catheter inserted via right femoral approach allows delineation of extent of lesion.

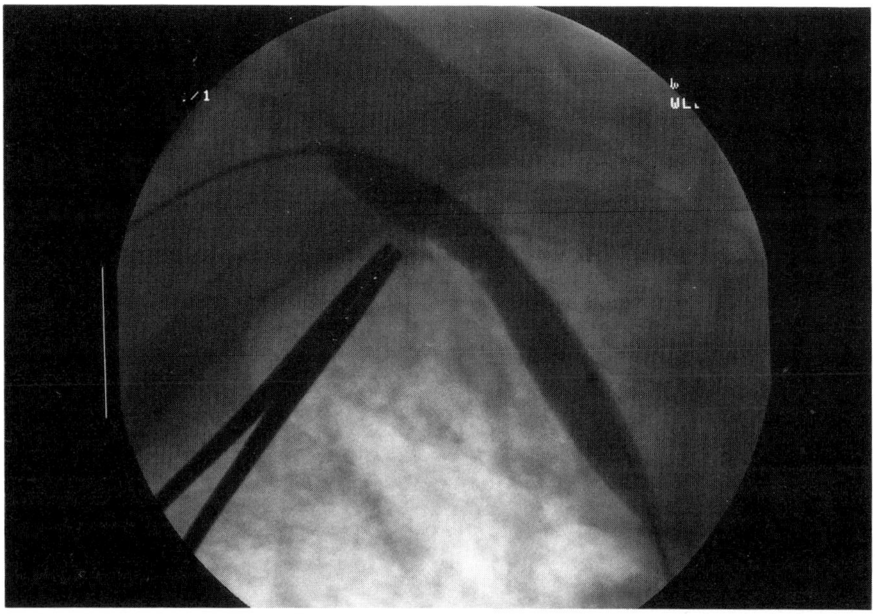

Figure 4-5C. After successfully crossing lesion with guide wire, balloon angioplasty was performed. Unfortunately, there was immediate recurrence of the occlusion.

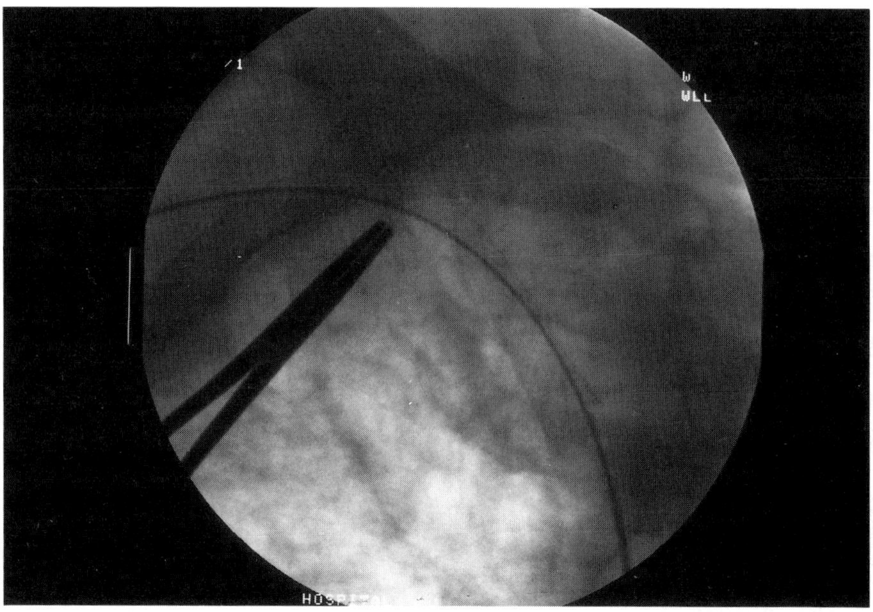

Figure 4-5D. Because of the extreme elasticity of the lesion, a Wallstent was placed.

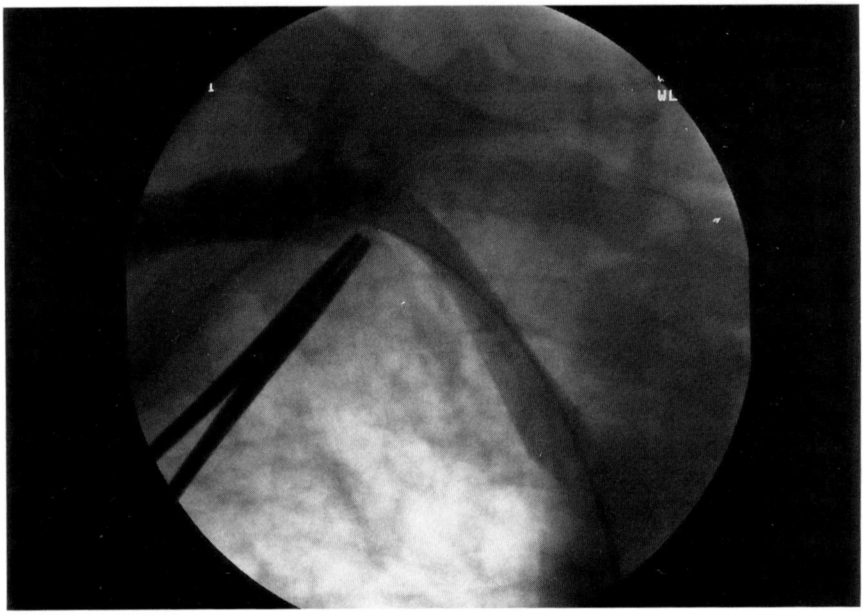

Figure 4-5E. Poststent angiographic result is excellent.

limb for months to years. Figures 4-5A–4-5E show use of a stent in central venous stenosis.

No comparative studies of stents to PTA in central venous stenosis have been performed, and most series describing central venous stents combine malignant indications with benign. Few large series describing central stents in hemodialysis access have been published. Quinn et al. stated that central stents appeared to suffer less restenosis than peripheral stents.[6] Vorwerk et al., describing brachial and central stents in 33 patients, had a 97% success rate with 40% one-year patency and 77% one-year assisted patency.[16] These and other limited and preliminary data indicate that although stents are initially effective in treating lesions no longer responsive to PTA, secondary intervention is neccessary in a substantial number of patients. Like peripheral lesions, re-stenosis is treated with repeat stent placement, PTA and/or use of the Simpson atherectomy catheter to cut out neointima ("neointimectomy"). Several observations regarding central stents are worth noting. It appears that Palmaz stents are poorly suited to treatment of central stenoses, as reports of stent migration[20] and compression[21] associated with this device have been published. Re-stenosis may be more significant with this stent in high-flow venous lesions (figure 4-6).[22] Since most central vessels are curved, the Wallstent is probably the stent of choice for these lesions, and the recently FDA-approved 12-mm diameter Wallstent may offer better patency by virtue of its larger initial lumen. Anticoagulation has been used by some investigators, but others give only aspirin or no medication at all, assuming that the high flow will prevent stent thrombosis in the short term.

The current protocol for stent placement at Indiana University Medical Center, Indianapolis, requires angioplasty to be used as the initial treatment modality for central venous stenosis. Primary stent placement is never performed. If angioplasty fails immediately (as indicated by persistent pressure gradient of 10 mm Hg or more

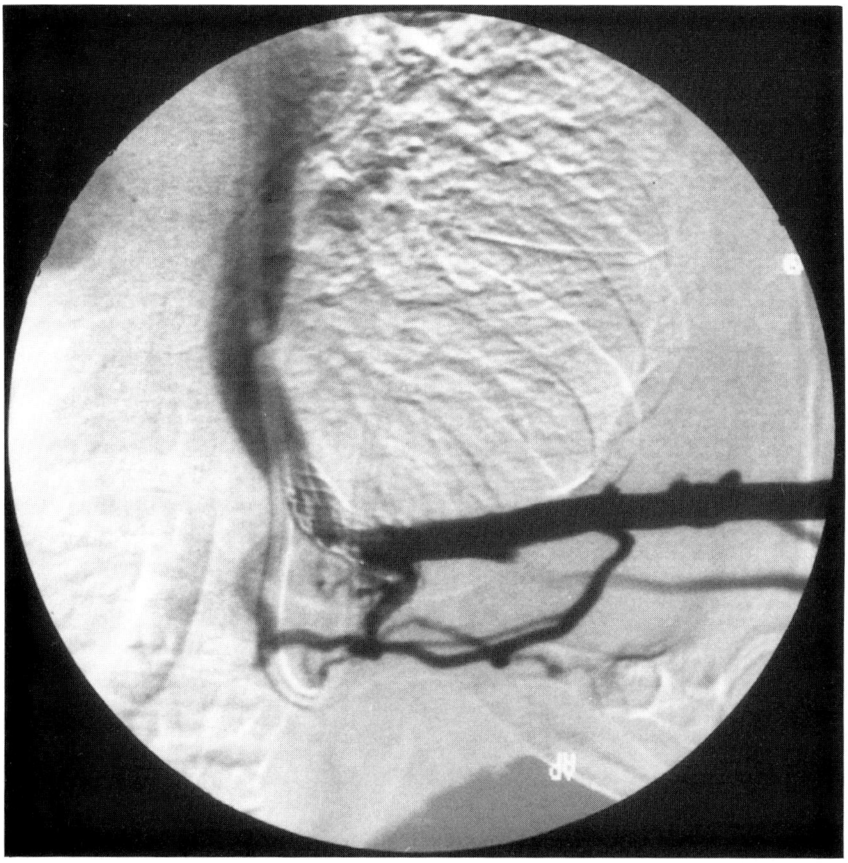

Figure 4-6. Re-stenosis in Palmaz stent used to treat central stenosis in patient with ipsilateral PTFE access graft. Note intimal hyperplasia within stent and collaterals. We currently avoid using this stent in hemodialysis access (see text).

and/or persistent of significant collateral vessels), or if re-stenosis occurs twice within a three-month period, stent placement is performed. Contraindica-tions to stent placement include active infection and inability to efface the waist on a high-pressure PTA balloon. Prophylactic antibiotics are given, as there has been at least one case of fatal sepsis associated with stent placement in a hemodialysis patient.[6] Venous access may be accomplished via the ipsilateral graft/fistula, common femoral vein, or, in difficult (especially right-sided) lesions, by both approaches using through-and-through technique. In general, every attempt is made to avoid crossing side branches that might be important for future access. The shortest stent possible is used. A Wallstent of suitable size and length is chosen to match the diameter of the adjacent normal vein with approximately 10% overdilation. Good stent contact with the adjacent vein is important but may not always be possible in veins larger than 12 mm. Once the stent is in place, it is dilated to the appropriate vessel size to ensure good contact. If low-dose anticoagulation can be tolerated by the patient, this is given for three months and then discontinued. Re-stenosis, as detected by recurrent arm swelling, access malfunction, or routine fistulography, is treated as described above.

Future Directions

It should be obvious from the preceding discussion that stents in hemodialysis access have been poorly studied to date, but are clearly not a panacea. Our initial enthusiasm for these devices has been tempered by the realization that they are much more prone to re-stenosis in this patient population than in the arterial or nonhemodialysis-related venous system. Future research concerning stents in this area will, it is hoped, lead to effective means of preventing re-stenosis, as well as stent designs that might be better suited to high-flow veins. These may include less metallic surface area, larger diameters, and stent coatings designed to avoid re-stenosis. Until that time, judicious use of these valuable devices in selected patients and lesions will allow us to reach the common goal of prolonging access life maximally.

References

1. Palder SB, Kirkman RL, Whittemore AD, Hakim RM, Lazarus M, et. al., Vascular access for hemodialysis. Ann Surg 1985; 202:235-239.
2. Brooks JL, Sigley RD, May KJ, Mack RM. Transluminal angioplasty versus surgical repair for stenosis of hemodialysis grafts. Am J Surg 1987;153:530-531.
3. Glanz S, Gordon DH, Butt KMH, Hong, J, Lipkowitz, GS. The role of percutaneous angioplasty in the management of chronic hemodialysis fistulas. Ann Surg 1987, 206(6): 777-781.
4. Gray, RJ, Dolmatch, BL, Buick, MK. Directional atherectomy in the treatment of stenotic dialysis access fistulas. JVIR 1990; 1:35-38.
5. Maeda M, Timmermans HA, Uchida BT, Uchida H, Keller FS, Rösch J. In vitro comparison of the spiral Z stent and the Gianturco Z stent. JVIR 1992; 3:565-569.
6. Quinn SF, Schuman ES, Hall L, et al. Venous stenoses in patients who undergo hemodialysis: treatment with self-expandable endovascular stents. Radiology 1992; 183:499-504.
7. Beathard G. Gianturco self-expanding stent in the treatment of stenosis in dialysis access grafts. Kidney Int 1993; 43:872-877.
8. Trerotola SO, Fair JH, Magee CA, Samphilipo MA. Comparison of stent designs in hemodialysis access grafts: Work in progress in an animal model (abstr). JVIR 1993; 4:57.
9. Maass D, Binswanger U, Rausis C, Uhlschmid GK, Largiader F. Intravenous spiral support for the prevention of outflow-tract stenosis in A-V-shunts for hemodialysis? Res Exp Med 1985; 185:63-68.
10. Zollikofer CL, Largiader I, Bruhlmann WF, Uhlschmid GK, Marty AH. Endovascular stenting of veins and grafts: preliminary clinical experience. Radiology 1988; 167:707-712.
11. Gunther RW, Vorwerk D, Bohndorf K, et al. Venous stenoses in dialysis shunts: treatment with self-expanding metallic stents. Radiology 1989; 170:401-405.
12. Vorwerk, D, Guenther, RW, et al. Follow-up results after stent placement in failing arteriovenous shunts: A three-year experience. Cardiovasc Intervent Radiol 1991; 14:285-289.

13. Antonucci F, Salomonowitz E, Stuckmann G, Stiefel M, Largiadèr J, Zollikofer CL. Placement of venous stents: clinical experience with a self-expanding prosthesis. Radiology 1992; 183: 493-497.
14. Zollikofer CL, Antonucci F, Stuckmann G, Mattias P, Bruhlmann WF, Salomonowitz EK. Use of the Wallstent in the venous system including hemodialysis-related stenoses. Cardiovasc Intervent Radiol 1992; 15:334-341.
15. Petar B, Tomislav I, Miodrag I, Snezana A. Strecker stent in stenotic hemodialysis Brescia-Cimino arteriovenous fistulas. Cardiovasc Intervent Radiol 1992; 15:217-220.
16. Vorwerk D, Guenther RW, Bohndorf K, Gladziwa U, Kistler D. Self-expanding stents in peripheral and central veins used for arteriovenous shunts: Five years of experience (abstr). Radiology 1993; 189 (P):174.
17. Turmel-Rodrigues L, Pengloan J, Blanchier D, et al. Insufficient dialysis shunts: Improved long-term patency rates with close hemodynamic monitoring, repeated percutaneous balloon angioplasty, and stent placement. Radiology 1993; 187:273-278.
18. Palmaz JC. Intravascular stents: tissue-stent interactions and design considerations. AJR 1993; 160:613-618.
19. Beathard GA. Percutaneous transvenous angioplasty in the treatment of vascular access stenosis. Kidney Int 1992; 42:1390-1397.
20. Gray RJ, Dolmatch BL, Horton KM, Romolo JL, Zarate AR. Migration of Palmaz stents following deployment for venous stenoses related to hemodialysis access. JVIR 1994; 5:117-120.
21. Bjarnason H, Hunter DW, Crain MR, Ferral H, Miltz-Miller SE, Wegryn S. Collapse of a Palmaz stent in the subclavian vein. AJR 1993; 160:1123-1124.
22. Ehrman KO, Reed JD, Gaylord GM, Harris VM. Use of the Palmaz balloon-expandable stent in subclavian/brachiocephalic vein stenosis (abstr). JVIR 1992;3(1):13.

5

CATHETERS: HOW TO MAKE THEM WORK

Robert Uldall, M.D.

VASCULAR ACCESS FOR HEMODIALYSIS increasingly relies on central venous catheter technology, not only in acute reversible renal failure, in which access is needed for only two to three weeks, but also, to an ever greater extent, in patients with end-stage renal disease (ESRD). Patients with ESRD are living longer, and in many cases their traditional access sites, which have been used for multiple arteriovenous (A-V) fistulas and grafts, have been destroyed. The depredations of intravenous (I.V.) infusionists have destroyed the dorsal forearm veins, and repeated subclavian cannulations have destroyed the proximal venous drainage of the arm as a result of subclavian vein stenosis and thrombosis. Diabetics, who now comprise more than 25% of the dialysis population in most centers, are especially problematic. Construction of grafts and fistulas may induce steal syndromes and lead to ischemia of the hands and gangrene of the fingers. Finally, there is an increasing number of elderly patients with impaired cardiac function who cannot tolerate the extra load caused by a high-flow fistula or graft that may increase the resting cardiac output by as much as 2 L/min.[1]

Central venous catheters do not increase cardiac output during dialysis or in the intervals between dialyses. We have seen many examples of elderly patients with borderline cardiac function whose left ventricular failure or unstable angina was dramatically relieved by ligating or dismantling an A-V fistula or graft.

For many years, subclavian cannulation has been the mainstay of temporary vascular access for hemodialysis.[2] Although it can probably still be justified in patients presenting with what appears to be predictably recoverable acute renal failure (who will probably never need long-term dialysis or an A-V fistula), it should now be discontinued completely in patients known to have ESRD.[3] The incidence of subclavian vein thrombosis (10-30%) [4-7] and stenosis (40-50%) resulting from subclavian cannulation [8-10] is too high to justify continuation of this practice. The new technology for jugular vein cannulation is now so good that subclavian vein cannulation is no longer necessary or justified in any patient with ESRD. The indications for femoral, subclavian, and jugular vein cannulation will be proposed herein. Methods for the safe and effective practice of these techniques will be described. Finally, the results of the first three years of percutaneous cannulation of the jugular veins with a new catheter from Cook Critical Care (Bloomington, Indiana) will be presented.

Femoral Catheters

Double-lumen Marhurkar-type tapered catheters should be used whenever only one dialysis is required for the management of severe poisoning by hemodialysis or hemoperfusion. It is important to avoid accidental femoral artery puncture when inserting a femoral vein catheter for hemoperfusion because hemoperfusion requires generous amounts of heparin to prevent clotting in the charcoal filter. Femoral catheters should also be used whenever a patient presents in renal failure with pulmonary edema and is therefore unable to lie flat. The same applies to any patient in respiratory distress in whom an accidental pneumothorax caused by a subclavian or jugular catheter could be a serious complication.[11]

Femoral catheters should always be at least 20 cm long to maximize blood flow and minimize recirculation.[12] In general, they should not be left in place for more than a week. Whenever a femoral catheter is removed after use, it is a wise precaution to listen with a stethoscope over the insertion site. A loud bruit may indicate an accidental traumatic A-V fistula at this site. This may otherwise remain clinically silent but at the same time be provoking left ventricular strain or failure because of the increase in cardiac output it causes.

Subclavian Catheters

Subclavian catheters are now rarely used in our program—and only for patients with predictably reversible acute renal failure and never in patients with ESRD who may need long-term hemodialysis in the future. The danger of creating subclavian venous stenosis and thrombosis, which interfere with the creation of A-V fistulas and grafts in the same arm, is just too great.[5] Subclavian cannulation is easy and convenient, but is always haunted by the danger of immediate or delayed perforation of the wall of the superior vena cava or right atrium if the semistiff tapered tip is incorrectly positioned.[14] Accidental perforation, which should be preventable by careful attention to positioning, is now nearly always attended by ligation if it occurs. The serious or fatal effects of perforation frequently occur at the onset of dialysis, when pumping of blood starts through the venous end of the catheter. They can still be prevented if hemodialysis nurses are trained to suspect the catheter when chest pain, hypotension, or breathlessness occur after the start of a dialysis run.

Subclavian vein thrombosis is often a silent event that goes undiagnosed clinically until it is too late, especially if there is not an A-V fistula in the same arm.[7] Once the thrombosis is organized, it is not amenable to heparin or thrombolytic treatment, and very few surgeons have attempted a reconstruction of the venous return by grafting. Hence, if we use subclavian catheters, we have an obligation to perform routine Doppler ultrasound examination as soon as the catheter is removed. Venograms should be carried out in positive or doubtful cases. Subclavian vein stenosis can be treated by angioplasty, but it nearly always recurs. The only way to maintain patency is by means of a stent,[15] but it is not always possible to use one because of the close proximity to the confluence with the internal jugular vein.

Jugular Catheters

Jugular vein cannulation is now generally accepted as the preferable access method for central venous catheters in all patients with ESRD.[3,16] This method, even if it results in jugular vein thrombosis, does not interfere with proximal venous return from the arm.

Physicians are reluctant to use jugular catheters for temporary vascular access because of the inconvenience and social embarrassment to the patient of having a semistiff Marhurkar-type catheter emerging from the side of the neck and secured with dressings close to the ear. In contrast, subclavian catheters are easy to conceal under clothing; this is important for outpatients.

Permacath (Quinton, Seattle, Washington), designed for surgical insertion in the jugular vein, is brought through a long subcutaneous tunnel to emerge on the anterior surface of the chest wall. It has proved reliable as a long-term access device for patients with refractory vascular access problems.[17,18] However, if it has to be removed it would be difficult to insert it surgically a second time in the same vein because of the extensive scarring that makes it difficult to dissect out the vein to obtain control above and below. Hence, the Permacath has limited usefulness as a temporary access device for repeated insertion in the same vein. Although it can be inserted percutaneously through a large peel-away sheath, the size of this sheath is calculated to frighten off most operators.[19]

Canaud in France has developed a technique using two cylindrical Silastic catheters side by side in the same jugular vein, each introduced through a separate peel-away, one reaching slightly farther down than the other.[20] He has had excellent results, but there is the disadvantage of two catheters and two separate exit sites.

We have developed a new double-lumen soft Silastic catheter in collaboration with Cook Critical Care with parallel cylindrical lumens to provide blood flows of 400 ml/min.[21] The essence of the device is that the distal portion of the catheter has a thin-walled lumen lying side by side with a thick-walled lumen. When compressed, the thin-walled lumen collapses to allow the catheter to be passed through a 13 Fr peel-away sheath. Once in the vein, both lumens are fully expanded and are interchangeable for withdrawal or return of blood. The upper part of the catheter has a smooth outer surface in keeping with its function of filling the opening in the vein wall and emerging at the exit site. The catheter has been fully described elsewhere, and the special points of technique for insertion, changing, and catheter maintenance have been previously described.[3] We now have three years' experience in the use of the catheters and have learned a great deal about how keep them functional.

Insertion of the Cook Catheter

None of the components of the insertion technique is particularly difficult, but there are some "tricks of the trade" that improve the success rate. Most of our procedures are done by nephrologists in a procedure room under a good light but without the aid of fluoroscopy, with the patient lying on a tipping stretcher. We use very strict aseptic techniques, and all new insertions are accompanied by I.V. administration of 1 g of cefazolin. We have found the following points to be of value:

- The right side is easier than the left, because without fluoroscopy it is easier to pass the guide wire reliably into the right atrium. We will also perform left-sided insertions without fluoroscopy, but occasionally the catheter may end up in the right innominate vein. If this happens, an interventional radiologist can access the femoral vein and, under fluoroscopic guidance, bring the catheter down into the superior vena cava with a hooked catheter. These occasional difficulties would not occur if all insertions were done with fluoroscopic guidance by interventional radiologists. We predict that in most centers, interventional radiologists will do most of the insertion and changing.
- Initial Doppler ultrasound examination is helpful to check the patency of the jugular vein as well as its exact location in relation to the heads of the sternomastoid muscle.[22] Initially, we did all these examinations in the ultrasound department. More recently, we have had a high success rate with a small, hand-held Doppler that allows one to hear the venous bruit. In doubtful cases, we insert a guide wire into the vein first before opening up the catheter tray. If the catheter is brought up through the tunnel first and it is then not possible to find the vein, the catheter ends up being wasted.
- The point of insertion into the vein should be at least 0.5-1.0 cm above the clavicle. If one gets too close to the upper border of the clavicle, it may be difficult to pass the upper, thicker part of the catheter through tough ligamentous tissue.
- We find that the catheter produces better flow rates if the tip is lying just inside the entrance to the right atrium rather than just above it in the superior vena cava. This is probably because the tip is more likely to become occluded by blood clots if it is lying against the vein wall. This is in contrast to the semistiff tapered catheters, which should never be allowed to protrude into the cavity of the right atrium, where they may cause right atrial perforation or thrombus formation.
- Closure of the skin wound over the anchoring grommet should be done with considerable care. The grommet should be located in a pocket above the clavicle, where the subcutaneous tissue has been deeply undermined. We always use subcutaneous catgut (absorbable) sutures to draw the subcutaneous tissues together, bury the grommet, and approximate the skin edges. The skin edges can then be closed without any tension, and there is no danger of the skin

edges coming apart to expose the grommet. Once this happens, the wound nearly always gets infected and the catheter may need to be removed. With careful skin closure, this latter complication should never occur.

Preventing and Treating Infection

The first essential is the use of good aseptic technique in inserting and changing the catheter. Chlorhexidine has been shown to be superior to povidone-iodine for skin preparation and also for cleaning the Luer-Lok connection at the start and end of dialysis. Gloves and masks probably are not necessary as long as one employs a meticulous no-touch technique. The manner of protecting the exit site is still controversial. We use a transparent adhesive sandwich dressing (Tegaderm, 3M, Minneapolis, Minnesota), but others in controlled studies have found dry gauze with povidone-iodine ointment to give superior results.[23] The new dressing, IV 3000 (Smith and Nephew), is permeable to water vapor and is useful for patients whose skin reacts to Tegaderm and for patients who perspire profusely. In our hands, IV 3000 was associated with lower infection rates than Tegaderm, and it also allows showering. For those not using IV 3000 who want to shower, we have developed a shower cape (obtainable from Cook Critical Care) that fastens snugly around the neck with Velcro (one size fits all) and protects the upper part of the chest from the direct impact of the shower jet. The advantage of the double transparent dressing technique is that it protects the exit site, at the same time helping to stabilize the catheter and preventing movement. It also allows the exit site to be visible at all times.

We have encountered the following types of infections:

- A skin exit site infection is characterized by a purulent discharge and a positive culture. It should be treated intensively and early with the appropriate antibiotic, and the catheter should be changed over a guide wire as soon as the purulent discharge disappears. Antibiotics should be continued for another two weeks. If the exudate does not clear up, there is no choice but to remove the catheter. *Staphylococcus epidermidis* is the more common causative organism. In our hands, these infections occur about once every 12 patient months.
- Blood stream infections are diagnosed by the presence of both a positive blood culture and fever not explained by infection at some other site. These should also be treated with antibiotics and changing the catheter over a guide wire after 48 hours, by which time the temperature is usually normal.[24] An antibiotic, usually vancomycin 1g given after every alternate dialysis, should also be given for two weeks after the change has been performed. The most common organism is *Staphyloccus aureus*, and the eradication rate from this regimen is better than 90%. With *S. aureus* septicemia, we advocate the concurrent use of Rifampin 300 mg orally twice daily. Our rate of blood stream infection is one in 30 patient months.[25] Both of the above types of infection can usually be treated without hospitalizing the patient.
- The third and most serious type of infection is that in which a blood stream infection is accompanied by pus at the exit site. When one encounters this combination, the correct management is antibiotics followed as soon as possible

by complete catheter removal. Any delay is dangerous. The most common cause is *S. aureus*, and the risk of delay is death from staphylococcal shock.

- Finally, one may encounter redness and tenderness of the skin around the exit site without fever or exudate. This usually responds to antibiotics alone without changing or removing the catheter.

Controversy still surrounds the matter of staphylococcal nasal carriage. If carriers can be identified by culturing the nares and treating with antibacterial ointment, can one reduce the incidence of staphylococcal exit site infections? The problem is that nasal carriers appear to be a changing population. Individuals found to be carriers one month may, even in the absence of treatment, not be carriers the next. The next month it is a different group of patients. There is a school of thought advocating the use of Mupirocin (antistaphylococcal ointment) in both nostrils twice a day during five days of every month in all patients. We have the clinical impression, not backed by controlled trials, that the use of chlorhexidine-containing detergent for daily showering and shampooing reduces the incidence of exit site infections in those who seem especially prone.

Occasionally, blood stream infections seem to arise from another organ system (e.g., *Escherichia coli* infections in patients with an active urinary tract infection). When this happens, it is, of course, necessary to treat the underlying infection, but it can be assumed that the organism has also invaded the catheter. The catheter will then perpetuate the infection if it is not also changed.

Thrombus Obstruction and Reduced or Absent Blood Flow

Obstruction of the catheter by a thrombus is undoubtedly the most frustrating problem of central venous catheter access. Although this is less of a problem in open-ended, blunt-tipped catheters than in tapered catheters with side-holes, it is frequent enough to be a nuisance and may lead to inadequate or delayed dialysis. Clots within the lumen of the catheter are readily prevented by an adequate heparin lock. Some operators, worried about the danger of heparin, have used a concentrated solution of citrate in the catheter lumen that appears to be equally effective.[26] The real problem seems to be clots that adhere to the outer surface of the catheter like a sheath. These may even hang in fronds that can be seen on venograms.[27] The thrombus acts like a valve by being sucked against the open end of the catheter. If reversing the direction of the flow does not solve the problem, the most effective treatment is an I.V. bolus of urokinase (UK) (250,000 U), which causes systemic thrombolysis.[28] The maximum activity is reached within 20 minutes, and it remains active for about three hours.[29] If one dose is not effective, it should be followed by another dose three hours later; occasionally, a third dose may be necessary three hours after the second. We administer UK in two clinical settings:

- The obstruction is so severe that dialysis cannot be started. In this case, we give UK and wait an hour. Often, after an hour the dialysis can be started without difficulty.

- Dialysis is started, but the blood pump speed cannot be raised above 200-250 ml/min. Dialysis is continued while UK is injected into the venous blood line;

usually, within a short time blood flow is adequate. It should be remembered that prolonged administration of UK in combination with heparin may cause widespread spontaneous bleeding. For this reason, we usually use the heparin once the UK has been given. Whether this is necessary for the short duration of a dialysis we do not know, but we err on the side of safety.

UK must not be given to any patient who has had a surgical procedure or an arterial puncture in the previous 24 hours. We would not use it for at least 48 hours after a renal biopsy. Patients need not be admitted for administration of UK, but they should be observed for three hours after each dose. It is not safe to inject it and send the patient straight home. If repeated doses of UK are not effective, or if UK must be used before every dialysis, one should suspect the possibility of a superior vena cava stenosis.[30] Angioplasty of the stenosis and a stent in the SVC may solve the problem.

Mild reactions to UK occur in a significant proportion of patients, taking the form of shivering and sometimes a slight fever. They can be partially prevented by prior administration of I.V. antihistamine (chlorpheniramine 10 mg) or by meperidine 25 mg. Either or both of these drugs can be given to reduce the severity of the reaction after it occurs.

Streptokinase, an equally effective thrombolytic agent (widely used for thrombolysis after myocardial infarction) can also be used for thrombus obstruction of catheters. It can be used for any individual patient only once because of its allergenicity. Repeated doses may be associated with serum sickness reactions or even anaphylaxis, and it is not worth the risk. Since most patients who need thrombolysis for catheter obstruction will need it more than once, we have scrupulously avoided the use of streptokinase. Occasionally, one encounters the dilemma of venous thrombosis in the presence of bleeding elsewhere. Heparin and thrombolytic agents are therefore contraindicated. In this situation, the problem may be solved by I.V. administration of ancrod, a derivative of viper venom. This substance has the ability to remove thrombus from within veins while not provoking bleeding elsewhere. The dosage is controlled by regular monitoring of fibrinogen levels. We have found it extraordinarily effective for treating deep vein thrombosis in the presence of a bleeding ulcer or within a short time after bleeding from a renal biopsy site. Theoretically, it should also be effective for thrombus around a catheter if thrombolytic agents cannot be used.

Only a proportion of patients with central venous catheters seem to suffer from thrombus obstruction (in our experience, about 25%), and it appears to be the same patients each time. Rather than having to resort repeatedly to expensive UK injections accompanied by delays in the start of dialysis, we put these patients on long-term anticoagulation with warfarin.

Warfarin is known to reduce fibrin formation on I.V. catheters[31] and almost certainly does so even in subtherapeutic doses (1-1.25 mg/day) that do not prolong the international normalized ratio (INR).[32] We have developed a system in which any patient who needs UK more than once is started on warfarin 1.25 mg (half of a 2.5-mg tablet) each day. If this is not effective in preventing thrombus obstruction, we raise the warfarin dose to bring the INR to between 1.5 and 2.0. If thrombus obstruction still occurs, we raise the INR to 2.0-2.5. In a very few patients, we may have to increase the INR to 2.5-3.0, but it has not been necessary to go higher than this. With this conservative approach, we have had no serious bleeding complications at our institution during the past year and a half. It goes without saying that all patients should be warned against the use of unprescribed drugs (e.g., aspirin) that will suddenly prolong the INR and may cause spontaneous bleeding.

It is quite safe to administer I.V. urokinase to patients already established on warfarin as long as the INR is being regularly monitored. Blood samples for INR should be drawn once a week predialysis through the catheter itself, first taking care to remove the heparin in the catheter with a heparin washout.[33] The heparin washout, held in a 30-cc syringe, is given back to the patient once the INR sample has been taken. A simultaneously estimated activated partial thromboplastin time, if it gives a normal result, serves as assurance that all traces of heparin have been removed and that the INR result can be deemed accurate.

Do Jugular Vein Catheters Damage the Veins?

Clearly, it is highly advantageous to avoid subclavian cannulation in patients with ESRD and thus preserve the proximal venous drainage of the arm. But if one uses jugular catheters for temporary access as well as for long-term access in patients (in whom fistula and graft construction is no longer possible), what will be the incidence of jugular vein thrombosis? We have just completed a Doppler ultrasound study of 101 veins, some of which were cannulated for two or three separate periods of hemodialysis (i.e., two or three separate times in each vein for variable periods). We have found a 2% incidence of jugular vein thrombosis with the Cook catheter.[34] This is clearly much less than the incidence of thrombosis in subclavian veins, and even if it occurs, it does not damage the venous drainage of the upper limb.

The Extreme Problem of Destroyed Jugular Veins

Occasionally, one may encounter a patient whose jugular veins have been destroyed by surgical insertion of Permacaths or repeated use of semistiff tapered catheters. In this case, the Cook catheter can be inserted for long-term use in the femoral vein with the exit site 10 cm below and lateral to the insertion site in the inguinal ligament (emerging on the anterior aspect of the thigh). We have had good long-term results in six patients with this technique. The catheter should be at least 32 cm long to ensure that it reaches up to the inferior vena cava.

Summary and Conclusions

Central venous catheter technology is assuming increasing importance in vascular access for hemodialysis. Femoral catheters should still be used in cases of poisoning and for unstable patients who are breathless. Subclavian catheters are still justified in acute reversible renal failure as long as precautions are taken to avoid accidental perforating injuries.

The new technology for percutaneous insertion of soft Silastic catheters in the jugular vein allows safe and effective access for temporary or prolonged hemodialysis in all ESRD patients. There should be no patients in whom reliable vascular access is not possible. Subclavian catheters should now be abandoned for all patients with ESRD.

References

1. Ahearn DJ, Maher JF. Heart failure as a complication of hemodialysis arteriovenous fistula. Ann Intern Med 1972; 77:201-204.
2. Uldall PR. Subclavian cannulation for hemodialysis: the present state of the art. Artif Organs 1982; 6:73-76.
3. Uldall PR. Subclavian cannulation is no longer necessary or justified in patients with end-stage renal failure. Semin Dialysis (in press).
4. El Nachef MW, Rashad E, Ricanati ES. Occlusion of the subclavian vein: a complication of indwelling subclavian venous catheters for hemodialysis. Clin Nephrol 1985; 24:42-46.
5. Vanherwegem JL, Yassine T, Goldman M, et al. Subclavian vein thrombosis: a frequent complication of subclavian vein cannulation for hemodialysis. Clin Nephrol 1986; 26:235-238.
6. Glaze RC, McDougall ML, Weigmann TB. Thrombotic arm edema as a complication of subclavian vein catheterization and arteriovenous fistula formation for hemodialysis. Am J Kidney Dis 1986; 7:439-441.
7. Brady HR, Fitzcharles B, Goldberg H, Huraib S, Simons M, Uldall PR. Diagnosis and management of subclavian vein thrombosis occurring in association with subclavian cannulation for hemodialysis. Blood Purif 1987; 7:210-217.
8. Barrett N, Spencer S, McIvor J, Brown EA. Subclavian stenosis: a major complication of subclavian dialysis catheters. Nephrol Dial Transplant 1988; 3:423-425.
9. Clark DD, Albina JE, Chezan JA. Subclavian vein stenosis and thrombosis: a potential serious complication in chronic hemodialysis patients. Am J Kidney Dis 1990; 15:256-268.
10. Spinowitz BS, Galler M, Golden RA, et al. Subclavian vein stenosis as a complication of subclavian catheterization for hemodialysis. Arch Intern Med 1987; 147:305-307.
11. Tapson JS, Uldall PR. Avoiding deaths from subclavian cannulation for hemodialysis. Int J Artif Organs 1983; 6:227-230.
12. Kelber J, Delmez JA, Windus DW. Factors affecting delivery of high efficiency dialysis using temporary vascular access. Am J Kidney Dis 1993; 22:243-249.
13. Holt S, Kirkham N, Myercough E. Hemothorax after subclavian vein cannulation. Thorax 1977; 32:101-103.
14. Tapson JS, Uldall PR. Fatal hemothorax caused by a subclavian hemodialysis catheter. Arch Intern Med 1984; 144:1685-1687.
15. Uchida BT, Putnam JS, Rosch J. Modifications of Gianturco expandable wire stents. Am J Radiol 1988; 150:1185-1187.
16. Cimochowski GE, Worley E, Rutherford WE, Sartain J, Blodin J, Harter H. Superiority of the internal jugular over the subclavian access for temporary dialysis. Nephron 1990; 54: 154-161.
17. Shusterman NH, Kloss K, Mullen JL. Successful use of double-lumen silicone rubber catheters for permanent hemodialysis access. Kidney Int 1989; 35:887-890.
18. Blake PG, Huraib S, Wu G, Uldall PR. The use of dual-lumen jugular venous catheters as definitive long-term access for hemodialysis. Int J Artif Organs 1990; 13:26-31.

19. McDowell DE, Pillai L, Goldstein RM. A simplified technique for percutaneous insertion of permanent vascular access catheters in patients requiring chronic hemodialysis. J Vasc Surg 1988; 7:574-576.
20. Canaud B, Saumier F, Beraud JJ, Joyeux H, Mion C. La cannulation jugulaire interne avec deux catheters silastic. Une nouvelle methode d'access vasculaire pour hemodialyse. Nephrologie 1986; 7:57-61.
21. Uldall PR, DeBruyne M, Besley M, McMillan J, Simons M, Francoeur R. A new vascular access catheter for hemodialysis. Am J Kidney Dis 1993; 21:270-277.
22. Denys BG, Uretsky BF, Reddy PS, Ruffner RJ, Sandhu JS, Breishlatt WM. An ultrasound method for safe and rapid central venous access.
23. Levin A, Mason AJ, Jindal KK, Fong IW, Goldstein MB. Prevention of hemodialysis subclavian vein catheter infections by topical povidone-iodine. Kidney Int 1991; 40:934-938.
24. Carlisle EJF, Blake PG, McCarthy F, Vas S, Uldall PR. Septicemia in long-term jugular hemodialysis catheters: eradicating infection by changing the catheter over a guide wire. Int J Artif Organs 1991; 14:150-153.
25. Mustata S, Less P, Uldall PR. Further experience with a percutaneously inserted double-lumen Silastic catheter for end-stage renal failure patients with refractory vascular access problems. Am Soc Artif Intern Organs 1994; p. 114.
26. Buturovic M, Boh R, Ponikvar M, et al. Filling of hemodialysis catheters in interdialysis period: Heparin V citrate V Haemaccel. Prospective randomized study. Am Soc Artif Intern Organs, 1994; p. 119.
27. Ratcliffe PJ, Oliver DO. Massive thrombosis around subclavian cannulas used for hemodialysis. Lancet 1982; 1:1472-1473.
28. Uldall PR, Besley ME, Thomas A, Salter S, Nuezea LA, Vas M. Maintaining the patency of double-lumen silastic jugular catheters for hemodialysis. Int J Artif Organs 1993; 16:37-40.
29. McNichol GP. The fibrinolytic enzyme system. Postgrad Med J 1973; 49:10-12.
30. Khanna S, Sniderman K, Simons M, Besley ME, Uldall PR. Superior vena cava stenosis associated with hemodialysis catheters. Am J Kidney Dis 1993; 21:278-281.
31. Ryan JA Jr, Abel RM, Abbott WM, et al. Catheter complications of total parenteral nutrition: a prospective study of 200 consecutive patients. N Engl J Med 1974; 290:757-760.
32. Bern MM, Lokich JJ, Wallach SR, et al. Very low doses of warfarin can prevent thrombosis in central vein catheters. Ann Intern Med 1990; 112:423-428.
33. Besley ME, Thomas A, Salter S, Sang YY, Vas M, Uldall PR. Control of oral anticoagulation in patients using long-term internal jugular catheters for hemodialysis access. Int J Artif Organs 1992; 15:277-280.
34. Agraharkar M, Mendelssohn D, Zevallos G, Uldall PR. Does percutaneous jugular vein cannulation for hemodialysis access cause jugular vein damage? Am Soc Artif Intern Organs 1994; p. 114.

DISCUSSION

Moderator:
Ronald M. Ferguson, M.D., Ph.D.
Panelists:
Arnold Miller, M.D., Ch.B.
Scott O. Trerotola, M.D.
Robert Uldall, M.D.

Dr. Ferguson: Dr. Dickerman presented an algorithm predominantly based on primary loop A-V PTFE grafts and then how to salvage those. We have come full circle. The techniques described by Dr. Uldall could make all of those kinds of access obsolete by a long-term permanent catheter for dialysis. Is that a real possibility?

Dr. Uldall: I have been asked this before, and I do not think so. I agree with Dr. Miller that for patients with end-stage failure, using a native A-V fistula created at the wrist, preferably well in advance of need, is the absolute gold standard. The problem is that if you do not make a native A-V fistula, then you must fall back on your next best alternative. Linn, a practitioner in New York, believes that a good central jugular catheter may be comparable to and perhaps cause less trouble in the long term with fewer days in the hospital and fewer interventions and procedures than PTFE grafts. One or two prospective studies comparing PTFE grafts with permanent catheters have shown that there is not too much difference in terms of lost days and interventions and so on. I think that with the new technology, the percutaneously inserted catheter, it will be very interesting to see what the long-term comparison will be and how well catheters measure up to PTFE grafts as an alternative.

Discussant: You may be right in the sense that there will not be as many infectious complications or clotting with a catheter, but what about the flow rate? Can you expect to provide adequate dialysis?

Dr. Uldall: If we are not getting a flow rate of 350 ml/min, I get pretty upset. When they are working well, most catheters will permit a flow rate of 400 ml/min. I have a conspiratorial plan to persuade the Cook company to design the next catheter with a slightly bigger internal lumen, because we have plenty of leeway to do that in view of the compressibility of the catheter. I think we should be aiming for a catheter with a flow rate that can provide 500 ml/min, but you should be able to get 400 ml/min with this one.

Dr. Henry: I have two questions for Dr. Miller. The first has to do with creating antecubital fistulas. In my experience, if you leave the basilic vein wide open, resistance in the basilic system is much less than that in the cephalic system, just due to size. It then tends to mature rather than the cephalic vein. We have tied these deep branches off, to allow flow out the cephalic system, which works pretty well. Have you had any problems with the basilic system maturing rather than the cephalic system? The second question: When you go back and use the basilic system, do you transpose that into the subcutaneous position?

Dr. Miller: We were worried about that, but it has not turned out to be a major problem. In fact, if the cephalic vein is of good quality, it almost invariably matures just as well as the basilic vein. There were five patients that we transposed. One had a cephalic vein that was ligated, two had cephalic veins that occluded, and there were two in our early experience in whom the nurses kept saying they could not use the vein. We did fistulograms and found it was a beautiful vein, but it was too deep because sometimes the cephalic vein runs beneath the deep fascia or close to the deep fascia. In the last few cases, where we have had any difficulty, we have outlined the vein with ultrasound and marked it exactly on the skin; cannulation then becomes easy. Our biggest fear was that we were doing the wrong thing, developing the wrong vein. It doesn't happen. The advantage, if you run into problems with a cephalic vein, is that you have a beautiful matured vein that you can then transpose subcutaneously (which we do). Another advantage is that the anastomosis to the radial artery remains patent, so you plug it into the proximal cephalic vein in a simple procedure. Dialysis can be started the same or the next day.

Discussant: Dr. Uldall, how are you mixing up the urokinase concentration? Is that just 10 cc or what kind of volume concentration are you mixing to place in the catheter?

Dr. Uldall: I suspect that it is not critical, but we put it in 20 ml of normal saline and we put half down through each lumen of the catheter. That is probably not necessary either, as long as it gets into the systemic circulation. As soon as the urokinase is in, then we re-heparinize the catheter just to keep some heparin within the lumen itself. Now we use it under two circumstances. In the first, if you cannot get the dialysis going at all, then we let the patient sit and wait with urokinase working systemically. It works with a maximum effect within 20 minutes and lasts for three hours. Often you need to wait only an hour before being back in business dialyzing the patient. The other setting in which we use it is after dialysis has started and we have a poor flow rate that we are not satisfied with. Most people are not satisfied with 200 ml/min. So if you are bumbling along with 150-200 ml/min, continue dialyzing, put the urokinase directly into the venous blood line, and at that point switch off the heparin.

Discussant: Another question for Dr. Uldall. Are you doing any work with primary fibrin sheath stripping and, if so, how does that compare with urokinase therapy? I know it has been in the interventional literature, but do you have any feeling how that compares with the thrombolytic therapy?

Dr. Uldall: We have not really tackled that, mainly because urokinase seems to be so convenient. It does not require any intervention other than the injection, and then we let the patient wait for a while.

Dr. Trerotola: I can address that. Fibrin sheath stripping, where you use a snare put up from a femoral approach to strip the clot off the wire, is an extremely cost *in*efficient way of cleaning dialysis catheters. One group recently reported an average cost of $1,800 per procedure. Urokinase works fine, and fibrin sheath-stripping is a complete waste of money. One thing I should point out, though, is if you use Dr. Uldall's single-dose bolus on a patient with a recently placed graft, you may get bleeding because they are systemically lytic. An alternative, which we use, is a lower-dose infusion of 20,000 units per hour per lumen for a total of six hours. Why is that the magic number? That is one vial of urokinase. That works very well and can be done in the dialysis unit. The staff arrives at 6 a.m. to get it started, and then they are ready to dialyze at noon. It works very well and has a greater then 90% success rate. We use it after a single dose of 5,000 units of urokinase has failed.

Discussant: I would like to suggest to Dr. Miller that we would take that basilic vein and elevate it from under the fascia and leave it under the subcutaneous tissue, under the skin and not have to do another anastomosis at all. As a matter of fact, we have done 100 such cases. Dr. Uldall, we introduce our Permacaths through the external jugular vein, which, of course, goes into the subclavian vein, but we have the impression that this does not cause subclavian vein stenosis. Would you comment, please?

Dr. Uldall: I did a lot of those, and putting a Permacath in through the external jugular is obviously much easier than going to the internal jugular. We found that in a number of our patients, the external jugular wasn't adequate for that. Now that we have the new percutaneously inserted catheter, it takes an average of 35 minutes just to put it in because it is compressible and goes through a relatively small sheath. If you have to take it out, you can always put it back in again. If you have to take out the Permacath from the external jugular, how successful will you be in using the same vein again?

Dr. Miller: In reply to the comment about elevating the basilic vein, we have not used that technique because I personally have not had any experience with it. But the people who taught me the procedure and who did it for many years always had difficulties, particularly in a primary basilic vein. There must be some trick to the technique, but we found that the patients complained of severe wound problems when we mobilized big flaps to get the wound anterior enough so that we could get the basilic vein in an accessible area. Simply tunneling it has the advantage that we can now have a much longer piece of vein that we can plug into the cephalic vein proximally in order to have a long, easy, gentle loop that is very accessible for dialysis.

Dr. Trerotola: I would like to comment about jugular versus subclavian approach for dialysis catheters. One of the comparisons that Dr. Uldall showed was percutaneous versus surgical placement. Obviously, there is a big difference. Interventional radiologists are doing more and more percutaneous placements. We did a series of more than 200 patients with subclavian vein insertions of a 13.5 Fr Davall dialysis catheter, which is round and has a small sheath. It is radiologically and fluoroscopically guided for insertion though an axillary vein puncture. We found only an 11% central venous abnormality, and only a couple of those were stenoses. I think that with the percutaneous approach and radiologic guidance, we can hold complications to a very low rate. Jugular catheters are associated with innominate vein stenoses. Don't think that doesn't happen, because it certainly does.

Discussant: I have a couple of questions for Dr. Uldall and one for Dr. Miller. Dr. Miller, how long do you wait to let your fistulas mature before you allow them to be used?

Dr. Miller: I leave that to nephrologists. We have a first-class nephrologist who decides, and it is quite variable. We try to wait as long as we can, usually around two months. Occasionally, if it is a very big vein, particularly in the upper arm, we can use it much earlier, even at three or four weeks, but I hate to do that. The vein is fragile and the incidence of infiltration and bleeding is high. So I prefer to wait as long as we can, somewhere around two to three months.

Discussant: Because the incidence of infection and other complications is high if a temporary is left in for two months, do you put in a Permacath or temporary catheter while waiting for the fistula to mature?

Dr. Miller: That has been the biggest argument for not going straight to PTFE. But if you look in retrospect at what happens to the PTFE patient, he does very well for the first six months. Then he starts with his revision process and you look at the time that he has his Permacath put in afterwards. You add up that time and compare it to the time you would have had if you put it in primary waiting for your vein to mature, and there's not much difference. I'm not sure about the morbidity, but Dr. Uldall probably has much more experience with that and can comment on it.

Discussant: Dr. Uldall, I would like to ask you a couple of questions. The first one is very simple. How much heparin do you put in each port between dialyses? There are a lot of different opinions on that. There is also a group that now advocates putting two catheters side by side instead of one Permacath, claiming that this produces better flows with fewer complications. I wish you would also comment on that.

Dr. Uldall: The first question about the heparin lock. We use 5,000 units in a total volume of 1.5 ml in each lumen, and that seems to work very well. Actually, because the dead space of each lumen is slightly less than 1.5 ml, you will have a certain amount of heparin leaking into the systemic circulation. I became concerned about it because of the possibility of bleeding in somebody who is going to the O.R. after coming off dialysis. I instructed the nurses to use the same amount of heparin but to cut down the total volume to 1.2, so that it would just fill the catheter and no more. We have a clinical impression that the problems of thrombus obstruction have increased since we did that. That still has to be resolved. There is a group that believes that heparin in the catheter itself in between dialyses is unnecessary and it is potentially dangerous because somebody can come along and start up an I.V. on the catheter and forget that there is heparin in there. They use a 4% solution of citrate in each lumen, which of course is harmless, and they say it is just as good as heparin. We, in fact, intend to take a look at that. Your other question was about using two catheters instead of one. The main supporter of that is Bernard Canno, who developed a double catheter technique in Montpelier. I was there recently and I saw his results, and they are really quite impressive. The nice thing about them is that each catheter is put in percutaneously, one beside the other. The problem is that there are two punctures and two exit sites to look after. We feel that because we have the new Cook catheter and the results with it are so good, we have not felt compelled to go to the two-catheter technique.

Discussant: Our centers have experienced difficulty with diabetic patients maturing autogenous fistulas. Do you have any suggestions or ideas on ways to enhance and optimize the success rate in these patients?

Dr. Miller: As you saw in our series, 40% of our patients are diabetic. The same question was raised in peripheral vascular surgery, and for many years the myth was that the diabetic patient was different from the nondiabetic patient. We now have a series of patients in which the incidence of diabetes is 80%, and our results are comparable with anyone's. I do not think there is an inherent problem with the veins in diabetic patients, but these patients tend to be hospitalized more frequently than other patients. Their arm veins are traumatized iatrogenically for the various antibiotics and infusions, so you are dealing with a poorer quality vein. If you are going to try to do arteriovenous fistulas in this patient population, you must know the quality of the vein. If you do it blindly, you will have a high failure rate and many fistulas that do not mature because they have stenoses somewhere higher up. I would like to encourage you to look at that vein with an angioscope. It really will make a tremendous difference in your selection and your intraoperative decision making. Our early failure rate for autogenous fistulas is about 12% now, but I am sure that with our experience over the last couple of years it is dropping dramatically. It is rare that we see a vein that does not mature. If it does not mature now, there is an inflow problem, stenosis at the anastomosis, or perhaps arterial disease itself.

Discussant: A question for Dr. Uldall. I have put in about 100 Permacaths percutaneously over the past couple of years, and I share your experience that if they are removed you can re-cannulate the internal jugular vein, usually without any problem. The problem I have had is that in about five patients who had long-term dialysis access through the Permacath, for one reason or another it had to be removed. The second time around I could get into the internal jugular vein; however, it will not advance secondary to superior vena cava or innominate vein. My question is, What is the incidence of this and does that decrease your enthusiasm for leaving Permacaths in for a very long time?

Dr. Uldall: As you heard me say, we have now abandoned Permacaths. We have not assessed the incidence of innominate and superior vena cava stenosis caused by these long-term catheters, but I suspect that it is greater than we think. Up to this time, it has not interfered with our ability to use these catheters long-term. The soft Silastic catheters have not been particularly liable to cause intimal vein damage and stenosis and trauma. We have not seen a great deal of that, and most of the cases of SVC stenosis we described in the *American Journal of Kidney Diseases* were caused mainly by previous semistiff tapered catheters introduced by the subclavian that had been rubbing on the wall of the innominate or the superior vena cava. If you start with a new patient who has not had previous semistiff tapered catheters, I would suspect that the incidence of innominate vein stenosis and SVC stenosis is fairly low. I would like to hear Dr. Trerotola's views on this.

Dr. Trerotola: Because most of these patients have had a semistiff catheter at some point, it is hard to separate what is the cause from what is not. I suspect that what you are seeing is just an effect of thrombosis around the catheter; I would be interested in knowing at what level you are putting the tip of the catheter. Do you concentrate more for an atrial position or at the cava/atrial junction?

Discussant: We started keeping the tip at the junction of the SVC and the atrium and found that the further in it is, the better the flows. We use 40-cm Permacaths on most patients, all inserted into the internal jugular, a technique that seems to work very well. I have not put in a subclavian line in more than two years. We found that the farther down the tip is, the better the patient does.

Dr. Uldall: I agree that if you arrange to have the tip of the Permacath or Cook catheter just inside the entrance to the right atrium rather than just above it, the flow characteristics tend to be better.

Discussant: We have seen innominate stenoses in patients who have never had anything but an internal jugular Permacath placed. We have also seen complete iliac vein or external vein occlusion or stenosis in patients who have never had anything but a femoral Permacath placed. I suspect that it is not the tip that causes the problem but rather the fibrin sheath along the catheter in the midportion of the catheter. This sets in motion a thrombophlebitis in the vein and an acute injury that turns into a chronic scar. I do think that no matter what kind of catheter you place or where you place it, you are going to induce inflammation. The point is that you need to minimize the use of these catheters if the patients are going to need grafts or fistulas long-term.

Dr. Ferguson: If Dr. Uldall is correct, and he has his 2% incidence of thrombosis and stenosis, he has something that might be extraordinarily useful in the future. I think it is one of those things that we are going to have to follow.

Discussant: I think it does matter what type of catheter you use. We have gathered most of the permanent catheters and all of the temporary catheters on the American market and hooked them to a dialysis pump in our laboratory and measured catheter motion. Various lumen configurations have a dramatic impact on how much pump-induced motion you get with the various catheters. Twelve hours a week of a catheter slamming wall-to-wall in a vein is different from a catheter that is still during dialysis. So I think what kind of catheter is used does make a substantial difference.

Dr. Uldall: You did not say which was better.

Discussant: All of the coaxial designs are far superior. The side-by-sides have much more motion unless both lumens are cut off flush at the tip and both jets go out straight, but then recirculation becomes a problem.

SECTION III

6

VASCULAR ACCESS SURGERY AS AN OUTPATIENT PROCEDURE

Ralph H. Didlake, M.D., and Edna T. Curry, R.N., B.S.N., C.N.N.

Since hemodialysis became widely available in the late 1960s, the dialysis-dependent-population in the United States has steadily increased. When the federally funded end-stage renal disease (esrd) program began in mid-1973, some 11,000 patients were being dialyzed.1 According to the 1993 annual data report of the United States Renal Data System, by 1990 the number of esrd patients had grown to 210,000, an almost 20-fold increase representing an increase of 10,000 new patients per year.2 If this trend continues, the esrd population will number 300,000 by the end of the century and there is no indication that this trend will change. By preference, by necessity of circumstance, or owing to the limited supply of organs for transplantation, the great majority of these patients will remain on hemodialysis for life.

Although the technology for hemodialysis therapy has improved dramatically over the past decade, the technology for providing chronic high-flow access to the blood stream for such therapy has not kept pace. Currently available hemo-access methods remain the most primitive and vulnerable element of hemodialysis therapy. The vulnerability of available access devices to complications requiring operative intervention is a source of significant morbidity for ESRD patients.

Appropriate surgical management of access-related pathology is a large and important part of the care of chronic dialysis patients. In the early 1980s, Hirschman reported that the most common cause of hospitalization among ESRD patients was access dysfunction, which accounted for 26% of all hospital admissions in a population of 1,049 patients followed for one year.[3] This review

The technical support of Elouise Farrar, Virginia Keith, Jackie Jordon, and Buffy Wiltcher is gratefully acknowledged.

included many individuals using first-generation access technology. In 1984, however, well after the introduction of expanded polytetraflouroethylene (ePTFE) grafts, Carlson et al. also reported that access dysfunction was the leading cause of hospitalization for ESRD patients, accounting for 17% of admissions in 830 individuals over a one-year period.[4]

More recently, Feldman et al. confirmed that dialysis access dysfunction remains the leading indication for hospital admission among dialysis patients[5]. This group reviewed the Medicare database and found that 16.5% of hospital stays were associated with vascular access–related morbidity. Risk factors identified for hospitalization due to access malfunction in this group were female sex, black race, advanced age, and diabetes. Lazarus et al. reported almost identical findings in their review of more than 25,000 dialysis patients in the National Medical Care, Inc., database.[6] Vascular access morbidity was responsible for 16.2% of all hospitalizations in this group of patients over a five-year period.

The overall size of the hemodialysis population and the frequency of access-related problems make access dysfunction a significant financial expenditure. The estimated total of direct costs for all ESRD care in the United States for 1990 was $7.26 billion.[2] Of this total, $5.2 billion is paid by the Medicare ESRD program. A recent report estimates that 6% of ESRD expenditure is associated with vascular access placement and maintenance.[7]

The cost of dialysis access dysfunction involves not only that associated with its therapy but also certain less obvious expenses that are not easily estimated. Major among these indirect costs is interruption of established dialysis schedules, which in turn leads to inadequate dialysis therapy, further reduction of patient productivity, additional strain on the patient's personal and emotional resources, and inefficient use of dialysis unit resources.

An examination of the costs associated with hemodialysis access and its maintenance is appropriate at a time when all of the costs and delivery mechanisms of American health care are being reevaluated. Many of the forces impelling the current health care reform effort have direct application to surgical procedures for hemodialysis access, including convenient access to care, patient choices in their care, rapidly increasing health care costs, the ultimate responsibility for these costs, and appropriate assessment and control of quality of care.

An established and effective strategy for achieving these goals is the conversion of operative procedures from the inpatient to the outpatient setting, a trend that over the past 15 years has significantly changed the surgical landscape. In 1979, 14% of hospital surgery was performed on outpatients.[8] By 1992, fully 50% of all surgical procedures in the United States were being performed on an outpatient basis.[9] This trend toward ambulatory surgery has led to the development of new venues in which operations are performed. Not only have hospitals provided ambulatory, same-day, or outpatient access to conventional hospital-based operating rooms, but also freestanding surgical facilities have developed and flourished by providing operating rooms dedicated to the outpatient. During the decade of the 1980s, the number of these freestanding surgical facilities increased by more than 300%.[10] Facilities of this type are attracting an increasing share of total outpatient surgery cases.[11]

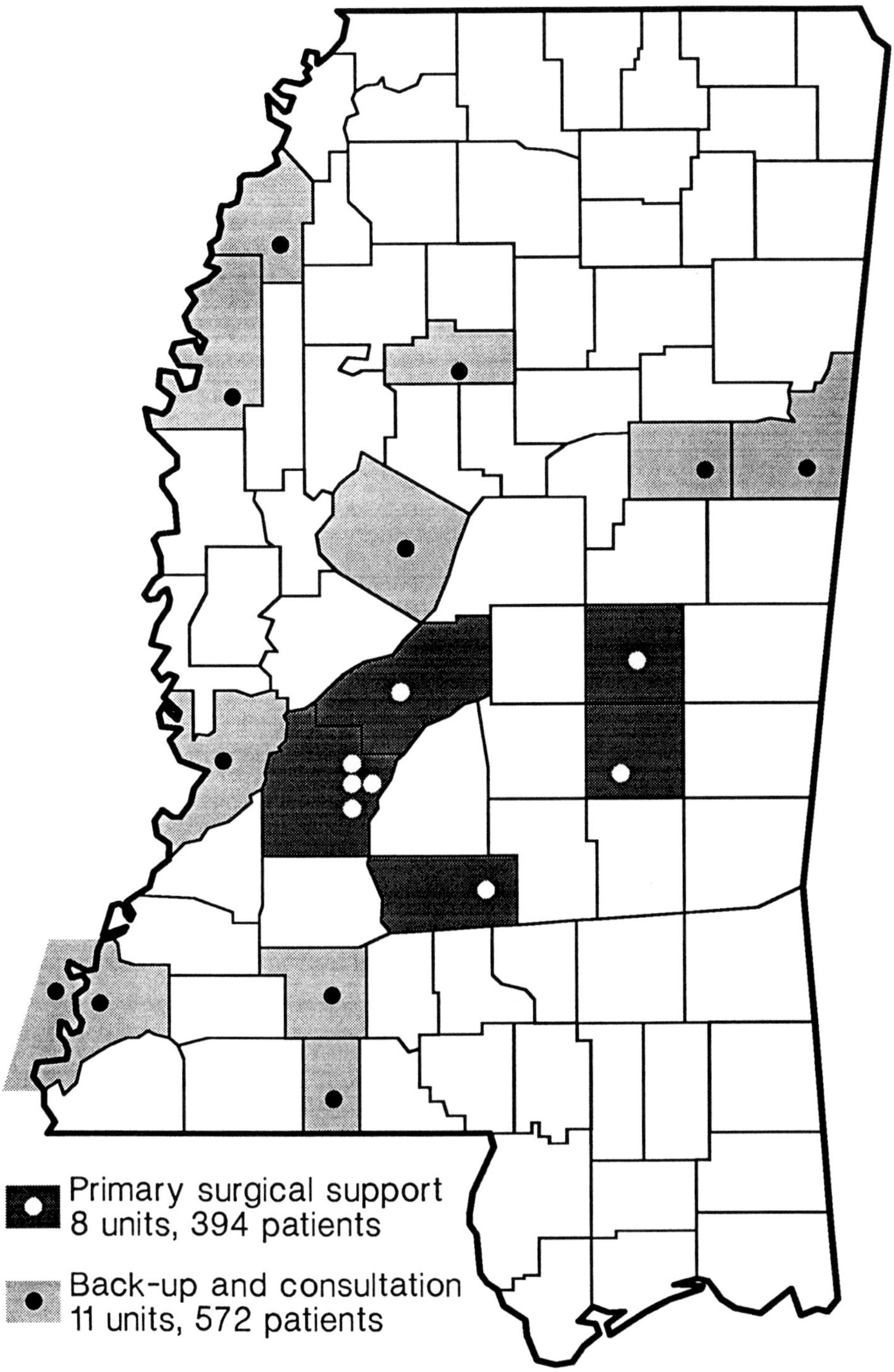

Fig. 6-1. Geographic distribution of dialysis patients for whom surgical care is provided by the University of Mississippi Medical Center.

Materials and Methods

The present interest of our institution in efficient mechanisms of surgical care stems from the fact that the surgical service of the University of Mississippi Medical Center provides dialysis access support services for much of central Mississippi. This support includes primary surgical care for 394 dialysis patients in eight dialysis units. Backup surgical care and consultation services are provided for an additional 532 patients in another nine dialysis units. These patients are located in a 145-mile radius of our facility (figure 6-1).

Demographically, this population is largely undereducated, lives predominately in rural areas, and has limited financial resources. These factors limit rehabilitation and are frequent barriers to optimal dialysis care. When access dysfunction occurs in this population, demographics and geography combine to make it necessary for the patient to travel significant distances for surgical care, to disrupt dialysis schedules, and to place additional strain on already thin resources.

It was through the mechanism of converting procedures to an ambulatory setting that the nephrology and surgical services of our institution sought to improve the accessibility to care for ESRD patients with hemo-access problems while simultaneously reducing cost and maintaining quality of care. Within this setting, it was believed that providing immediate outpatient services for access dysfunction would allow the patient to return immediately to his or her primary dialysis unit with minimal disruption in dialysis routine. Another potential advantage of an immediately available ambulatory surgical facility for ESRD patients with access dysfunction is reduction of the need for temporary access catheter placement. Dual-lumen dialysis catheters are exceptionally useful in providing temporary hemo-access for patients with maturing or dysfunctional access grafts, but it is now clear that subclavian and innominate vein stenosis and occlusion are associated with the use of these catheters.[12-14]

The facility our group developed to accommodate ambulatory dialysis access surgery has been described in detail.[15] This facility is unique in its location and in that it is dedicated to vascular access procedures. Although it is apparent that such a facility may not be practical or appropriate for many practices, some lessons for other settings can be derived from our experience by reviewing the unit's function over the past five years. Certain aspects of the operation of this facility can be applied both to conventional hospital-based outpatient surgery units and to freestanding surgical facilities.

Our facility is located adjacent to a hospital-based 16-bed acute and chronic dialysis unit. It consists of a single operating room with adjacent patient pre- and post-operative observation and instrument preparation areas. The O.R. is equipped with standard O.R. lighting, a conventional operating table, dynamic EKG monitor, automated blood pressure monitor, pulse oximeter, and pneumatic tourniquet. The facility is staffed by a registered nurse who monitors the patient during the procedure. This individual has surgical experience and is also a certified nephrology nurse. Surgical technicians serve as instrument nurse and circulator.

Table 6-1. Access Procedures Performed, November 1988–December 1993

Artificial kidney unit–based operating room	
Inpatient	521
Outpatient	2,372
Main hospital O.R.	
Inpatient	72
Outpatient	252
Total	3,217

Table 6-2. Procedures Performed in an Artificial Kidney Unit–Based Operating Room, November 1988–December 1993

Procedure	Inpatient	Outpatient
Thrombectomy	63	878
Thrombectomy with revision	29	628
Procedure for infection	70	255
Procedure for pseudoaneurysm	28	114
Access graft placement	255	324
A-V fistula creation	29	74
Other	47	99
Total	521	2,372

Results and Discussion

A five-year experience with the artificial kidney unit (AKU)–based operating room has now been compiled and as of December 1993 included 2,893 vascular access procedures. This number represents 89.9% of all vascular access cases performed by our group during this time period (table 6-1). These procedures are stratified in table 6-2, which shows that 2,372 (82%) of these operations were performed on outpatients. Only 6.7% of simple thrombectomies were performed on inpatients, and seldom was access thrombosis alone the indication for these patients' admission to the hospital. More frequently, these individuals were hospitalized for other medical problems, and the thrombosis was either incidental or the result of other pathology for which the patient was receiving inhospital treatment, e.g., cardiac failure, volume depletion, or hypotension.

Thrombectomy procedures requiring surgical revision of the access were also most commonly performed as outpatient operations, with 628 (95.6%) of a total of 657 thrombectomy/revision procedures being performed on nonhospitalized patients. Similarly, most procedures for infection (78.5%) were performed on an outpatient basis. The proportion of operations for infection was smaller than that seen for procedures for thrombosis, however, reflecting the need to admit some patients with access infection for treatment of systemic sepsis.

In contrast, only 56% of access graft placement procedures were performed on outpatients. The relatively lower proportion of outpatients in this category reflects the nature of our patient population. Many of our patients present very late in their disease process and often require placement of a prosthetic vascular access device at

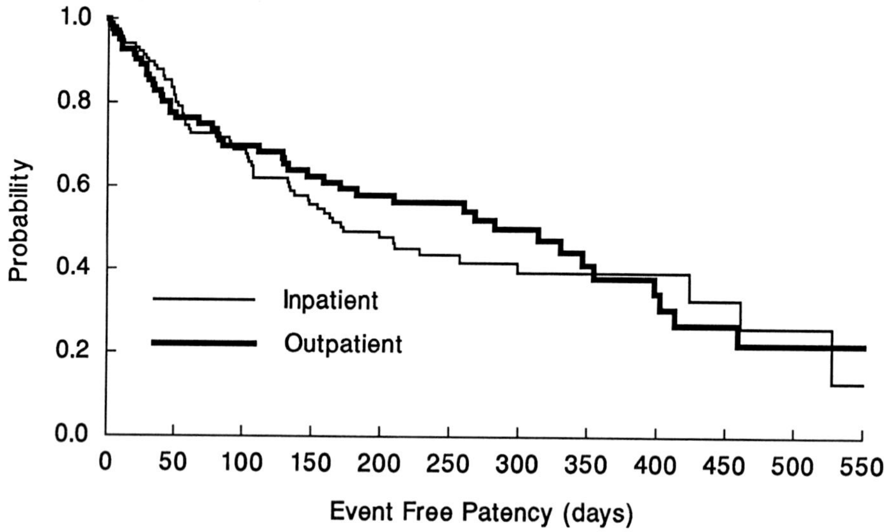

Fig. 6-2. Event-free patency analysis of 160 grafts placed in inpatients and 156 grafts placed in outpatients.

the time of their initial hospitalization and diagnosis. In the stable adult patient, however, placement of a conventional forearm access can almost always be performed on an outpatient basis.

Our initial 28 months of experience with this facility demonstrated that a traditional surgical setting was not necessary for quality access graft placement or for the management of most access complications in the ambulatory patient.[15] Event-free patency and postoperative complications, including perioperative infection, early thrombosis, and unanticipated admission following outpatient placement of primary PTFE grafts, were not different between a group of 173 outpatients operated on in a conventional O.R. environment and 98 outpatients operated on in an AKU-based surgical facility.

This initial review compared only the two types of ambulatory surgery settings and did not address the issue of outpatient versus inpatient procedures. Data collection since that report has allowed direct comparison of outpatient and inpatient procedures for the placement of prosthetic access grafts in previously unoperated forearms. Figure 6-2 represents a Kaplan-Meier analysis of event-free patency (EFP) for 316 dialysis access grafts placed in such patients. EFP is defined as the interval, in days, from graft placement to the first event requiring surgical intervention. Comparison of EFP curves using Cox's Proportional Hazard's model for 160 inpatients who underwent graft placement and 156 outpatients who underwent the same procedure showed no statistical difference in patency between the two groups. The events that occurred in this population of patients are shown in table 6-3.

The proportion of patients in the outpatient group who experienced thrombosis, infection, pseudoaneurysm formation, or who died with a functional graft was not different from the inpatient group. Significantly more grafts in the outpatient group remained event-free ($p=0.01$). The higher number of event-free grafts in the outpatient group probably reflects the fact that hospitalized patients undergoing graft

Table 6-3. Events Occurring in 316 Vascular Access Grafts Placed in Previously Unoperated Forearms

Event	Inpatients	Outpatients	P value
Thrombosis	69	56	ns
Infection	6	7	ns
Pseudoaneurysm	5	3	ns
Seroma	2	0	ns
None	57	82	0.01
Death	17	12	ns
Total	156	160	—

placement are more likely to have comorbid conditions that predispose to access problems.

A similar pattern was noted in a group of 93 patients who underwent placement of Medtronic Atrium (Plasma TFE) grafts (Medtronics, Inc., Minneapolis, Minnesota). Of the total, 54 grafts were placed in outpatients and 39 in hospitalized patients. Kaplan-Meier analysis of EFP for these two groups is shown in figure 6-3. Comparison of these curves revealed no statistically significant difference ($p=0.459$) in EFP between the procedures performed on inpatients and those performed on outpatients, and no difference was noted in the number of infections, pseudoaneurysms, or the number of grafts that remained event-free.

We have developed four indications for requesting either general anesthesia or regional block in patients undergoing vascular access surgery. We also use these indications to determine the necessity to use a conventional O.R. environment rather than our AKU-based vascular procedure room. The first is dissection above the middle one-third of the humerus. Frequently, we revise the venous outflow of a salvageable forearm access to an above-the-elbow position for patients in whom patch angioplasty or interposition revision distal to the elbow is inappropriate. This operation is performed by tunneling externally supported GORE-TEX (FEP-ringed) across the anteromedial aspect of the joint from the antecubital incision to a second incision in the upper arm through which the basilic vein is isolated.

If for any reason this upper arm incision must be placed above the middle one-third of the humerus, the dissection and exposure of the basilic vein can become difficult under local anesthesia. At this level, the median nerve and bicep muscle may require retraction to achieve proximal and distal control of the vein for anastomosis. Such retraction can be very uncomfortable for the patient, and general anesthesia or proximal regional block is not only appropriate for patient comfort but also greatly facilitates the procedure.

The second indication for the services of an anesthesiologist and a conventional O.R. setting is operation for pseudoaneurysm of the brachial or proximal radial artery. These aneurysms are most often due to infected artery-to-graft anastomoses and occasionally involve formal reconstruction of the brachial artery, which demands appropriate exposure to effect safe repair or bypassing of this vessel in order to maintain distal limb perfusion. In contrast to aneurysmal lesions in the region of the antecubital fossa, pseudoaneurysms at the wrist are managed in our vascular procedure room under local infiltration anesthesia and pneumatic tourniquet control.

The third indication is significant debridement of infected tissue. The efficacy of lidocaine and, to some extent, bupivacaine is pH-dependent. The chronic tissue

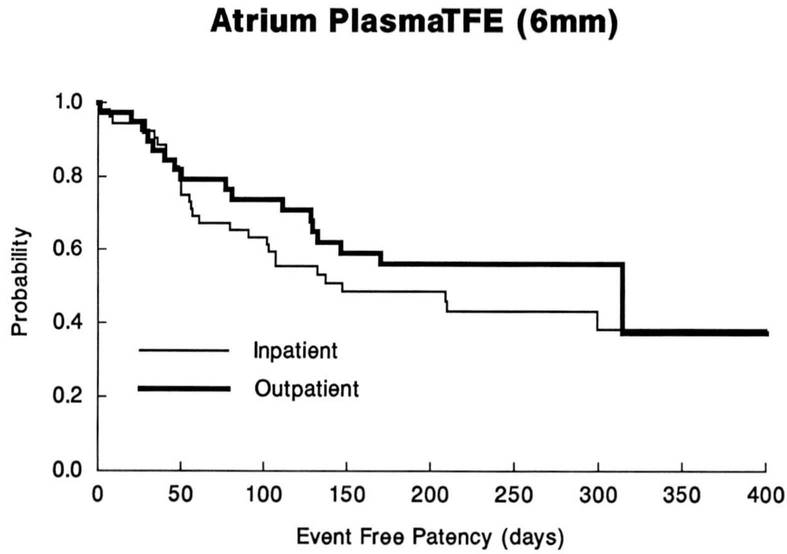

Fig. 6-3. Event-free patency analysis of 93 Atrium Plasma TFE grafts.

acidosis of uremia, coupled with the local acidosis of bacterial infection, dramatically reduces the efficacy of local infiltration anesthesia. Therefore, we do not use local anesthesia to achieve adequate tissue debridement of extensive infections. These three indications for using anesthesia modalities other than local infiltration do not, however, constitute indications for hospital admission.

The fourth indication for general anesthesia in the ESRD patient undergoing access surgery is placement of a prosthetic access graft in the femoral position. Spinal anesthesia is also quite adequate for this operation. Although the femoral vessels at the groin can be safely exposed and controlled under local anesthesia, adequate local infiltration anesthesia for tunneling the graft in the thigh is difficult. It has been our practice to admit these patients to the hospital for observation and assistance with ambulation for 24 to 48 hours.

Hospital admission of ESRD patients with access dysfunction is also indicated in certain other situations. Evidence of systemic sepsis in patients with access infection mandates admission for appropriate monitoring and management of comorbid conditions. It must be recognized, however, that access infection or the need for I.V. antibiotics alone does not dictate admission of ESRD patients who can receive excellent I.V. antibiotic therapy during dialysis. It is frequently our practice to complete a course of antibiotic therapy during routine outpatient dialysis in a patient who was admitted briefly for acute management of an extensive access infection complicated by sepsis.

Questionable perfusion of an extremity in which an access has been placed is a second indication for inhospital care. Any acute change in hand perfusion that manifests in a functional or dysfunctional dialysis access or after any access operation generally demands admission for observation even if immediate surgical intervention is not planned. We have found that observation can be facilitated by the use of pulse oximetry, which provides a constant index of digital perfusion. Compartment syndromes are exceptionally rare in access-bearing extremities, but any evidence of neuromuscular dysfunction that suggests elevated pressure in the subfascial compartments of the forearm warrants hospital admission.

The patient with chronic steal syndrome manifesting as pain on dialysis can usually be evaluated and surgically managed on an outpatient basis. Applying the above-described indications for hospital admission, we have performed 2,624 (81.67%) of the total of 3,217 vascular access cases on an outpatient basis. Again, many—if not most—of the primary access placement procedures performed in hospitalized patients could have also been provided on an outpatient basis, but were performed during initial hospitalization for the convenience of the patient.

Summary

For the foreseeable future, surgery for placement of vascular access grafts and management of their complications will continue to be a central feature in the care of the patient with ESRD. The expanding dialysis population and the high frequency of access-related problems requiring surgical intervention make dialysis access dysfunction costly to both the patient and society. Providing vascular access surgery on an outpatient basis is a strategy by which most hemo-access operations can be performed safely and effectively while simultaneously reducing costs, optimizing patient productivity, efficiently utilizing ESRD resources, and maintaining a high standard of care.

References

1. Evans RW, Blagg CR, Bryan FA Jr. Implications for health care policy; a social and demographic profile of hemodialysis patients in the United States. JAMA 1981; 245: 487-491.
2. U.S. Renal Data System. USRDS 1993 Annual Data Report. Bethesda, MD.: The National Institutes of Health, National Institute of Diabetes and Digestive and Kidney Diseases, March 1993.
3. Hirschman GH, Wolfson M, Mosimann JE, Clark CB, Dante ML, Wineman RJ. Complications of dialysis. Clin Nephrol 1981; 15:66-74.
4. Carlson DM, Duncan DA, Naessens JM, Johnson WJ. Hospitalization in dialysis patients. Mayo Clin Proc 1984; 59:769-775.
5. Feldman HI, Held PJ, Hutchinson JT, Stoiber E, Hartigan MF, Berlin JA. Hemodialysis vascular access morbidity in the United States. Kidney Int 1993; 43:1091-1096.
6. Lazarus MJ, Huang WH, Lew NL, Lowrie EG. Contribution of access-related disease to morbidity of hemodialysis patients. In: Henry ML, Ferguson RM, eds. Vascular access for hemodialysis—III. Chicago:WL Gore & Associates, Inc., and Precept Press, 1993: 3-13.
7. Kallich JD, Litwin MS, Markovich M. Vascular access procedures for end-stage renal disease Medicare beneficiaries. RAND/ UCLA/Harvard Center for Health Care Financing Policy Research (DRU-420-HCFA). Santa Monica:Rand Corp., 1994.
8. Rutkow IM, ed. Socioeconomics of Surgery. St Louis:CV Mosby, 1989.

9. Detmer DE, Gielijns AC. Ambulatory surgery: a more cost-effective treatment strategy? Arch Surg 1994; 129:120-127.
10. Hospital Statistics: 1992-93 Edition. Chicago:American Hospital Association, 1992:xxxiii-xxxviii.
11. Ambulatory care trendlines. Chicago:American Hospital Association, 1992. (xxxiii-viii.)
12. Barrett N, Spencer S, McIvan J, Brown EA. Subclavian stenosis: a major complication of subclavian dialysis catheters. Nephrol Dial Transplant 1988; 3: 423-423.
13. Spinowitz BS, Galler M, Golden RA, Pascoff JH, Schecter L, Held B, Claryton C. Subclavian vein stenosis as a complication of subclavian catheterization for hemodialysis. Arch Intern Med 1987; 157:305-307.
14. Fant GF, Dennis VW, Quarles LD. Late vascular complications of the subclavian dialysis catheter. Am J Kidney Dis 1986; 7:225-228.
15. Didlake R, Curry E, Rigdon EE, Raju S, Bower J. Outpatient vascular access surgery: Impact of a dialysis unit-based surgical facility. Am J Kidney Dis 1992; 19:39-44.

7

THE ROLE OF PERCUTANEOUS INTERVENTION IN TREATING HEMODIALYSIS INSUFFICIENCY

Stephen R. Ramee, M.D.

Introduction

SINCE THE INCEPTION OF EXTRACORPOREAL DIALYSIS in 1944 by Kolff, a variety of techniques for maintaining vascular access for hemodialysis have been developed.[1-8] Failure of dialysis access remains one of the most frequent causes of hospitalization in the dialysis population.[9] In addition to the patient's need for temporary dialysis access when permanent access fails, dialysis access insufficiency with inadequate dialysis over a prolonged period also correlates with early mortality in this patient population. Early detection and treatment of access problems can play an important role in preventing dialysis access failure and may improve the long-term survival of dialysis patients by improving dialysis efficiency. Percutaneous transluminal angioplasty (PTA) has become an accepted technique for avoiding repeated surgical revision and prolonging the useful life of existing dialysis access sites.[10-14] In our institution (Ochsner Medical Institutions, New Orleans, Louisiana), angioplasty has become the treatment of choice for selected patients with dialysis access dysfunction.[15] The technique of angioplasty as well as several new experimental treatments will be discussed in this paper.

Types of Hemodialysis Access

The two types of hemodialysis access that are most commonly used are the endogenous arteriovenous (A-V) fistula developed by Brescia in 1966 and the polytetrafluoroethylene (PTFE of GORE-TEX, W.L. Gore & Associates, Flagstaff, Arizona) A-V graft. The endogenous A-V fistula is most often placed in the wrist using the radial or ulnar artery in a side-to-side anastomosis with a neighboring vein (figure 7-1). The PTFE grafts are preferentially placed between the brachial artery and brachial or cephalic vein with a loop tunneled subcutaneously in the forearm (figure 7-2). If this site has previously been used, PTFE grafts may be placed between any major artery and vein in the forearm, upper arm, or thigh. Physical examination will readily distinguish between the two types of access.

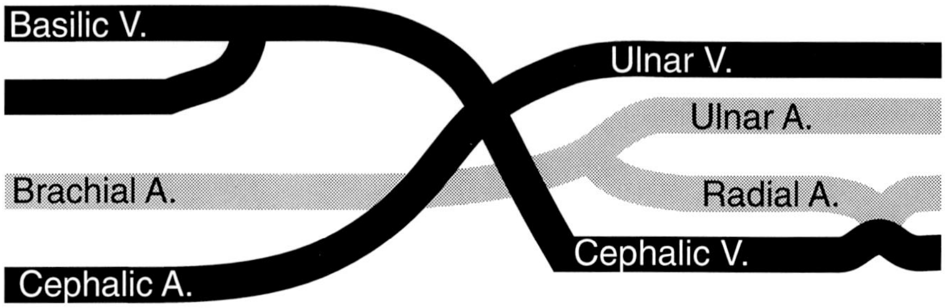

Figure 7-1. Endogenous A-V fistula.

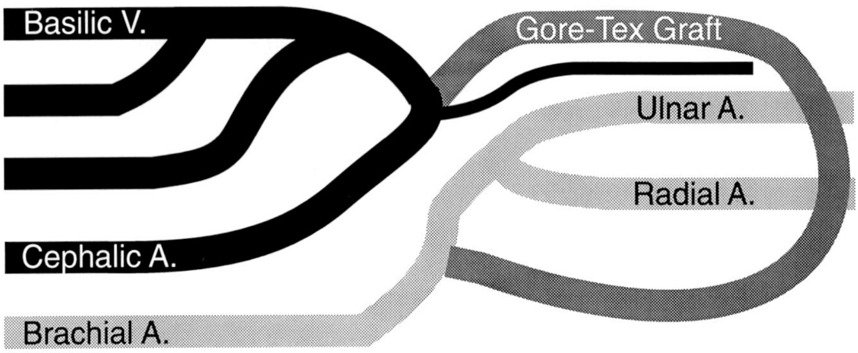

Figure 7-2. Synthetic PTFE (GORE-TEX) graft.

Detection of Dialysis Access Failure

Both types of dialysis access sites have similar long-term patency rates. Unfortunately, all access sites tend to become compromised with time, with patency rates of about 60-70% at one year and nearly 50% at four years (figure 7-3). One of the most common causes of access failure is thrombosis. Although this can occur spontaneously, the development of a stenosis in the arterial inflow or venous outflow is the usual precipitating event. Histopathologic examination of surgical specimens has shown that neointimal hyperplasia and fibrosis are responsible for the development of these stenoses.[16]

LESION LOCATION

The site of the stenosis can be predicted based upon the type of access. PTFE grafts show a predilection for development of stenosis at or near the venous anastomosis or in the draining venous system. A-V fistulas tend to develop stenoses at the A-V anastomosis or in the draining veins. Patients with either type of dialysis access can develop stenosis of the subclavian vein. In our experience, subclavian vein stenoses have always been associated with preexistingindwelling subclavian or jugular venous lines. In most cases, patients have had long-term temporary dialysis catheters placed in their subclavian vein.

EARLY DIAGNOSIS

Early diagnosis of dialysis access malfunction requires close surveillance of the patient by the nephrologist and dialysis nurse. If stenosis is not detected early,

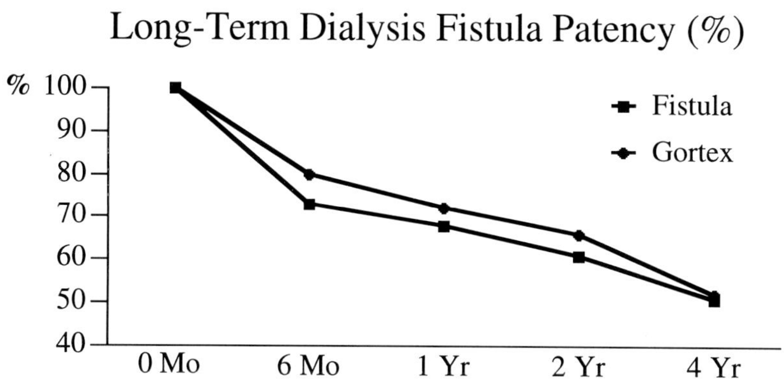

	N	6 Mo	1 Yr	2 Yr	4 Yr
Fistula	594	73	68	61	51
Gore–Tex	336	80	72	66	52

Figure 7-3. Dialysis patency, pooled surgical series.

thrombosis can occur with loss of pulsatile flow through the fistula or graft. Depending on the location of the stenosis, early access failure can be manifested in several ways, including an increase in the recirculation fraction (RF) above 20% [where RF = (serum BUN - inflow BUN) ÷ (serum BUN - outflow BUN)], decrease in dialysis efficiency (increase in dialysis time), high pressure on the venous return line, arterial line "sucking," aneurysm formation, and extremity edema.

NONINVASIVE EVALUATION

The history and physical examination can provide important clues as to the location of the stenosis in a patient with malfunctioning dialysis access. In patients with PTFE grafts, a thrill is usually present at the arterial and venous anastomoses. A localized thrill within the graft or at a distal site remote from the graft in the draining veins often signifies a significant stenosis. The quality of the pulse within the graft may indicate the location of the stenosis. A stronger-than-usual pulse commonly accompanies graft outflow obstruction, and a weak pulse may signify inflow obstruction. Arterial line "sucking" usually indicates proximal anastomosis stenosis and is most commonly encountered with A-V fistulas, not PTFE grafts. Increased dialysis time and increasing recirculation fraction both mean that there is poor flow through the fistula, but do not help with localization of the site of stenosis because they occur with either inflow or outflow lesions. Most lesions are found somewhere in the venous drainage at or beyond the distal anastomosis. Of 63 lesions in patients undergoing percutaneous transluminal angioplasty, 73% were in the venous drainage, 17% were in the fistula or graft, and 10% were artery or proximal lesions.

Color flow Doppler can be used to clarify the location and number of stenoses in cases in which the physical examination is ambiguous. This may be especially helpful in cases of suspected peripheral arterial steal.

Methods

Angiographic and Hemodynamic Assessment

In otherwise healthy dialysis patients, angiography and PTA can be performed on an outpatient basis. The optimal site for vascular entry is determined by the history and physical examination so that all suspected stenoses may be successfully dilated. A 6 Fr sheath is used to obtain access for angiography, hemodynamic assessment, and intervention. In PTFE grafts, the venous limb of the graft is the most common entry site. In endogenous A-V fistulas, the brachial artery is commonly used. Because stenoses are often multiple, it is important to angiographically study the entire graft and its venous drainage to the superior vena cava. We usually perform a hemodynamic assessment of the entire system as well, making certain to check the gradient across all suspected stenoses.

Angioplasty Technique

After documenting the number and location of significant stenoses, a steerable wire is then negotiated across the lesions and an angioplasty balloon is inserted over the guide wire. In our early experience, 3,000 U of heparin were given; however, in the dialysis population the activated clotting time (ACT) was commonly longer than 200 seconds after such a small dose of heparin. Other investigators have documented the safety of performing PTA in these patients without the need for heparin, so except in unusual circumstances (preexisting thrombosis, hypercoagulable state, stenting, or intense arterial spasm), we have abandoned the routine administration of heparin.

High-pressure balloons may be required because the venous outflow lesions often require high pressures (10 atmospheres or greater) before dilating completely. It is not uncommon for 10-16 atmospheres to be required for eliminating the waist on the balloon. The balloons are sized to match the diameter of the vessels being dilated. The most common size for PTFE grafts placed in dialysis patients is 6.0 mm, so we use the diameter of the graft as a reference in choosing balloon sizes in these patients. In patients with proximal anastomosis PTFE graft lesions and with lesions at the arterial anastomosis of endogenous A-V fistulas, a smaller balloon is generally used because of the smaller size of the inflow artery. In patients with lesions of the subclavian or innominate veins, balloons of 10 mm or larger diameter may be required. After successful angioplasty, angiography is repeated and a pressure pullback is again performed. The sheath is removed immediately after the procedure in the catheterization suite.

Definitions of Success

Success can be measured angiographically, hemodynamically, and clinically. Angiographic success is defined as <50% residual stenosis after angioplasty

Table 7-1. Dialysis Access Angioplasty Results

Re-stenosis post-PTA		
Patients	8/44	18%
Lesions	14/61	32%
Repeat angioplasty		
Patients	7/8	88%
Lesions	13/14	93%

with brisk contrast flow. Although the hemodynamic definition of success is still evolving, we generally can abolish or ameliorate the gradient at each lesion. Clinical success can be determined by improvement in dialysis after angioplasty, with resolution of the clinical problem that led to the initial referral. A recirculation fraction of <15% is desirable for long-term hemodialysis, and a high recirculation fraction after the procedure suggests an inadequate clinical response to PTA.

Results

We have performed PTA in more than 250 dialysis patients with failing dialysis access. In our first 16 months of performing angioplasty for dialysis insufficiency, we dilated 63 lesions in 45 patients. Thirty-four had PTFE shunts and 11 had endogenous fistulas. The distribution of lesions is shown in table 7-1. Angioplasty was successful in 96% of patients, 97% of lesions.

Only one complication occurred in these patients. Shunt thrombosis occurred in a patient who intentionally did not receive heparin. This complication was successfully treated with re-dilation and anticoagulation without requiring thrombolysis or surgery.

Re-stenosis occurred in 18% of patients and 32% of lesions at six months with 100% follow-up (table 7-2). There were no hemodynamic or angiographic predictors of re-stenosis. Most of the patients with re-stenosis were treated with repeat angioplasty, so that the six-month patency with one or more angioplasties was 90%. These patency rates compare favorably with the results from surgical series and other angioplasty series that have been published.[2-8] Totally occluded veins, even long ones, can usually be crossed successfully and then dilated. We use a hydrophilic wire (Glidewire, Meditech, Watertown, Massachusetts) to cross the lesion and then a standard angioplasty balloon to dilate.

When a graft has thrombosed, there are two options for recanalization: (1) surgical thrombectomy, or (2) thrombolysis. Because of the ease and low morbidity with which thrombectomy can be performed, this has been our treatment of choice. Immediately after thrombectomy in the outpatient surgery suite, the patient is heparinized, and angiography is performed in the catheterization laboratory to locate the culprit lesion or lesions that predisposed the patient to graft thrombosis. After undergoing PTA, the patients can generally be sent home after a short period of observation in the outpatient recovery area. Hospitalization is rarely required.

Thrombolysis

Percutaneous recanalization using a short course of intra-graft urokinase has also been used successfully in patients who were unwilling or unable to have surgical thrombectomy. The results of this technique are also good; however, patients either must remain on the catheterization table for 45-60 minutes during the infusion or return to the catheterization suite when the infusion is complete. After thrombolysis, the underlying stenosis is dilated with balloon angioplasty.

Rheolytic and Aspiration Thrombectomy

We have recently begun a trial of percutaneous thrombectomy using a Rheolytic thrombectomy catheter (Possis, Minneapolis, Minnesota). This catheter, which can be inserted through a 6 Fr sheath over an 0.018-in. guide wire, uses the Venturi phenomenon to aspirate and remove large amounts of thrombus from occluded vessels and grafts. Initial results with this device in nine patients have been extremely promising. Seven patients have been treated by percutaneous thrombus aspiration using a large-lumen catheter and a simple vacuum, also with good results. As with thrombolytic therapy, angioplasty, atherectomy, or stenting is then performed to treat the underlying stenoses after thrombectomy.

Some lesions will not dilate with nominal or even high balloon inflation pressures. Intentional rupture of the balloon is never our goal; however, it commonly occurs in stubborn stenoses and has not caused vessel rupture in our experience. But there are several reports in the literature of vessel rupture, so caution is advised. We have encountered several lesions that would not dilate despite pressure sufficient to rupture the balloon. In these patients, we have successfully performed directional atherectomy using a Simpson atherectomy catheter (PSG, Santa Clara, California).

Endogenous A-V fistulas tend to be technically more difficult to treat because of the need for antegrade brachial or radial artery access, the massive dilation that can occur in the recipient veins due to repeated venipuncture, and the difficulty in crossing lesions in a retrograde manner against the intact venous valves. With proper equipment selection, however, most stenoses and many total occlusions can be successfully dilated.

Some lesions will not adequately dilate despite repeated balloon inflations. A persistent high-grade stenosis demonstrated angiographically or a persistent pressure gradient across a stenosis may indicate elastic recoil. This can occur at any location, but is especially common in the venous drainage lesions. These patients require either surgical revision or stenting.

Stent Implantation

We deployed intravascular stents in 31 hemodialysis patients (34 lesions) with suboptimal results after PTA.[17] Indications for angiography in 31 patients were increased recirculation fraction (22 patients), increased dialysis time (7), and high venous pressure (2). This patient group consisted of 14 males and 17 females whose ages were 56.6 ± 12.6 years. Mean vessel diameter was 8.1 ± 3.3 and lesion length 24.1 ± 21.3. A single nonarticulated Palmaz stent (Johnson & Johnson Interventional Systems, Warren, New Jersey) was deployed in 12 (35%) lesions and

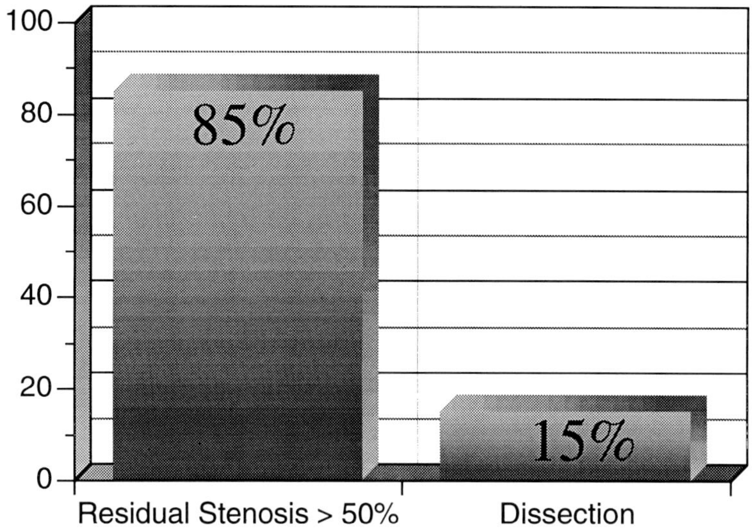

Figure 7-4. Dialysis access PTA, type of stent deployed.

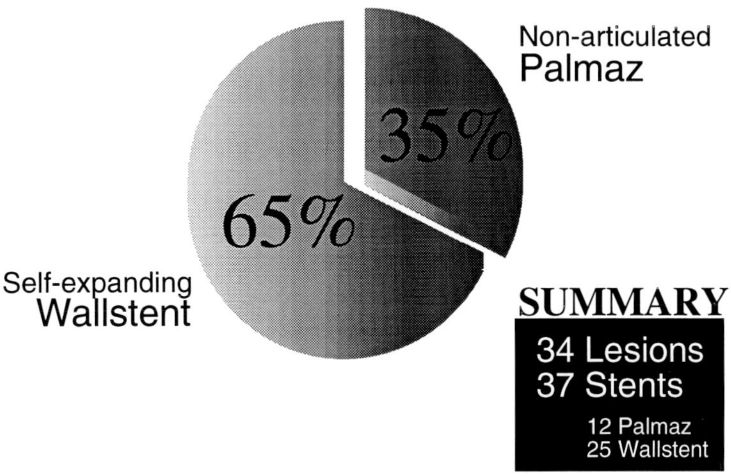

Figure 7-5. Indications for stenting.

Table 7-2. Location of Stent Implantation

Anastomotic Lesions	N
Venous Side	11
Arterial Side	1
Draining Vein	**N**
Basilic or cephalic	10
Subclavian or brachiocephalic	12

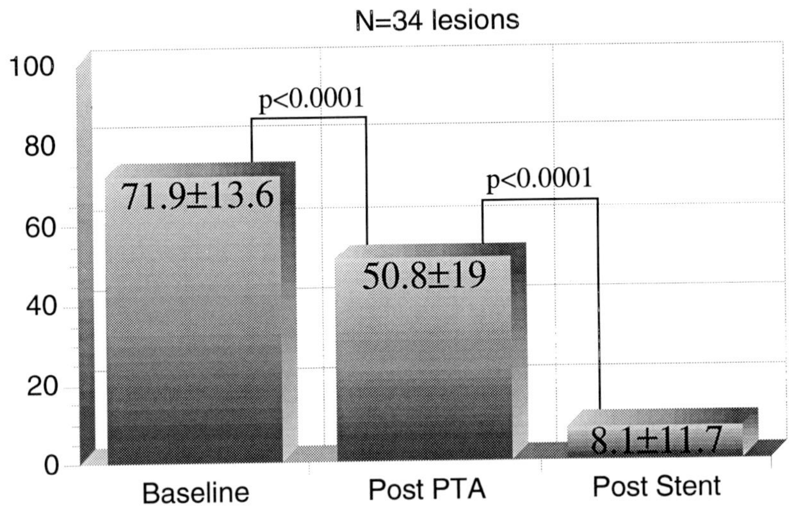

Figure 7-6. Minimum luminal diameter.

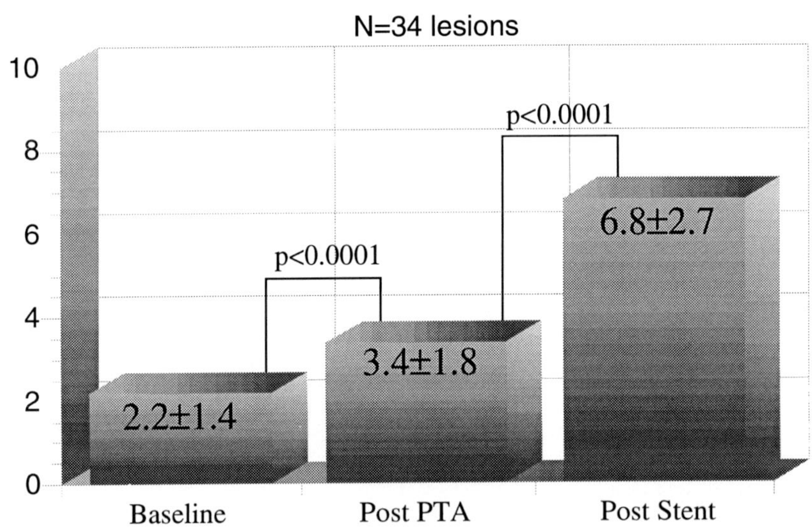

Figure 7-7. Percent diameter stenosis postintervention.

a self-expanding Wallstent (Schneider, Minneapolis, Minnesot) in 22 (65%) lesions (figure 7-4). Indications for stent deployment included persistent angiographic diameter stenoses of more than 50% after balloon angioplasty in 29 (85%) patients and flow-limiting dissections in five (15%) patients (figure 7-5). Stent locations are shown in table 7-2, with the majority being placed in the venous drainage. Multiple stents were placed in three patients. No anticoagulants were administered after stent implantation.

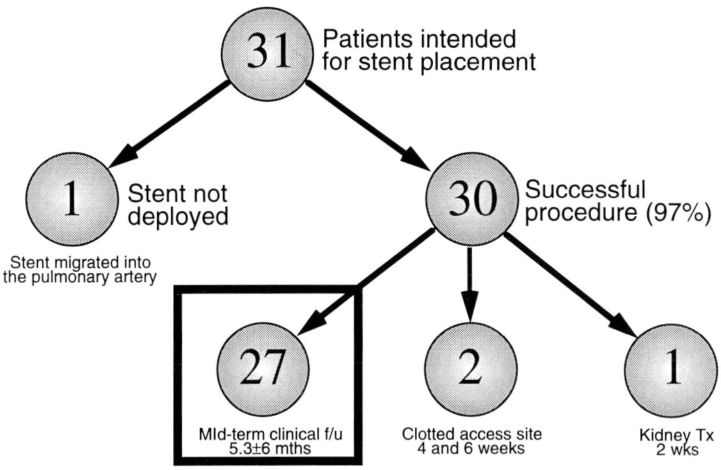

Figure 7-8. Short-term results of intervention.

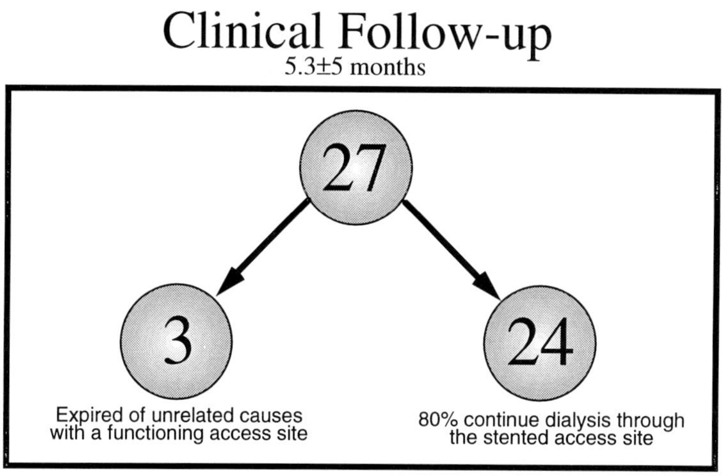

Figure 7-9. Clinical results of stent placement.

Residual stenosis was significantly reduced by stent implantation after failed PTA. Successful stent delivery was accomplished in 30 (97%) of 31 patients. One complication occurred in a patient where the stent migrated into the pulmonary artery without sequelae. The remaining 30 patients obtained immediate clinical benefit and were able to be dialyzed through the stented access site within 24 hours. The minimum lumen diameter and percent diameter stenosis showed significant improvement after stent implantation (figures 7-6 and 7-7). Upon clinical follow-up (mean time = 5.3±5 months), 27 (90%) of the 30 patients continued dialysis through the stented access site (figure 7-8). Of the three patients who did not continue dialysis, one underwent kidney transplantation and two required a new access site within one month due to stent thrombosis (figure 7-9). There were no instances of bleeding, infection, or stent-related death. During the follow-up period, three patients expired of unrelated causes with a functioning access site.

We concluded that stent deployment is a safe and effective nonsurgical treatment strategy for failed PTA in hemodialysis access sites. The lack of anticoagulation and the ability to dialyze the patients immediately renders stent implantation an attractive adjunct to balloon angioplasty. Although our early experience with stent implantation in these vessels has been promising, it remains an experimental technique, and long-term follow-up is needed.

Summary

Angioplasty is a reasonable alternative to surgical revision in patients with failing dialysis access, with a high success rate and low complication rate. The technique is very similar to that of peripheral artery angioplasty; however, some differences do exist. Hemodynamic assessment can be helpful in determining lesion severity and location in these patients. Although the long-term clinical results of angioplasty in these patients appear to be quite good, there is a 20-30% incidence of re-stenosis. It is to be hoped that the development of newer techno-logic approaches (stents and atherectomy) for opening stenotic lesions will lead to improvement in the re-stenosis rate in patients with dialysis access insufficiency.

References

1. Kolff W, Berk H. The artificial kidney: a dialyzer with a great area. Acta Med Scand 1944; 117:121.
2. Brescia M, Cimino J, Appel K, et al. Chronic hemodialysis using created arteriovenous fistula. N Engl J Med 1966; 275:1089-1092.
3. Kinnaert P, Vereerstraeten P, Toussaint C, Van Geertruyden J. Nine years experience with internal arteriovenous fistulas for hemodialysis: a study of some factors influencing results. Br J Surg 1977; 64:242-246.
4. Tellis V, Kohlberg W, Bhat D, et al. Expanded polytetrafluro-ethylene graft fistula for chronic hemodialysis. Ann Surg 1979; 189:101-105.
5. Jenkins A, Buist T, Glover S. Medium-term follow-up of forty autogenous vein and forty polytetrafluoroethylene (Gore-Tex) grafts for vascular access. Surgery 1980; 88:667-672.
6. Palder S, Kirkman R, Whittemore A, et al. Vascular access for hemodialysis: Patency rates and results of revision. Ann Surg 1985; 202:235-239.
7. Rohr M, Browder W, Frentz G, McDonald J. Arteriovenous fistulas for long-term dialysis. Arch Surg 1978; 113:153-155.
8. Munda R, First M, Alexander W, et al. Polytetrafluoroethylene graft survival in hemodialysis. JAMA 1983; 249:219-222.
9. Hunter D, Castaneda-Zuniga W, Coleman C, et al. Failing arteriovenous dialysis fistulas: Evaluation and treatment. Radiology 1984; 152:631-635.
10. Gordon D, Glanz S, Butt K, et al. Treatment of stenotic lesions in dialysis access fistulas and shunts by transluminal angioplasty. Radiology 1982; 143:53-58.
11. Saeed M, Newman G, McCann R, et al. Stenoses in dialysis fistulas: treatment with percutaneous angioplasty. Radiology 1987; 164:693-697.

12. Glanz S, Gordon D, Butt K, et al. The role of percutaneous angioplasty in the management of chronic hemodialysis fistulas. Ann Surg 1987; 206:777-781.
13. Gmelin E, Winterhoff R, Rinast E. Insufficient hemodialysis access fistulas: Late results of treatment with percutaneous balloon angioplasty. Radiology 1989; 171:657-660.
14. Rodriguez-Perez J, Maynar M, Rams A, et al. Percutaneous transluminal angioplasty as best treatment in stenosis of vascular access for hemodialysis. Nephron 1989; 51:192-196.
15. Ramee S, Rees A, Husserl F, et al. Percutaneous angioplasty for preservation of dialysis access: Immediate results and follow-up (abstr). Circulation 1991; 84(suppl II):292.
16. Stehbens W, Karmody A. Venous atherosclerosis associated with arteriovenous fistulas for hemodialysis. Arch Surg 1975; 110:176-180.
17. Escobar A, Karsan A, Collins T, et al. Hemodialysis access angioplasty: Stent deployment for suboptimal balloon angioplasty results (abstr). JACC 1994; 23(suppl A):470A.

8

ROUTINE ANGIOSCOPY FOR VASCULAR ACCESS SURGERY

Arnold Miller, M.D., Ch.B., Thomas J. Hölzenbein, M.D., and Michael N. Gottlieb, M.D.

VASCULAR ENDOSCOPY, OR ANGIOSCOPY, is now an established technique for providing the surgeon with information that enhances the results of surgery performed for lower extremity revascularization.[1-4] The role of routine angioscopy in vascular access surgery appears to be very similar, essentially providing the surgeon with useful information on the remote, unexposed vasculature or graft. This allows rational intraoperative decisions based on accurate information rather than on one's "clinical" experience, thus often simplifying and minimizing the surgical procedure.[5,6]

Improved management of end-stage renal disease (ESRD), together with the limited number of available transplant organs, has resulted in an ever-increasing population of chronic hemodialysis patients. The maintenance of functional vascular access in these patients is becoming more and more complex. Decisions regarding the establishment of a primary vascular access or its revision often play a critical role in the patient's ultimate survival.

We have previously described the techniques of intraoperative angioscopy in detail, with particular reference to techniques of saline irrigation to clear the visual field.[5,7-9] We have also described the specific techniques for vascular access surgery.[5] In this chapter, we will review the indications for angioscopy in vascular access surgery and our experience with routine angioscopy, then describe a modified and simple approach to the occluded vascular access.

Indications and Techniques

Indications and techniques for the routine use of angioscopy vary with the type of access—autogenous arteriovenous fistula (A-VF) or synthetic bridge graft

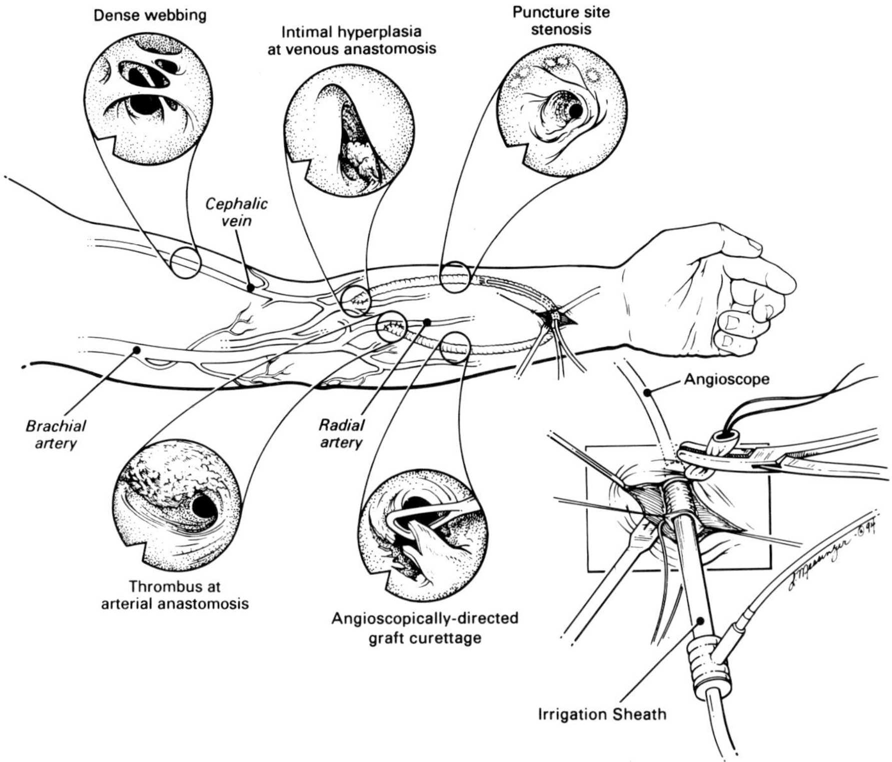

Figure 8-1. Technique of angioscopy to evaluate a failed vascular access graft. The angioscope is inserted through a small skin incision and a transverse graft arteriotomy and directed toward the venous and arterial anastomosis to evaluate the graft, both anastomoses and native vessels. If additional sites of pathology are localized, direct limited exposure is facilitated by the light of the angioscope shining through the skin. Occlusive lesions can be removed under direct vision with a Kevorkian-Young curette. (Printed by permission of Hölzenbein et al [ref 6])

A-V fistula (BGF)—and whether the surgery is primary (to establish the procedure) or revision (to salvage the failed or failing vascular access). In primary surgery for A-VF, angioscopy is used for systematic inspection of the "outflow" vein before the arterial anastomosis is performed. Depending on the proposed site of the anastomosis, this allows inspection of the forearm cephalic vein and the cephalic and basilic veins of the upper arm. The axillary vein generally is not examined, as clearing this large vein of blood would require a larger volume of irrigation fluid than can be safely tolerated by these patients. In revision surgery for A-VF, the "outflow" vein is evaluated for completeness of thrombectomy, with special attention given to the needle-stick sites for dialysis and the overall quality of the vein.

In the primary bridge graft fistula (BGF), in addition to the systematic examination of the outflow vein, the venous anastomosis is routinely monitored for presence of technical deficits. Routine angioscopy for revision surgery of the BGF has resulted in a new approach to the occluded BGF (see below). Angioscopy allows (1) assessment of the venous and arterial anastomoses for the presence of stenosis, residual thrombus, or technical abnormalities; (2) complete examination of the synthetic bridge graft for the presence of residual intraluminal and mural thrombus after balloon thrombectomy, as well as the diagnosis of midgraft stenosis or other abnormalities so common at the needle-stick sites; and (3) the assessment of both the runoff vein and inflow artery.

Techniques for angioscopy during vascular access surgery are similar to the techniques for intraoperative angioscopy during infrainguinal bypass grafting. The angioscopes we use range in size from 0.8 to 2.2 mm in external diameter (Olympus Corporation, Lake Success, New York). We seldom use an angioscope with an irrigating channel, because these angioscopes tend to be larger and more rigid; also, they often do not provide sufficient flow to clear the visual field completely of blood, particularly when arterial inflow is being examined. Clearing blood from the visual field is a prerequisite of successful angioscopy and remains the limiting factor to performing angioscopy.

For autogenous A-VF surgery, the angioscope is inserted either through an irrigation sheath inserted into the open distal end of the outflow vein, or collateral to a smaller irrigation needle or catheter. *In situ* inspection of the unexposed vein is performed with the same technique described for harvesting of arm vein for infrainguinal bypass grafting.[2] In the failing or occluded autogenous A-V fistula, the angioscope is introduced into the vein through a venotomy at a site where the cause of failure is most likely determined either by clinical examination or preoperative fistulogram. The angioscope is introduced in both antegrade and retrograde directions, allowing inspection of the runoff veins of the forearm and upper arm, as well as the proximal vein and anastomosis.[6]

In primary surgery for the BGF, the angioscope is inserted through the open end of the graft after completion of the venous anastomosis, usually after tunneling the graft. Again, irrigation is provided either with an irrigation sheath or collateral catheter. The outflow vein and the anastomosis are inspected.

The techniques of angioscopy unique to revision surgery in the occluded synthetic bridge graft are illustrated in figure 8-1. A small incision is made, usually at the apex of the loop graft. A few centimeters of synthetic graft are freed up to allow placement of fine occluding clamps after reestablishing flow. Rummel tourniquets are placed to prevent leakage of irrigation fluid around the angioscope once it is inserted. A transverse opening is made in the anterior wall of the graft. Thrombectomy of the venous limb is generally performed first to take advantage of the lack of bleeding from the occluded arterial limb. The arterial limb is approached only after completion of all manipulations on the venous limb. The angioscope is then introduced through an irrigation sheath and passed through the graft, anastomosis, and into the runoff vein. The extent and location of any endoluminal pathology, completeness of the thrombectomy, or other endoluminal intervention is determined. Repeat angioscopic examination after each manipulation may be performed. On occasion, the light of the angioscope shining through the skin may serve as a guide to direct further exposure of the graft of autogenous vessel at the site of a particular abnormality. This allows much of the revision procedure to be performed through separate small skin and graft incisions, limiting surgical exposure of the graft and the extent of the surgery and eliminating the

Table 8-1. Clinical Characteristics of 51 Patients Undergoing 84 Vascular Access Surgical Procedures with Intraoperative Angioscopy*

Average age, 63.5 (range 28.9—84.6); male, 19; female, 32		
Reason for vascular access		
Renal failure		49
Diabetic nephropathy	19	
Atherosclerosis/ischemia	10	
Glomerulonephritis	8	
Polycystic disease	5	
Miscellaneous	7	
Familial hyperlipidemia (plasmaphoresis)		2
Primary		
Autogenous arteriovenous fistula		36
Radio-cephalic (wrist)	18	
Radio-midcubital (elbow)	9	
Radio-cephalic (elbow)	2	
Brachio-basilic (elbow)	1	
Basilic vein transposition	6	
Bridge graft fistula		7
Radio-cephalic (loop ePTFE)	6	
Radio-basilic (straight ePTFE)	1	
Revision		
Autogenous arteriovenous fistula		7
Radio-cephalic (wrist)	4	
Radio-cephalic (elbow)	3	
Bridge graft fistula		34
Forearm		
Radio-cephalic (loop, bovine)	1	
Radio-cephalic (loop, ePTFE)	16	
Radio-basilic (loop, ePTFE)	14	
Radio-brachial (loop, ePTFE)	1	
Upper arm		
Radio-axillary (straight, ePTFE)	1	
Radio-brachial (straight, ePTFE)	1	

*Printed with permission of Hölzenbein et al. (ref 6)

need for general anesthesia. In addition, to monitor thrombus removal with the various thrombectomy catheters, angioscopy may be used to direct removal of the excessively thickened intimal lining causing stenosis of the graft with a curette or any other interventional device.

Techniques to Reduce Irrigation Fluid

Various techniques are used to minimize the volume of irrigation fluid used during angioscopy. A standard tourniquet may be applied to the upper arm preoperatively and inflated to occluding pressures during the angioscopy. This is particularly useful for the more prolonged procedures where repeated angioscopically directed

Table 8-2. Size of Angioscope (outer diameter) and Volume of Irrigation Fluid and Occlusion Techniques Used during 84 Vascular Access Procedures Monitored with Angioscopy*

	Primary		Revision	
	A-VF n = 36	BGF n = 7	A-VF n = 7	BGF n = 34
Angioscope (OD) mm				
0.8	2	—	1	2
1.4	28	1	5	13
2.2	6	6	1	19
Irrigation fluid (ml)				
Tourniquet	220 (n = 11)	—	—	432 (n = 8)
No tourniquet	281 (n = 18)	242 (n = 7)	221 (n = 7)	309 (n = 22)
Endoluminal balloon	—	—	—	309 (n = 2)
External compression	123 (n = 7)	—	—	300 (n = 2)
Mean irrigation fluid volume (range: 30-518 ml)	235	242	221	309

*Printed with permission of Hölzenbein et al. (ref 6)

interventions such as curetting the lining of the graft or repeated thrombectomy are performed. Simple digital pressure of the upper arm to compress the veins or directly on inflow artery to control arterial bleeding or intraluminal balloon occlusion are useful adjuncts that are frequently applied.

Clinical Experience

We recently reviewed our experience with 51 patients undergoing 84 vascular access procedures with angioscopy.[6] The clinical details are summarized in table 8-1. The average age was 63.5 years, with a predominance of females, and a 54.5% incidence of diabetes mellitus as the underlying cause of renal failure. Of the 43 primary procedures, 83.7% were autogenous A-VFs and 16.3% were synthetic BGFs, all with polytetrafluoroethylene (PTFE). Of the 41 revision procedures performed for the occluded or failed vascular access, 82.9% were for BGF and 17.1% for A-VF.

The size of the angioscope, the volume of irrigation fluid, and technique used to minimize the irrigation fluid volumes are shown in table 8-2. For evaluation of autogenous fistula, the smaller angioscopes (1.4 mm or less) were most commonly used, while in the synthetic BGF the larger, steerable angioscopes were most useful. The average volume of irrigation fluid per angioscopy study was 274 ml (range: 30 ml-518 ml). Prewarmed normal saline solution without potassium, heparin, or papaverine was used in all patients. In primary access surgery, there was no difference in the average volume of irrigation fluid in A-VF (220 ml) and BGF (281 ml). In revision surgery for failed BGF, an upper-arm tourniquet was frequently used, particularly when angioscopically directed endoluminal thrombectomy or curettage was performed. In these cases (n=8), the total irrigation volumes averaged 432 ml (range: 175-508 ml) per angioscopy. Without the

Table 8-3. 67 Abnormal Angioscopy Findings in 84 Operations for Vascular Access Monitored with Angioscopy*

	Primary		Revision	
	A-VF	BGF	A-VF	BGF
No. of procedures	36	7	7	34
"Webs," vein stenosis	5	1	—	2
Vasa vasorum / vein sclerosis	2	—	1	—
Thrombus	1	—	2	19
Midgraft / puncture site stenosis	—	—	3	15
Anastomotic stenosis	—	—	—	7
"Irregular" surface, flaps	—	—	—	9
Total abnormal findings	8	1	6	52

*Printed with permission of Hölzenbein et al. (ref 6)

tourniquet, where the procedure was often less prolonged, the irrigation fluid volume averaged 309 ml (range: 200-500 ml) per angioscopy (n= 22). Manual compression was often done in cases in which the tourniquet could not be applied, such as in anterior transposition of the basilic vein and in situations in which minimal irrigation fluid was required. In seven of these cases, irrigation fluid averaged only 123 ml (range: 30-200 ml).

No complications were encountered that were directly related to angioscopy. All patients tolerated the additional fluid load, and in no patient was angioscopy abandoned or urgent hemodialysis instituted as a result of acute fluid overload. The quality of the angioscopic studies was excellent in 85.7% (72/84), fair in 11.9% (10/84) and poor in 2.4% (2/84).

The 67 abnormal angioscopy findings in the 84 vascular access operations are shown in table 8-3. Similar to our experience for arm vein bypass surgery, the most frequent abnormality found in the primary surgery group was segmental recanalization.[2] In the revision graft, the residual thrombus following what appeared to be adequate thrombectomy was the commonest finding in both A-VF and BGF. Unsuspected midgraft stenosis was found in 15 (44.1%) and stenosis of the venous anastomosis in only seven (20.%) of the 34 occluded BGFs.

Table 8-4 summarizes the surgical decisions and interventions. Curettage for unsuspected midgraft stenosis and re-thrombectomy were the most common interventions resulting from angioscopic findings. Only one patient for whom a primary A-VF was planned had a PTFE graft inserted when the superficial veins were found to be to severely affected by segmental recanalization.

Patency of the 84 vascular access procedures monitored with angioscopy is shown in table 8-5. Early uncorrected secondary (<30 days) patency after revision procedures for all BGFs was 55.9% (19/34 grafts). In BGFs where endoluminal pathology noted on angioscopy was corrected, the 30-day patency was 66.6% (16/24). In contrast, if no correction of the angioscopically demonstrated pathology was performed, the 30-day patency was only 33.3% (3/9). This difference is statistically significant ($p \leq 0.012$, Fisher exact test). At three months, the patency for all revision procedures in BGFs was 38.2% (13/34). Where endoluminal pathology detected on angioscopy was corrected, the patency at three months was 41.7%; when not corrected, 33.3%. This did not reach statistical significance.

Table 8-4. 32 Surgical Interventions and Decisions in 84 Operations for Vascular Access, Monitored with Angioscopy

	Primary		Revision	
	A-VF	BGF	A-VF	BGF
No. procedures	36	7	7	34
Graft curettage	—	—	—	15 (13 + 2)*
Redo thrombectomy	—	—		17
Redo venous anastomosis	—	—	—	4 (2 + 2)*
Redo arterial anastomosis	—	—	1	2
Interposition graft	—	—	1	—
Change procedure	—	1	—	—
Total	0	1	3	28 (24 + 4)*

*Four procedures with two interventions. (Printed with permission of Hölzenbein et al. [ref 6])

Table 8-5. Patency of 84 Vascular Access Surgical Procedures with Angioscopic Monitoring

	Primary		Revision	
	A-VF	BGF	A-VF	BGF
No. procedures	36	7	7	34
Patency (%)				
30 days	100	71.4	85.7	55.9
90 days				
Primary	91.7	57.1	85.7	38.2
Secondary	97.2	71.4	—	—

Comment

The advantages of angioscopy during access surgery are, in general, similar to those in vascular surgery and in other areas where the greatest benefit has been with vein conduit preparation,[2,10,11] monitoring technical success, [1,3,7] or intraluminal manipulations such as valvulotomy,[10] thrombectomy, or thrombolysis.[4] Our study shows that angioscopy of A-V fistulas and bridge grafts is technically feasible and can be performed with safety and with high-quality studies, even in anuric patients. With careful planning and technique, we were able to limit the irrigation fluid volume to <300 ml in primary access surgery and to about 500 ml during revision surgery.

Angioscopy provides the surgeon with additional information on the macroscopic intraoperative findings in unexposed areas of the hemodialysis fistula that otherwise would be inaccessible without surgical exploration. The angioscope is a most effective and valuable tool with which to monitor and assess the amount and localization of residual thrombus, intimal hyperplasia, or other pathological changes within the autogenous vein, anastomosis, or synthetic graft. This is particularly important in the revision surgical procedure where routine angioscopy may detect the underlying cause of graft failure and ensure the completeness of thrombectomy. Although our study is not randomized and is too small to reach clear conclusions

Table 8-6. Patency Following Correction of Abnormal Angioscopic Findings during Revision Surgery for the Failed or Failing Bridge Graft Vascular Access (n = 36)

	Corrected	Uncorrected	
No. procedures	24	9	
Patency			
30 days	18 (66.8%)	3 (33.3%)	p<0.012
90 days	10 (41.7%)	3 (33.3%)	ns

about the effectiveness of angioscopy in improving the overall patency of primary vascular access surgery, review of the results of patients undergoing revision surgery shows where the underlying problem could be identified and corrected intraoperatively. In addition, the 30-day patency improved from 33.3% to 66.6% (p=0.012, Fisher exact test, table 8-6).

It is generally believed that the commonest cause of failure of synthetic BGFs is stenosis due to intimal hyperplasia at the venous anastomosis.[12,13] In this study, however, stenosis in the midgraft at the needle puncture site of the venous or arterial limb was more frequent. We have observed the various stages of this phenomenon endoluminally with the defect in the graft caused by the needle stick, the ingrowth of a tissue "plug" and their confluence to form a midgraft stenosis. These findings are similar to the report on explanted PTFE vascular access grafts showing disrupted graft at the needle puncture sites sealed by ingrowth of fibrous tissue cork.[14] In the autogenous vein, we have noted loss of vessel wall, thinning, and aneurysmal dilation. In the BGF, the high occurrence of midgraft stenosis also leads us to suspect that in acute occlusion of the BGF, pseudointimal dissection following needle puncture at the time of dialysis may be a more common cause of acute occlusion than is generally appreciated.

Angioscopy also allows directed interventions. Unlike routine blind curettage of the midgraft as described by Puckett and Lindsay,[15] routine angioscopy allows selective curettage only when midgraft stenosis is present. Directed curettage prevents excessive removal of the pseudointima with bleeding or graft disruption and avoids the problem of leaving large intraluminal flaps, which may cause early reocclusion.

Finally, routine angioscopy for revision surgery simplifies the approach and surgical technique for failed synthetic BGFs. Exposure of the graft at its midpoint and examination of both limbs and anastomoses of the graft endoluminally is less demanding than exposing the venous anastomosis through the previous surgical incision. Accurate assessment of the adequacy of thrombectomy and precise definition of the underlying problem frequently minimizes the extent of a corrective surgical procedure.

References

1. Miller A, Stonebridge P, Jepsen S, et al. Continued experience with intraoperative angioscopy for monitoring infrainguinal bypass grafting. Surgery 1991; 109:286-293.
2. Marcaccio E, Miller A, Tannenbaum G, et al. Angioscopically directed interventions improve arm vein bypass grafts. J Vasc Surg 1993; 17:994-1004.

3. Miller A, Marcaccio E, Tannenbaum G, et al. Comparison of angioscopy and angiography for monitoring infrainguinal bypass vein grafts. J Vasc Surg 1993; 17:382-398.
4. Hölzenbein T, Miller A, Tannenbaum G, et al. Role of angioscopy in reoperation for the failing or failed infrainguinal vein bypass graft. Ann Vasc Surg 1994; 8:74-91.
5. Miller A, Marcaccio E, Goodman W, Gottlieb M. The role of angioscopy in vascular access surgery. In: Henry M, Ferguson R, eds. Vascular access for hemodialysis—III. Chicago:W.L. Gore & Associates and Precept Press, 1993.
6. Hölzenbein T, Miller A, Gottlieb M, Gupta S. The role of angioscopy in vascular access surgery. J Endovasc Surg 1994 (in press).
7. Miller A, Campbell D, Gibbons G, et al. Routine intraoperative angioscopy in lower extremity revascularization. Arch Surg 1989; 124:604-608.
8. Miller A, Jepsen S. Angioscopy in arterial surgery. In: Bergan J, Yao J, eds. Techniques in arterial surgery. Philadelphia: Saunders, 1990; 409-416.
9. Kwolek C, Miller A, Stonebridge P, et al. Safety of saline irrigation for angioscopy: results of a prospective randomized trial. Ann Vasc Surg 1992; 6:62-68.
10. Miller A, Stonebridge P, Tsoukas A, et al. Angioscopically directed valvulotomy: a new valvulotome and technique. J Vasc Surg 1991; 13(6):813-821.
11. Stonebridge P, Miller A, et al. Angioscopy of arm vein infrainguinal bypass grafts. Ann Vasc Surg 1991; 5:171-175.
12. Raju S. Grafts for hemodialysis access: techniques for insertion and management of complications. Ann Surg 1987; 206:666-673.
13. Etheredge E, Haid S, Maester M, Sicard G, Anderson C. Salvage operations for malfunctioning polytetrafluoroethylene hemodialysis access grafts. Surgery 1983; 94:464-470.
14. Delorme J, Guidoin R, Canizales S, et al. Vascular access for hemodialysis: pathologic features of surgically excised ePTFE grafts. Ann Vasc Surg 1992; 6:517-524.
15. Puckett J, Lindsay S. Midgraft curettage as a routine adjunct to salvage operations for thrombosed polytetrafluoroethylene hemodialysis grafts. Am J Surg 1988; 156:139-143.

DISCUSSION

Moderator:
Mitchell L. Henry, M.D.
Panelists:
Ralph A. Didlake, M.D.,
Alvaro Escobar, M.D.
Arnold Miller, M.D., Ch.B.

Discussant: Dr. Didlake, I want to compliment you on a very fine presentation. I, too, do most of my access procedures on an outpatient basis. What local anesthesia do you use? I cannot treat these patients under regular local anesthesia. I need sedation, and when I sedate them, I need somebody monitoring them. I would rather have somebody from the anesthesia department, but I wonder how you handle that.

Dr. Didlake: We do sedate these patients a bit. We give them Demerol and Versed, but we have a policy that all sedation is given I.M. in our outpatient unit. If we are going to do I.V. sedation, we go to the main hospital operating room and have anesthesia standing by. We are in a unique situation in that the nurses who monitor the patients in our outpatient unit are certified nephrology nurses with extensive O.R. experience. Every patient is monitored with a dynamic EKG, a pulse oximeter, and an automated blood pressure monitor. We have been very happy with I.M. Demerol and Versed, even though the anesthesiologists tell us that I.M. Versed has no real function. A significant number of our patients will sleep through at least a portion of the procedure. For local anesthetic, we use lidocaine. Obviously that is a problem if you are working in infected or inflamed tissues where pH is a problem. Also, we have noticed, if the patient has had a long interval between dialyses and may have local tissue acidosis, lidocaine frequently doesn't work. If we reach a 60-ml limit on our lidocaine dosage, we go to Marcaine, which we have found to be quite effective. It has been interesting to watch the evolution over time. Dialysis patients communicate with one another very effectively, and it has been a bit like the phenomenon of laparoscopic cholecystectomy. This has become a patient-driven thing. They are now requesting to be treated in this way.

Discussant: Do you use epinephrine in your lidocaine or your Marcaine?

Dr. Didlake: No, we have never used epinephrine in these patients.

Dr. Didlake: We also heparinize virtually everyone with about 5,000 units. And we seldom, if ever, reverse it.

Discussant: Our anesthesiologists have recently called our attention to a block that has just been described in their literature. This is a pure sensory block of the forearm in which two sites are blocked. It is a very simple block, and we have been very impressed with the extent of sensory block without any motor block. That was published within the last six months in *Anesthesia*. Dr. Escobar, regarding the subclavian vein stents, what do you tell these patients and your colleagues about subsequent subclavian puncture in those who have these stents?

Dr. Escobar: That is an absolute contraindication. Patients should not have subclavian catheters wherever their stent is placed. I do have one case in which they put a catheter across the stent and the stent thrombosed. We believe that after a subclavian stent is inserted, that vein should not be punctured percutaneously again.

The stent may be crushed and may subsequently thrombose.

Dr. Henry: Or migrate, as we heard yesterday.

Dr. Escobar: Yes, but after the stent has been in for at least five weeks, this would be unusual.

Dr. Henry: Maybe this is a new trend. We should put tattoos under the subclavian area with a big X through the words "No Stick." It would be very fashionable.

Discussant: I have performed more than 3,000 new and revision procedures, all with the patients under local anesthesia. Eighty percent of the patients were outpatients—ambulatory surgery patients—and we have not had any problems with any of them. I want to ask Dr. Miller what is the total cost of angioscopy equipment .

Dr. Miller: The cost of angioscopy equipment varies. In the old days, when we started angioscopy, nobody in the O.R. knew what a monitor or a video camera was. Now those devices are part of laparoscopic surgery and are available in the O.R. The only necessary additional equipment is the pump and an angioscope, and these are not very expensive. The costs to get started are certainly below $10,000. All you need to do is to buy the appropriate angioscope and a pump and you can be on your way.

Dr. Henry: The angioscope needs to be gas sterilized, so you can't reuse it the same day.

Dr. Miller: That is true. As scope prices are coming down, there are some disposable units that are reusable about 10 times, and there are others that can be used for about 40 times. You get good life from them once you know how to handle them. The problems occur in the beginning when people don't handle them correctly and a lot of breakage occurs. Angioscopy takes technique and requires a learning curve, so don't get frustrated in the beginning. You have to persist for a little while, but the rewards are worthwhile.

Discussant: Central lesions are a big problem. Because there is really no good surgical option, we think stents are a very good solution. The medical/legal problem of having a stent is a difficult one in terms of a future central line. We have tried telling that to patients, but that doesn't seem to work. Since many patients do not really understand what you are trying to say, we have been recommending Medic Alert bracelets to those with central vein stents. The bracelet merely says, "No central lines." The doctor who is caring for the patient can call a central national number to learn the details.

Discussant: Dr. Miller, how aggressive are you with the residual flaps that you see in the graft and around the anastomoses? How long do you persist in trying to remove those, and do you feel that doing so adds anything to the long-term patency in these grafts?

Dr. Miller: That is a good question and a very important one for angioscopy. In all endoscopy, the closer the endoscope is to the subject, the larger it looks. The farther away the scope is, the smaller the subject looks, and to truly quantitate it is extremely difficult technically. There is a certain amount of judgment to apply to what you are seeing. Some flaps look extraordinarily large if you are very close, and as you move back a little bit they look smaller. So you have to try to judge the size of the flap in terms of the diameter size of the entire vessel. We don't worry much about the smaller flap that is nonobstructive and does not obstruct the lumen. In our experience, if the flap is simple and is occluding the lumen more than 25%, we would probably try to get rid of it. If it is less than that, we would not worry too much.

Discussant: Are you using anything besides the curette to try to remove those flaps?

Dr. Miller: We have different instruments that we have been playing with, but there is really nothing available that is good. One of the problems with all the available instruments is that they are forward biting, or cutting, or grabbing, and when you put an angioscope behind them you are basically obscuring what you are doing. We have not found any really good solution yet, but there are some in the making.

SECTION IV

9

EARLY USE OF THE GORE-TEX STRETCH GRAFT

Ingemar J. A. Dawidson, M.D., Ph.D., Aamer Ar'Rajab, M.D., Ph.D., L. Denise Melone, R.N., Timothy Poole, P.A., Dorothy Griffin, R.N., and Richard Risser, M.S.

THE GORE-TEX STRETCH VASCULAR GRAFT (W.L. Gore & Associates, Inc., Flagstaff, Arizona) is the latest addition in PTFE grafts used for hemodialysis. The new or added properties of this graft include its ability to stretch longitudinally. There is no lateral or radial distensibility. It also has some memory, and once fully stretched, the graft retracts somewhat.

The present study expands our previous preliminary report[1] of the overall outcome with the 4–7-mm Tapered GORE-TEX Stretch Vascular Graft for hemodialysis access. A second objective of the present study was to evaluate the feasibility of early graft cannulation.

Material and Methods

Between January 1, 1991, and December 31, 1993, 303 GORE-TEX Stretch 4–7-mm Tapered Vascular Grafts were placed. Thirty-three of the patients were lost to follow-up. This report, therefore, comprises 270 consecutive patients with the graft placed for the first time in the forearm loop configuration. The GORE-TEX Stretch Vascular Graft was used in all cases when a PTFE graft placement was indicated without exclusions. This study, therefore, contains some technically challenging surgical procedures. The graft was always placed in a loop formation in the forearm with both arterial and venous anastomoses in the antecubital fossa. The venous anastomosis was performed first and anastomosed to a superficial antecubital vein, usually the cephalic vein, in 81%, and to the deep concomitant vein in 19%. The arterial anastomosis was to the brachial artery in 40%, at the brachial/radial confluence in 36%, and to the proximal radial artery in 24%. Before the anastomosis was performed, the graft was pulled through the subcutaneous tunnel using a 6-mm, 25-cm long dilator in a two-step fashion exiting at one counter skin incision at the apex of the loop. This procedure creates a fairly tight tunnel, minimizing postoperative bleeding and swelling. No systemic heparinization was used; however, veins and arteries were locally flushed with heparinized saline. Both venous and arterial anastomoses were performed in a running fashion using permanent suture material (GORE-TEX Suture CV6, Needle TT-9).

When indicated, the grafts were used for hemodialysis within 14 days after placement. The lack of other access for hemodialysis was the usual indication in our early experience. Later, the indications were expanded to include patients needing dialysis rather than placing a dual-lumen percutaneous subclavian catheter, and this was the case in 96 cases (36%). Of these, 78 (82%) were cannulated within seven days and 21 (22%) within 48 hours. Accordingly, 174 patients (64%) were cannulated beyond 14 days postsurgery.

Statistical Methods

Survival estimates were derived using the Kaplan-Meier technique, and comparison of survival curves for early and late cannulation groups were made using the log rank test. Proportional hazards regression was also used to define the comparisons assessing differences over time. Demographic comparisons of the early and late cannulation groups were made with respect to sex using the chi-square test, with respect to race with the 2x4 Fisher exact test, and with respect to age using the Student's 2-sample *t*-test. Early and late cannulation groups were also compared for the incidence of thrombosis within one month and after one month of cannulation, for failures caused by infection and thrombosis, and for infection rates (early, late, and overall) using the Fisher exact test.

Results

The patient demographics for the 96 patients with early cannulation and the 174 patients with late cannulation, as well as the entire patient population, are shown in table 9-1. The two groups did not differ significantly in sex ($p=0.196$) or race ($p=0.905$). The relatively large proportion of minority patients accurately reflects the inner-city Parkland Memorial Hospital (Dallas, Texas) patient population. The early and late cannulation groups do differ in mean age ($p=0.002$), however, with the early cannulation group younger on average than the late cannulation group.

Graft survival, i.e., functional grafts, was significantly greater in the late cannulation group, estimated at 93%, 92% and 91% at one, two, and three years, respectively. In contrast, one-, two-, and three-year graft survival in the early

Table 9-1. Patient Demographics (Age, Sex, Race) in Comparison Study of Early versus Late Cannulation.

		Time of cannulation		Overall
		< 14 days	> 14 days	
N		96	174	270
Age (years ± SD)		45 (13)	52 (15)	50 (15) 6 – 89
Sex M/F (%)		49/51	41/59	44/56
Race (%)	Black	66	64	64
	White	16	19	18
	Latin	16	14	15
	Oriental	3	3	3
Minorities (%)		85	81	82

cannulation group was 80%, 78%, and 73%, respectively (p=0.0008) (figure 9-1A). Similarly, survival of grafts free from thrombosis formation was significantly higher in the late cannulation group, with 83%, 80%, and 75% versus 67%, 50%, and 40% for early cannulation at one, two and three years, respectively (p=0.0002) (figure 9-1B).

The overall patient survival was 96%, 93%, and 92% at one, two, and three years, respectively, with no difference among the groups. The overall graft survival at one year (89%) was essentially unchanged at two and three years (88% and 86%, respectively). Seventy-seven percent of the grafts were clot-free at one year, 72% at two years, and 64% at three years (figure 9-2).

The incidence of thrombosis within one month after cannulation was similar for early and late cannulation—6.3% and 6.9%, respectively (p=1.0). Beyond one month after cannulation, however, early cannulation was associated with a significantly higher incidence of thromboses for the entire follow-up period (p<0.001) (figure 9-3). Overall, of the 96 early cannulated grafts, 37 (39%) have thrombosed versus 37/174 (21%) of the late cannulated grafts (p<0.01) (table 9-2). Of the thrombosed grafts, the rate of successful declotting was similar for the two groups, or 86% and 84% for early and late cannulated grafts, respectively, with a 14% and 16% failure rate, respectively, requiring new grafts. Repeat declotting was required in 44% and 42% for early and late cannulation, respectively, with a higher failure rate than that for first-time declotting—57% and 46%, respectively.

The overall failure rate was 20/96 (21%) for early cannulation versus 14/174 (8%) for late cannulation (p=0.004). Failures caused by infection in the early cannulation group (7/96, 7%), were significantly greater than in the late cannulation group (2/174, 1%) (p<0.011). Failures caused by thrombosis were more common with early cannulation (13/96, 14%) than late cannulation (12/174, 7%), but the difference is not statistically significant (p=0.082).

Infections, although more common in the early cannulation group, also tended to occur later. Only 1/96 (1%) and 2/174 (1.1%) of the early and late cannulation groups, respectively, had infections within 30 days. Late infections, especially after two and three months, were more common with early cannulation (10.4%) compared to late cannulation (1.1%, p<0.001) (figure 9-4).

Hematoma, bleeding, and swelling associated with first-time cannulation for dialysis occurred in six (6%) cases in the early cannulation group versus one

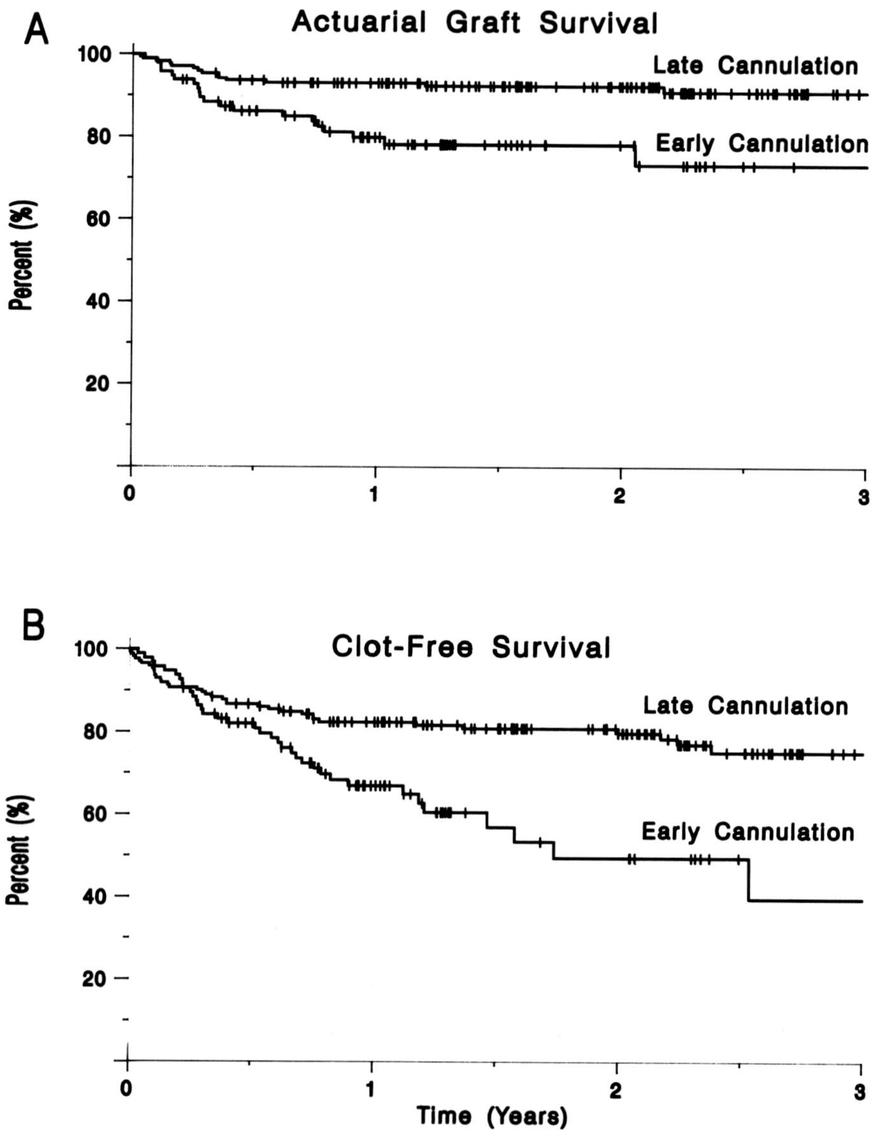

Figure 9-1. Actuarial one-, two-, and three-year graft survival (or secondary patency rate) (A) and clot-free survival (B) for 96 GORE-TEX Stretch Vascular Grafts cannulized <14 days (early cannulation) and for 174 grafts with cannulation >14 days (late cannulation) after placement.

(0.6%) in the late cannulation group ($p<0.05$) (table 9-3). No grafts failed or required surgical intervention for these complications.

Early cannulation has increased over time in the present study. In 1991 and 1992, only 23.4% of our patients were cannulated within 14 days, compared to 55.7% in 1993. This trend matches the change in indications from lack of any other access for hemodialysis to cannulation of any patient in need of dialysis, rather than inserting dual-lumen subclavian catheters. Our overall result

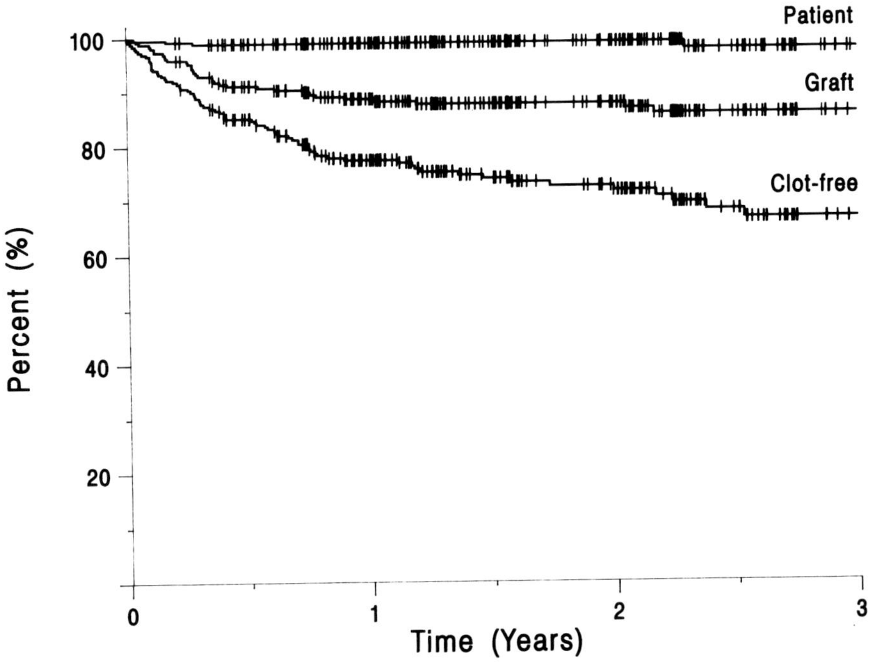

Figure 9-2. Overall actuarial patient, graft, and clot-free survival for one, two, and three years in 270 patients after placement of the GORE-TEX stretch graft.

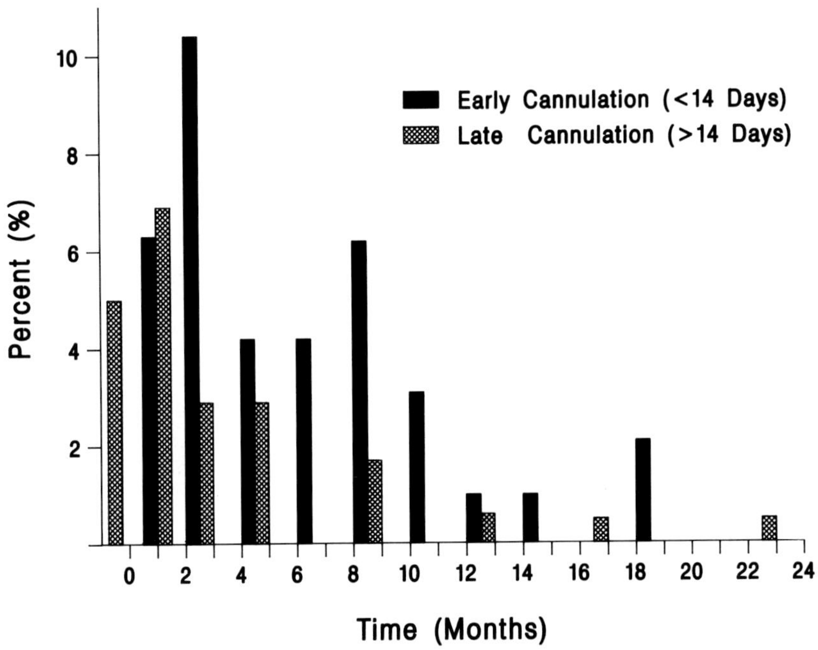

Figure 9-3. Percentage of graft thrombosis up to 24 months after placement for 96 grafts with early cannulation versus 174 grafts cannulized > 14 days after placement.

Table 9-2. Incidence of First and Repeat Graft Thrombosis and Failure Rate in 270 Patients, 96 of Them Cannulated within 14 Days

	Time of cannulation < 14 days	> 14 days	All patients
	N = 96	N = 174	N = 270
Thrombosed	37 (39%)	37 (21%)	74 (27%)
Declotted	32 (86%)	31 (84%)	63 (85%)
Failed	5 (14%)	6 (16%)	11 (15%)
Repeat declotting	14 (44%)	13 (42%)	27 (43%)
Failed	8 (57%)	6 (46%)	14 (52%)
Overall failure	20 (21%)	14 (8%)	34 (13%)
Thrombosed	13 (14%)	12 (7%)	25 (9%)
Infection	7 (7%)	2 (1%)	9 (3%)

Table 9-3. Bleeding Complications for 270 Patients, 96 of Them Cannulized within 14 Days

Type of Complication	< 14 days N = 96	> 14 days N = 174	270
Hematoma	1 (1%)	1 (0.6%)	1
Bleeding	2 (2%)	0	0
Swelling	3 (3%)	0	0
Total	6 (6%)	1 (0.6%)	0.4

indicates that early cannulation is related to poorer clot-free survival; accordingly, we anticipated poorer results in 1993 compared to 1991-92 in graft survival and clot-free survival. Using proportional hazards regression analysis, we have found, however, that there is a marginally significant interaction (p=0.082) between year and timing of cannulation for clot-free survival. This test indicates that the risk of early cannulation on clot-free survival is not equivalent in 1993 compared to the earlier grafts. In fact, in 1993, there was no significant difference in graft survival (p=0.26) or clot-free survival (p=0.77), whereas 1991-92 graft survival and clot-free survival both differ significantly (p<0.001) when early and late cannulation groups are compared.

The results from this analysis are in part due to shorter available follow-up for 1993 patients. The one-year survival data, however, depict the disparity in a direction counter to the general results. For 1991-92, early cannulation had 47% one-year clot-free survival compared to 82% for late cannulation. For 1993, however, comparable clot-free survival was 86% for early and 85% for late cannulation. Graft survival estimates follow this pattern, albeit without statistical significance. We had 75% graft survival with early cannulation in 1991-92 versus 93% with late cannulation, but in 1993, there was 83% graft survival in early cannulation compared to 93% with late cannulation.

Table 9-4 outlines dialysis staff opinions about the stretch graft versus the regular PTFE grafts in terms of the ease of locating the graft, the ease of cannulation, and

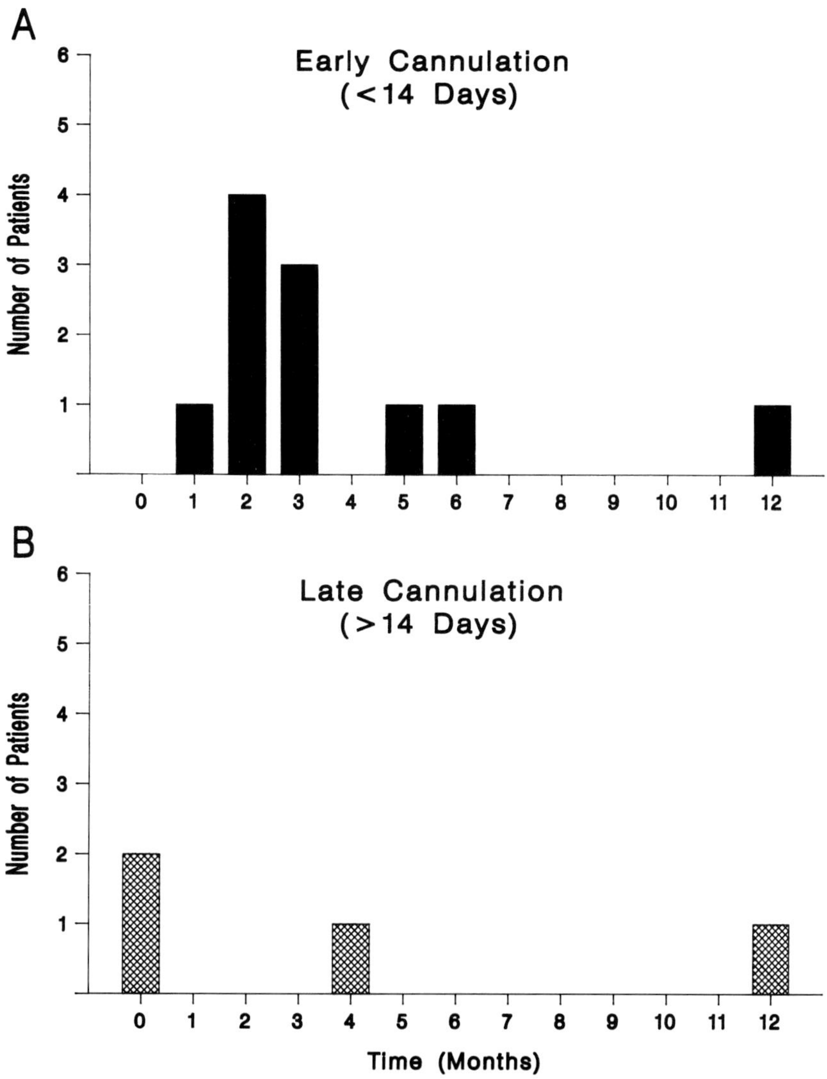

Figure 9-4. The incidence of infection was 11% (11/96) for early cannulation (A) versus 2.2% (4/174) when the cannulation was beyond 14 days after graft placement (B).

overall comparison. About 75% of dialysis unit staff members felt that the stretch graft had advantages over the regular PTFE grafts.

Discussion

The GORE-TEX Stretch Vascular Graft may represent an improvement over regular expanded PTFE grafts.[1,2] First, the intraoperative conformity seems to be better,

Table 9-4. Dialysis Staff Rating of Stretch Graft versus Regular PTFE Graft.

	Easier (%)	No difference (%)	Worse (%)
Locating graft	73	23	0
Cannulation	75	22	3
Overall	75	24	1

and by allowing early cannulation, the risks with dual-lumen catheters can be avoided.[3,4] The overall graft survival of 88% and 86% at two and three years equals or exceeds the best results reported in the literature with regular PTFE grafts.[5,6] Most published reports indicate graft survival in the 50-60% range at two years.[7-13]

Early use of the stretch graft was associated with significantly poorer outcomes. The incidence of graft thrombosis and infections with early cannulation occurred late or during the entire three-year follow-up period. In fact, within 30 days of use, the clotting and infection rates were identical for the two groups. Therefore, factors other than the early use of the graft seem to be responsible for late clotting and graft failure. The early cannulation group represents a selected patient population more likely to be in acute need of hemodialysis. In fact, the indication for using the graft early was a lack of other means of hemodialysis. In many cases, the graft was used in an urgent need for hemodialysis in a patient who had exhausted all access sites. These and other negative factors may affect long-term function of the graft. These aspects are currently being explored and will be reported later. The mortality rate in the 270 analyzed patients is surprisingly low, comparing favorably with the reported end-stage renal disease mortality rate in the United States of about 20% annually.[14]

The ability to safely cannulate grafts early may be related to the graft material[1] and surgical and dialysis techniques.[15,16] Factors that have been implicated in successful early use of the regular PTFE grafts is creation of a tight-fit subcutaneous tunnel.[14,15] Also, in the present study, gentle compression of the puncture sites for 20-30 minutes essentially eliminated hematoma formation after early cannulation.

References

1. Dawidson I, Melone D. Preliminary experience with a new PTFE graft for vascular access. In: Henry ML, Ferguson RM, eds. Vascular access for hemodialysis—III. Chicago: W.L. Gore & Associates, Inc., and Precept Press, 1992; 10:133-136.
2. Simoni E, Jain K, Munn J. Use of 6 mm stretch PTFE grafts for early use in hemodialysis. In: Henry ML, Ferguson RM, eds. Vascular access for hemodialysis—III. Chicago: W.L. Gore & Associates, Inc., and Precept Press, 1992; 11:142-145.
3. Parsa H, Freeman H. Precautions for long-term maintenance of central venous catheters: pt I. Surg Rounds 1992 (Nov); 967-974.
4. Parsa H, Freeman H. Precautions for long-term maintenance of central venous catheters: pt II. Surg Rounds 1992 (Dec); 1013-1017.
5. Palder SB, Kirkman RL, Whittemore AD, et al. Vascular access for hemodialysis. Ann Surg 1985; 202(2):235-239.
6. Puckett J, Lindsay S: Midgraft curettage as a routine adjunct to salvage operation for thrombosed polytetrafluoroethylene hemodialysis access grafts. Am J Surg 1988; 156:139-143.

7. Anderson CB, Sicard GA, Etheredge EE. Primary and secondary operations for vascular access. In: Bergan J, Yao J, eds. Evaluation and treatment of upper and lower extremities. New York: Grune and Stratton, 1983; chap 16.
8. Munda R, First R, Alexander J, et al. Polytetrafluoroethylene graft survival in hemodialysis. JAMA 1983; 249(2):219-222.
9. Rendi K, Prenner K. The redo-surgery of expanded polytetrafluoroethylene (PTFE) arteriovenous fistulas for hemodialysis. Vasc Surg 1984; 18(5):261.
10. Kherlakian G, Rodersheimer L, Arbaugh J, et al. Comparison of autogenous fistula versus expended polytetrafluoroethylene graft fistula for angioaccess in hemodialysis. Am J Surg 1986; 152:238-243.
11. Tellis V, Kohlberg W, Bhat D, et al. Expanded polytetrafluoroethylene graft fistula for chronic hemodialysis. Ann Surg 1979; 189:101-105.
12. Rizzuti R, Hale J, Burkart T. Extended patency of expanded polytetrafluoroethylene grafts for vascular access using optimal configuration and revisions. Surg Gynecol Obstet 1988; 166: 23-27.
13. Tordoir J, Herman J, Kwan T, et al. Long-term follow-up of the polytetrafluoroethylene (PTFE) prosthesis as an arteriovenous fistula for haemodialysis. Eur J Vasc Surg 1987; 2:3-7.
14. U.S. Renal Data Systems. 1993 annual data report. Washington, D.C.: Dept. Health & Human Services, 1993.
15. Haag B, Paramesh V, Roberts T, Taber T. Early use of polytetrafluoroethylene grafts for hemodialysis access.
16. Taucher L. Immediate, safe hemodialysis into arteriovenous fistulas created with a new tunneler: An 11 year experience. Am J Surg 1985; (150):212-215.

10

EXOTIC VASCULAR ACCESS

Richard C. Anderson, M.D., and
James R. DeBord, M.D.

KOLFF AND ASSOCIATES FIRST DEMONSTRATED a practical dialyzer for hemodialysis in 1944,[1] but lack of angio-access prevented its application as a therapeutic modality for reversible renal failure for two decades. In 1960, an internist, a surgeon, and an engineer finally developed the Scribner shunt, which permitted initial temporary hemodialysis for renal failure patients.[2] By far the greatest advancement in angio-access occurred in 1966 with the advent of the Brescia-Cimino primary arteriovenous fistula.[3]

The ultimate current treatment for chronic renal failure is kidney transplant surgery. While awaiting a transplant, or while on life-long hemodialysis, patients with renal failure will inevitably require declotting or revision of their angio-access grafts or fistulas. When an adequate superficial vein is not available for a primary arteriovenous (A-V) fistula, a bridged A-V fistula must be constructed. In most patients, expanded polytetrafluoroethylene (ePTFE) prostheses are recommended for the bridge graft A-V fistula. The placement of these conduits is conventionally in the upper extremities, preferably in the forearm and secondarily in the upper arm. When venous outflow obstruction and/or graft infection preclude the use of the upper extremities, even for revisions, surgeons are forced to turn to exotic vascular access.

The exotic vascular access procedures are limited only by the imagination of the vascular surgeon and the availability of adequate arterial inflow and venous outflow. The purpose of this paper is to review the surgical literature on creative and exotic, or unusual, vascular access techniques used to extend the hemodialysis life of patients with chronic renal failure and failed upper extremity dialysis grafts or fistulas.

Transposed Basilic Vein–Brachial Artery Fistula

Failure of the distal forearm venous collaterals to provide adequate cannulation sites or flow rates for dialysis following a primary radial-cephalic A-V fistula often leads directly to prosthetic bridge ePTFE A-V fistula construction in the ipsilateral

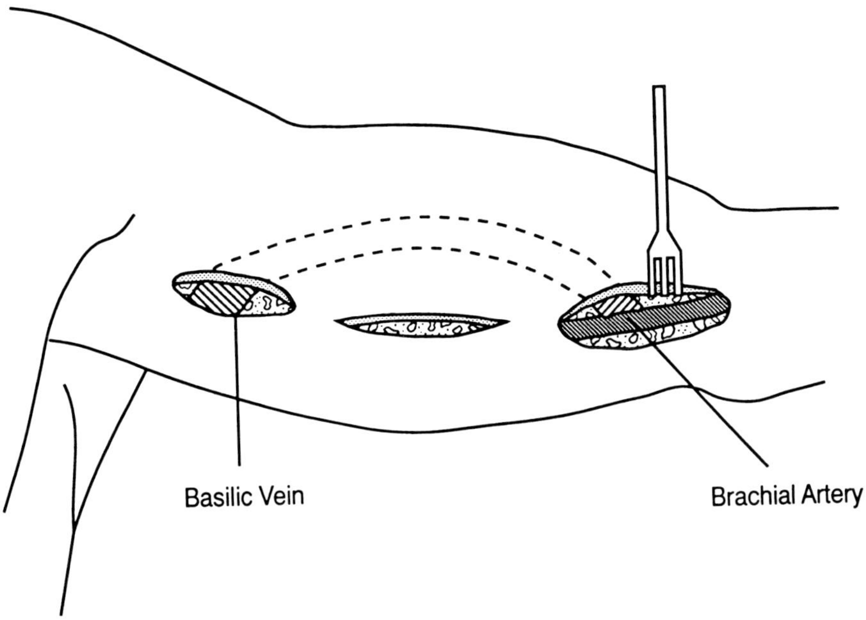

Figure 10-1. Transposed basilic vein–brachial artery fistula.

upper extremity. The basilic vein is often an undamaged vein that can be used for autologous angio-access because it is left protected in the medial upper extremity from repeated venipuncture and cannulation. This procedure, originally described by Cascardo et al. in 1970[4] and updated by reports from Dagher et al. in 1976,[5] LoGerfo et al. in 1978,[6] Hatjibaloglous et al. in 1992,[7] and Rivers et al. in 1992,[8] is an often overlooked but viable autologous fistula, requiring only one surgical anastomosis and providing adequate hemodialysis access.

The vein is mobilized from a longitudinal incision in the medial upper arm and divided distally at or near the elbow. The vein is "transposed" above the fascia to an accessible position under the skin where it can be easily felt by the dialysis technician for cannulation. The vein may be left in the medial arm or transposed into a more lateral position for easier and possibly more comfortable dialysis access (figure 10-1). Flow rates will easily support hemodialysis and will equal or exceed several hundred milliliters of blood per minute. One-year cumulative patency rates of 60-80% have been reported, with a 30-month cumulative patency rate of 49% reported by Rivers et al.[8]

The usual complications of vein stenosis—pseudoaneurysm formation and steal phenomenon—do occur and are manageable by standard techniques. However, when these autologous fistulas thrombose, they are difficult to thrombectomize compared to prosthetic EPTFE grafts, and patency postthrombectomy is decreased. Infectious complications are lower with autologous tissue versus prosthetic grafts, and the lack of a veno-venous surgical anastomosis is thought to be of benefit in the prolonged patency of this type of A-V fistula. Thus, when superficial vein failure

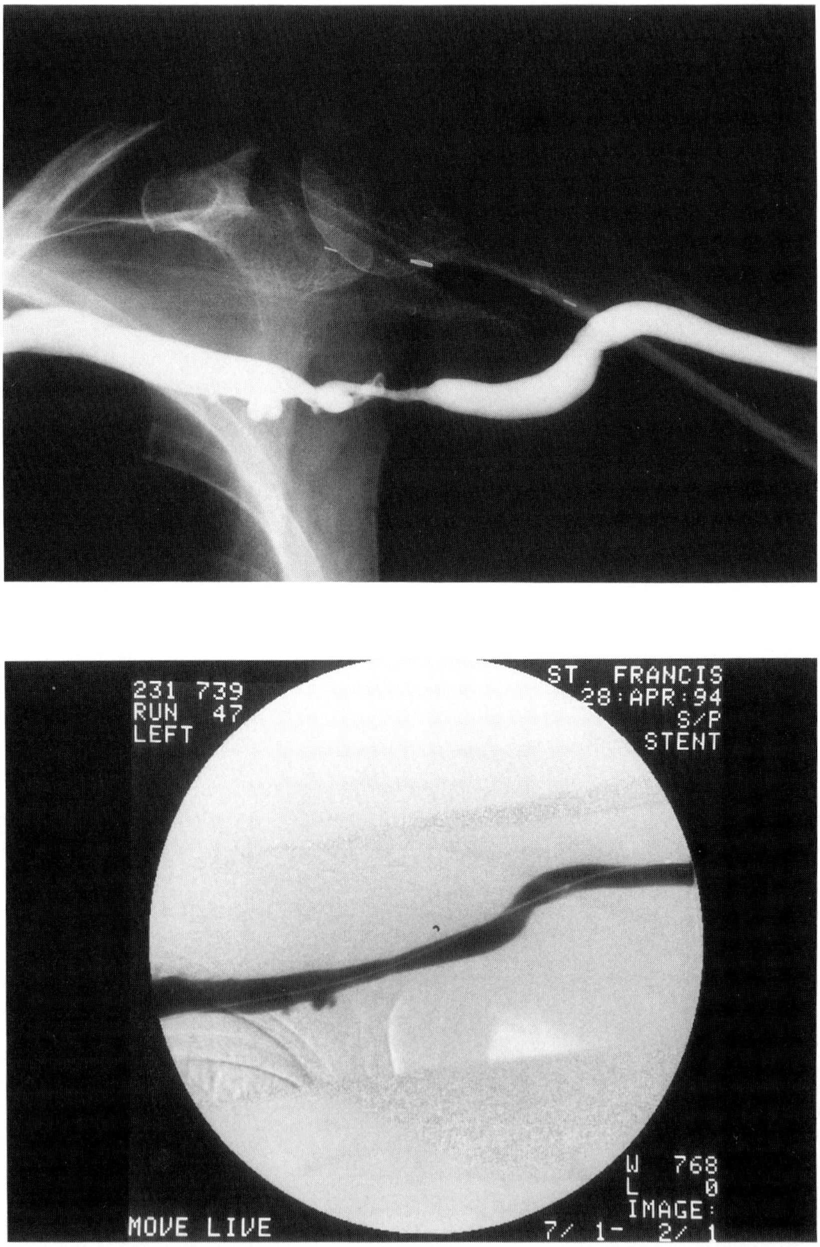

Figure 10-2. Balloon angioplasty—stent of subclavian vein stenosis. Top: before; bottom: after.

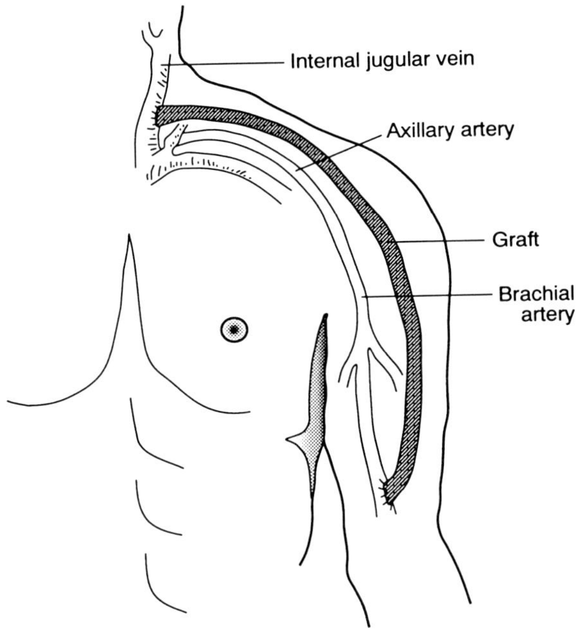

Figure 10-3A. Brachiojugular A-V graft.

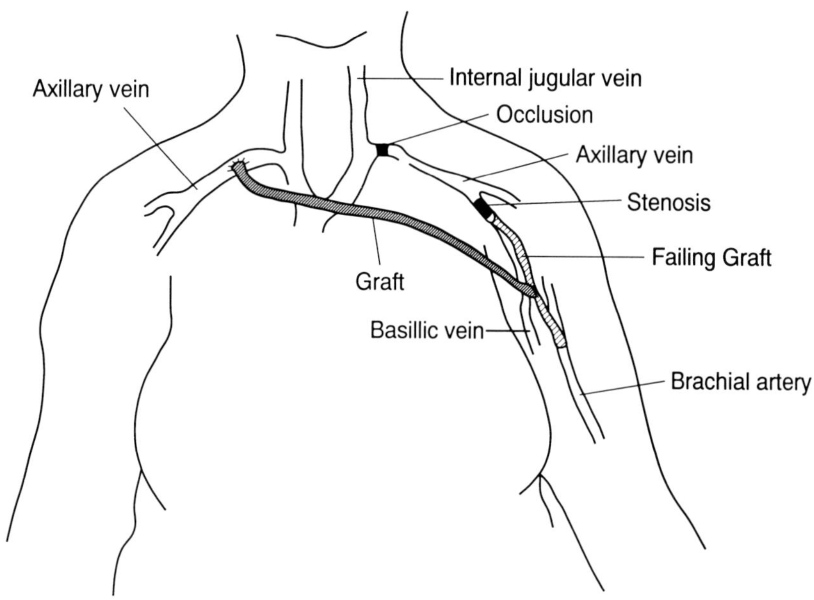

Figure: 10-3B. Brachiocontralateral axillary A-V graft.

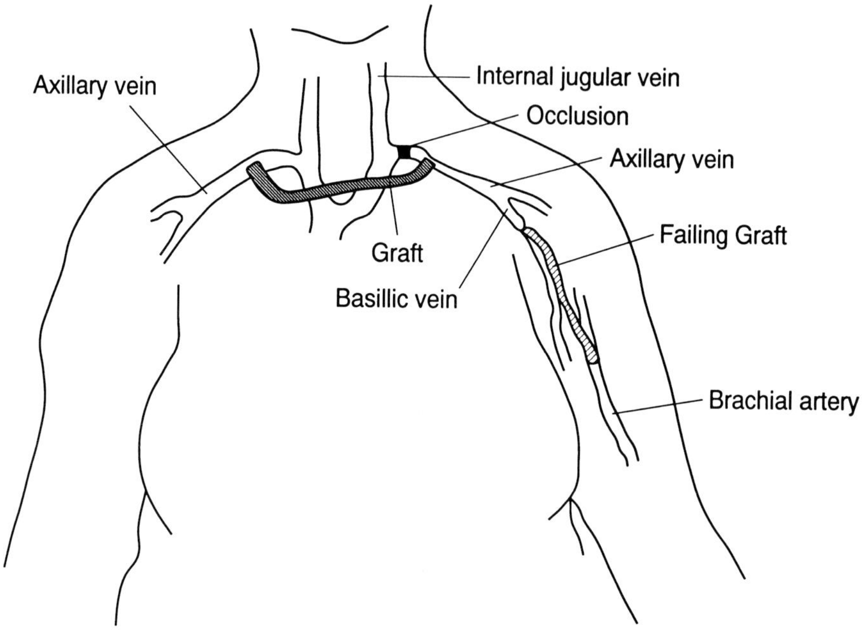

Figure 10-3C. Axillary-axillary venous graft to overcome proximal left subclavian vein stenosis.

will not permit a primary Brescia-Cimino A-V fistula, or results in its failure, use of the transposed basilic vein-brachial A-V fistula should be considered prior to constructing a prosthetic bridge A-V fistula. The use of this autologous fistula does not appear to compromise the later use of an ipsilateral prosthetic dialysis graft.

Brachiojugular and Brachiocontralateral Axillary A-V Grafts

The major and ultimate reason for failure of upper extremity angio-access is stenosis or occlusion of the ipsilateral axillary-subclavian vein with resultant venous hypertension and graft thrombosis. Direct repair of high axillary venous stenosis by patch angioplasty or medial extension of the venous anastomosis is sometimes possible, but proximal exposure is often problematic. Interventional radiological techniques using balloon angioplasty and stent placement can salvage otherwise functional grafts or fistulas in many of these patients (figure 10-2). When further interventional techniques are unsuccessful, exotic access grafting may be required. Patients with adequate arterial inflow are candidates for extension of their graft to the ipsilateral internal jugular vein as described by Haimov in 1982[9] or to the contralateral axillary or jugular vein.

Polo et al. have described their experience with ePTFE brachiojugular bridge grafts[10] (we refer the reader to this article for further review). In 1992, Jain and Simoni described their experience with two patients having significant arm swelling due to subclavian vein

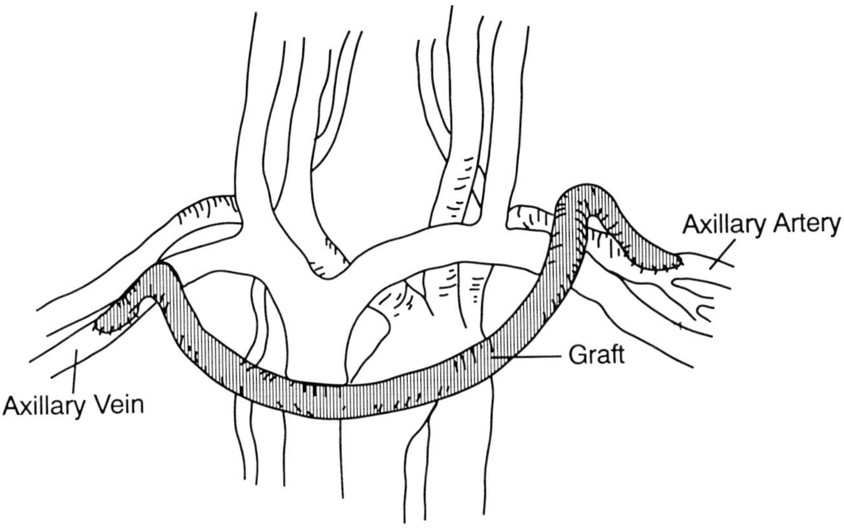

Figure 10-4A. Axillary-axillary A-V bridge fistula (cross-chest).

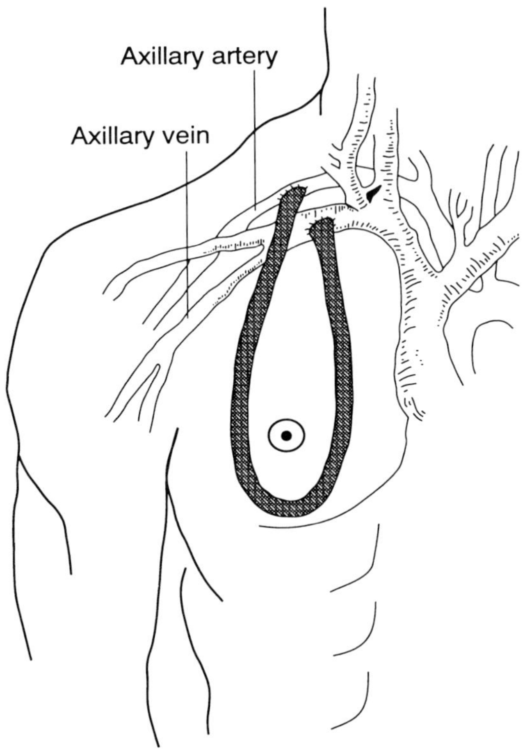

Figure 10-4B. Axillary-axillary A-V bridge fistula (ipsilateral loop).

occlusion who were managed either by extending the brachiobasilic graft to the contralateral axillary vein or by a direct ipsilateral-to-contralateral axillary-vein-to-axillary-vein graft interposition to overcome the proximal subclavian vein obstruction (figure 10-3).[11] Both patients experienced relief of their venous hypertension symptoms and achieved long-term functional salvage of their dialysis grafts. Proximal subclavian stenosis or occlusion is not an uncommon complication of indwelling venous catheters, whether for dialysis or simple I.V. access. Currently, with the frequent use of subclavian dialysis catheters for initial angio-access, we may see more and more proximal subclavian vein obstruction in the future. Familiarity with these direct and simple, though unconventional, graft extension routes to the jugular and opposite axillary vein will allow the vascular access surgeon to salvage these otherwise unusable A-V grafts.

Axillary-Axillary A-V Graft

When infection or inadequate arterial or venous anatomy precludes using the upper extremity at all for dialysis access, then extra-anatomic routes for ePTFE bridge A-V fistulas must be used. Axillary-axillary arterial bypass grafts for extra-anatomic vascular reconstruction of aortic arch disease is well established. A similar A-V ePTFE graft provides a relatively easy route for a subcutaneous large-diameter (6–8-mm) A-V fistula for hemodialysis. The graft may go from the left axillary artery to the right axillary vein or vice-versa, depending on surgeon/patient preference or on existing anatomic factors. The axillary artery and vein are easily located through bilateral infraclavicular incisions laterally that may be performed easily under local anesthesia with I.V. sedation. The clavicular and sternal heads of the pectoralis major muscle are separated bluntly, and the pectoralis minor insertion is transected at the coracoid process exposing the neurovascular bundle. With added local anesthetic and a bolus of I.V. sedation, a subcutaneous tunnel is developed between the two incisions and the graft is passed from one to the other across the anterior chest wall. End-to-side arterial and venous-to-graft anastomoses are then created with monofilament suture (figure 10-4). Garcia-Rinaldi and Von Koch described this technique in 1978 using a bovine carotid heterograft, but ePTFE is presently the preferred conduit.[12] This procedure has the following advantages: (1) technical ease of construction (for surgeon and patient); (2) the graft lies in a gentle curve and not in a loop; (3) the size of the vessels permits a larger graft (8 mm) than can be used in the forearm location; and (4) the graft is in a position that makes cannulation easy for the dialysis technician. Disadvantages include the need to use the thin-walled axillary vein and the fact that the graft is located across the upper anterior chest wall, which may produce an unwanted cosmetic result. Results reported by Garcia-Rinaldi and Von Koch showed 10/10 grafts patent up to 18 months with excellent flow for hemodialysis. The axillary-axillary A-V graft may also be positioned on one side of the chest as a loop graft, as described by Haimov.[9]

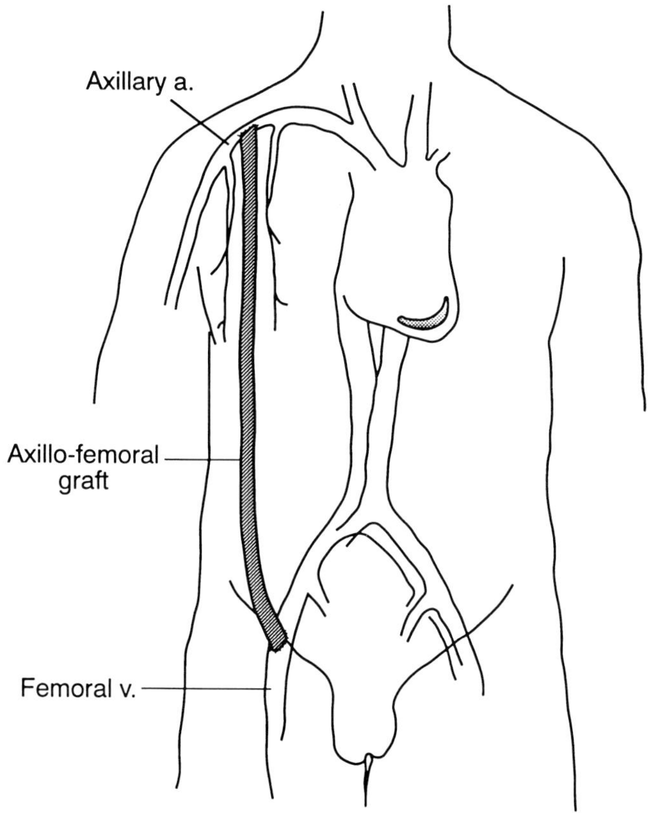

Figure 10-5. Axillary-femoral A-V bridge fistula.

Axillary-Femoral and Femoral-Axillary A-V Grafts

When the axillary-subclavian veins bilaterally are not adequate for the venous anastomosis of an A-V graft, alternate venous outflow must be sought. The axillary-femoral route, commonly applied in vascular reconstructive surgery, may also be used for A-V bridge fistulas for hemodialysis. The appropriate axillary artery (usually the right, in view of the propensity for left subclavian stenosis) is mobilized as described earlier for an axillary-axillary graft. The ipsilateral common femoral vein is isolated and mobilized via a groin incision, and a 6- or 8-mm ePTFE graft is tunneled between the two wounds in an identical fashion as for an axillary-femoral bypass graft (figure 10-5). The procedure may be done under general anesthesia or local anesthesia with I.V. sedation. While axillary-femoral arterial grafts are often externally supported along the chest-abdominal wall portion of the graft, this is neither necessary nor desirable for an A-V graft, since the external support rings would interfere with cannulation of the graft and the high flow rates would make compression thrombosis less likely. The longer length (50-60 cm) of these grafts makes graft deterioration from frequent needle puncture at the same site less likely. To avoid infection, cannulation close to the axilla or groin should be avoided, since these areas are more likely to be contaminated. In the reversed setting of axillary artery stenosis and adequate lower extremity inflow with patent axillary-subclavian veins, a

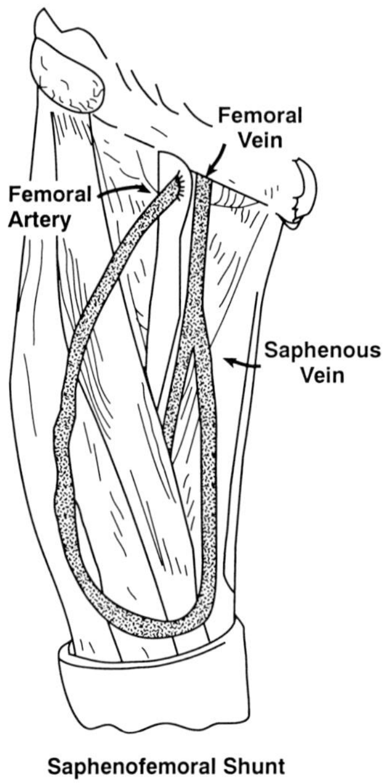

Figure 10-6. Loop sapheno-femoral shunt.

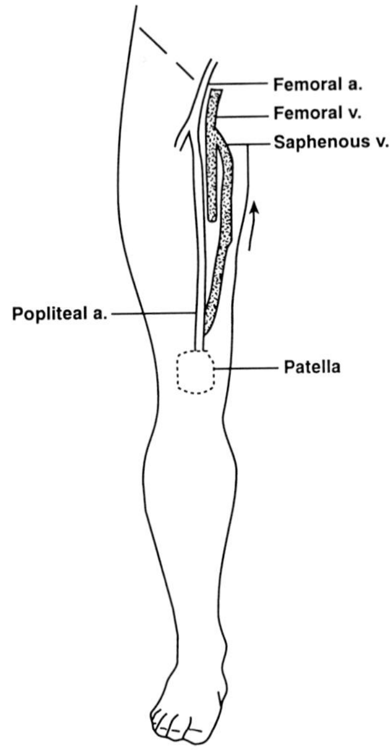

Figure 10-7. Straight popliteal-saphenous shunt.

femoral-axillary A-V graft may be placed with flow going in the opposite direction. Dialysis function should be just as adequate. In 1991, Rueckmann et al. reported on seven patients who received an axillo-femoral A-V graft. Six of seven grafts functioned well for dialysis, with flow rates of 300-1,700 cc/min, and one graft thrombosed to hypotension in a patient who expired.[13] Patients did not have unusual complaints related to these unconventional dialysis grafts, and in most cases the pain and edema associated with their subclavian vein stenosis resolved after dialysis access was changed to the axillary-femoral graft.

Femoral-Femoral A-V Grafts

The groin is clearly not a preferred site for angio-access grafts due to increased infection as well as patient discomfort and inconvenience. In extreme cases of upper extremity vascular or infectious complications, a loop thigh ePTFE or saphenous vein A-V graft may be constructed. A crossover femoral-femoral A-V graft may be designed that is analogous to a femoral-femoral bypass graft but more superficially placed for ease of cannulation. The techniques of placing these grafts are standard ones similar to loop or bridge grafts in the upper extremity. The same basic principles of vascular access surgery apply to all angio-access graft insertions. The use of the saphenous vein from the upper leg as a dialysis conduit in the thigh was popularized in the early 1970s either as a loop saphenofemoral shunt as described in 1972 by Firlit and Canning[14] (figure 10-6) or as a straight popliteal-saphenous graft as reported in 1974 by Blakeley[15] (figure 10-7). Both techniques involve transposing the arterialized saphenous vein to a more superficial location to facilitate use of the graft by the dialysis staff. While sporadic good results with autologous saphenous vein grafts for hemodialysis have been noted, the modern consensus is that due to stricture, pseudoaneurysm formation, and thrombosis, as well as the preferential preservation of the saphenous vein for peripheral and coronary revascularization, this autologous conduit is not recommended for hemodialysis access either in the leg or in the upper extremity as a bridge graft A-V fistula. When other options will not suffice, it is acceptable to use the lower extremity for ePTFE bridge or loop A-V grafts (figure 10-8). These lower extremity graft A-V grafts may originate from the common femoral artery, the superficial femoral artery, the popliteal artery above the knee, or from the deep femoral artery (profunda femoris artery) and drain into either the common femoral vein or the proximal saphenous vein.

External-Carotid-to-External-Jugular Primary A-V Fistulas

The most common sites of primary A-V fistula construction for hemodialysis access are the radial-cephalic fistula at the wrist or in the anatomical snuff box, the antecubital fistula, the brachiocephalic fistula, the brachiobasilic fistula, and the ulnar-basilic fistula (figure 10-9). Exotic primary fistula construction is limited by the need for an accessible, maturable venous bed and the greater propensity for proximal A-V fistulas using larger vessels to create a vascular steal. Shepherd et al. in 1973 described several cervical A-V fistulas using the external carotid artery or any of its larger named branches (4 mm or larger) to anastomose directly end-to-end with the external jugular vein[16] (figure 10-10). Their reported fistula function was good, but often the short length of the arterialized vein makes it preferable to use the fistula for arterial inflow only and to provide venous return via an adequate peripheral vein. No episodes of cardiovascular or cerebrovascular events have been reported, but a minor annoyance reported by patients is the low-intensity bruit that becomes noticeable when the patient lies on the side of the fistula. This exotic primary A-V fistula was conceived before the advent and popularity of ePTFE grafts for effective bridge A-V shunts, and its use has likely been preempted by the ready availability of more suitable forms of access even in the most complicated cases.

'Needleless' Access

In the early 1980s, two exotic devices were highly touted to improve angio-access. The Hemasite vascular access device (Renal Systems, Inc., Minneapolis, Minnesota) and the DiaTAP button (American Bentley, Irvine, California) both constructed of "space age" materials designed to resist infection and thrombosis, served as needleless angio-access devices secured to the vascular tree by an implantable ePTFE graft. Despite initial appearances of modest success, these devices succumbed to infection and other complications and are no longer available for use. The needleless approach to dialysis was warmly embraced by patients, but the success rate has not permitted continued use.

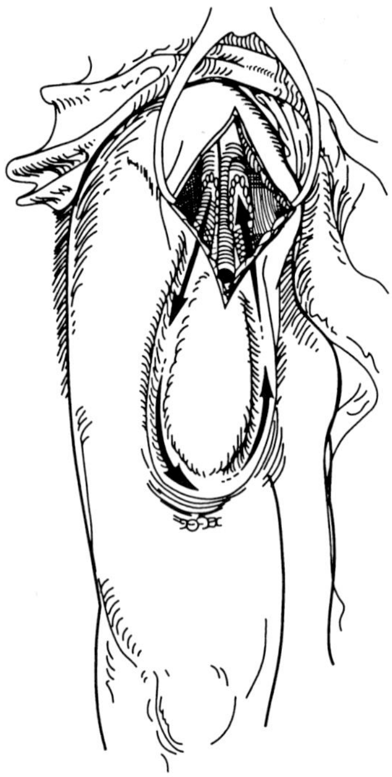

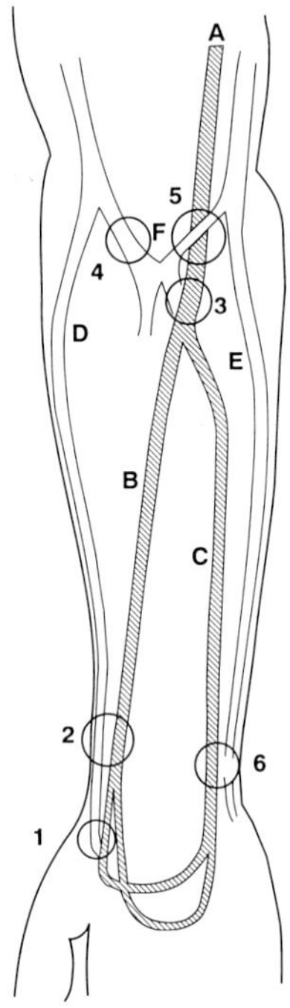

Figure 10-8. Prosthetic loop A-V graft in groin (above left).

Figure 10-9. Common sites of primary A-V fistulas (above right). 1 = snuff-box fistula; 2 = radiocephalic fistula; 3 = antecubital fistula; 4 = brachiocephalic fistula; 5 = brachiobasilic fistula; 6 = ulnarbasilic fistula; A = brachial artery; B = radial artery; C = ulnar artery; D = cephalic vein; E = basilic vein; F = cubital vein.

Stretch Grafts

Resolution of the problems of infection, thrombosis, and intimal hyperplasia continues to elude vascular access surgeons and provides fertile ground for continued research. These problems are as devastating to the renal failure patient with failed angio-access as they are to the vascular surgery patient with a failed bypass graft. Some early evidence exists that the new stretch ePTFE grafts have improved compliance and therefore have less propensity toward intimal hyperplasia. Research into decreasing the thrombogenicity of ePTFE grafts is ongoing, with studies using carbon bonding as well as antibiotic impregnation of prosthetic grafts to reduce infection.

Conclusion

Patients are being successfully maintained on hemodialysis for longer time periods, and providing access will continue to challenge the vascular access surgeon.

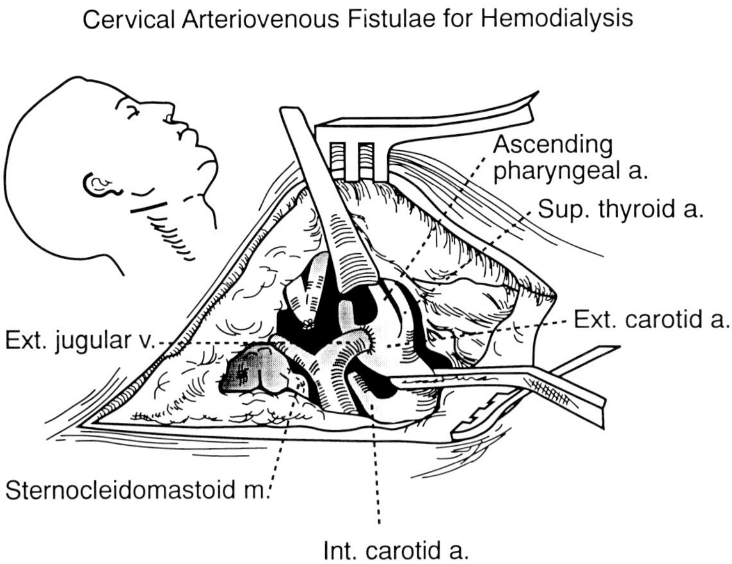

Figure 10-10. External carotid–external jugular primary A-V fistula.

A primary Brescia-Cimino A-V fistula at the wrist remains the initial procedure of choice for angio-access for hemodialysis. A more proximal brachiocephalic level fistula should be considered next or a transposed basilic-brachial fistula constructed to maximize autologous angio-access. A prosthetic bridge A-V graft of ePTFE in the nondominant forearm or upper arm is the next level of dialysis access to consider. Only after failure at this level of access does one proceed to the level of exotic vascular access. Exotic vascular access is limited only by the imagination of the surgeon and the anatomical restrictions of the patient.

References

1. Kolff WJ, Berk HTJ, ter-Welle M, van der Leg JW, Van Dijk EC, van Nordwijk J. The artificial kidney: a dialyzer with a great area. Acta Med Scand 1944; 117:121-134.
2. Quinton W, Dillard D, Scribner BH. Cannulation of blood vessels for prolonged hemodialysis. Trans Am Soc Artif Intern Organs 1960; 6:104-113.
3. Brescia MJ, Cimino JE, Appel K, Hurwich BJ. Chronic hemodialysis using venipuncture and a surgically created arteriovenous fistula. New Engl J Med 1966; 275:1089-1092.
4. Cascardo S, Acchiardo S, Beven EG, Popowniak K, Nakamoto S. Proximal arteriovenous fistulae for hemodialysis when radial arteries are not available. Proc Eur Dial Transplant Assoc Eur Ren Assoc 1970; 7:42-46.
5. Dagher F, Gelber R, Ramos E, Sadler J. The use of basilic vein and brachial artery as an A-V fistula for long term hemodialysis. J Surg Res 1976; 20:373-376.
6. LoGerfo FW, Menzoian JO, Kumaki DJ, Idelson BA. Transposed basilic vein-brachial arteriovenous fistula: a reliable secondary access procedure. Arch Surg 1978; 113:1008-1010.

7. Hatjibaloglous A, Grekas D, Saratzis N, et al. Transposed basilic vein-brachial arteriovenous fistula: An alternative vascular access for hemodialysis. Artif Organs 1992; 16:623-625.
8. Rivers SP, Scher LA, Sheehan E, Lynn R, Veith FJ. Basilic vein transposition: an underused autologous alternative to prosthetic dialysis angioaccess. J Vasc Surg 1993; 18:391-397.
9. Haimov M. Vascular access for hemodialysis—New modifications for the difficult patient. Surgery 1982; 92:109-110.
10. Polo JR, Sanabia J, Calleja J. Brachiojugular ePTFE grafts for dialysis (abstr). Symp on dialysis access IV, May 5-6, 1994. Orlando, Fla.
11. Jain KM, Simoni EJ. Cross-over bypass to axillary vein in hemodialysis patients. Eur J Vasc Surg 1992; 6:101-103.
12. Garcia-Rinaldi R, Von Koch L. The axillary artery to axillary vein bovine graft for circulatory access. Am J Surg 1978; 135:265-268.
13. Rueckmann I, Ouriel K, Berry C, Hoffart N. The synthetic axillofemoral graft for hemodialysis access. ANNA Journal 1991; 18(6):567-571.
14. Firlit C, Canning J. Saphenofemoral shunt—its application in long term hemodialysis. Arch Surg 1972; 104:854-855.
15. Blakeley W. Current surgical management of fistulae for dialysis: Methods and improvisations. Am Surg 1974; 40:168-171.
16. Shepherd RL, Ing TS, Magalhaes R, Economou SG. Cervical arteriovenous fistulae for maintenance hemodialysis. Nephron 1973; 11:7-11.

11

HEMODIALYSIS: A NURSING PERSPECTIVE

Deborah Joan Brouwer, R.N., C.N.N.

TO ACHIEVE ANY LONG-TERM SOLUTION TO THE ISSUES associated with vascular access, the team approach must be expanded beyond the current standards for end-stage renal disease (ESRD). This expansion must include the patient, nursing staff, nephrologist, radiologist, and the vascular access surgeon. A team-approach quality assurance tool is needed that can be implemented to track vascular access procedures and associated complications. Also needed is a vascular access surveillance protocol to maintain patency.

Once the vascular access surgeon has successfully created an arteriovenous (A-V) fistula, or implanted a polytetrafluoroethylene (PTFE) graft, the dialysis staff must correctly care for the access. A typical hemodialysis patient has two dialysis needles inserted per treatment, with three treatments per week. For each year on dialysis, the patient undergoes 312 needle cannulations. A typical dialysis nurse cares for four patients at a time, with a minimum of two patient shifts per day. In a typical workweek, a dialysis nurse will perform 64 needle cannulations, and in one year, 1,248. Needle cannulation experience increases quickly as a dialysis nurse is trained and completes one year of work, but experience does not equal expertise. Improperly performed needle cannulations can easily lead to access complications and/or failure. If access surgeons are familiar with the principles of correct cannulation techniques, they can work with the dialysis units to ensure that correct principles are taught to all dialysis staff.

Before a graft can be correctly cannulated, the direction of the arterial blood flow must be clearly determined and documented. If a graft has been implanted too deeply, it may be difficult to locate and determine the direction of blood flow. When a graft for hemodialysis has needles placed incorrectly, the percentage of recirculation can be greatly increased. A patient who undergoes long-term dialysis with incorrect needle placement in relation to arterial blood flow direction may show signs and symptoms of uremia secondary to poor urea clearance. Dialysis-associated pericarditis, pericardial effusion, or pericardial tamponade are some of the severe complications of uremia that might occur through the simple error of not determining

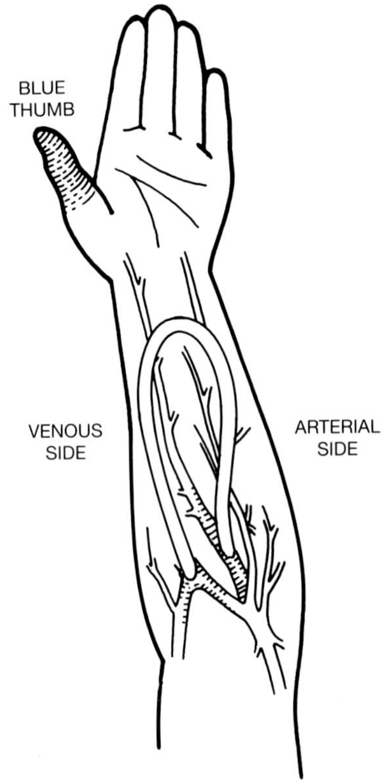

Figure 11-1. Regular graft, or "blue thumb."

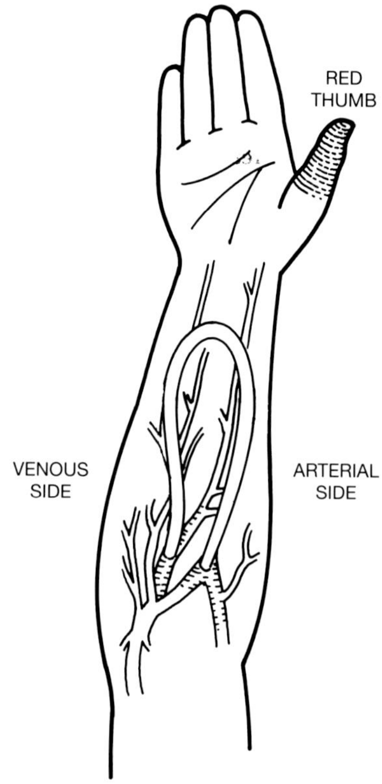

Figure 11-2. Reverse graft, or "red thumb."

arterial blood flow direction within a PTFE graft. These types of dialysis-associated complications can be avoided with good communication among the access surgeon, nephrologist, and dialysis nursing staff. Accurate operative reports should include a description of the arterial-to-venous blood flow direction. The terms to describe the direction of blood flow include "regular" or "reverse." Most PTFE grafts have the arterial inflow on the medial limb of the graft and the venous outflow on the lateral limb. This description of a regular graft implantation may also be referred to as a "blue thumb," due to the venous outflow limb on the same side as the thumb (figures 11-1 and 11-2).

Illustrating graft blood flow direction in the operating room progress note or drawing it on the graft manufacturer illustration can prevent any confusion in distinguishing the direction of blood flow within a patient's access. Several simple evaluation techniques can be used to determine blood flow direction in a PTFE graft. Prior to graft cannulation, apply pressure to the middle of the graft using two fingers to briefly occlude the blood flow. Palpate both sides of the graft to feel for the stronger pulse of the arterial side. A stethoscope may also be used to listen for the bruit on the arterial limb of the graft. Another technique is to cannulate the graft with two dialysis needles and briefly occlude the midsection of the graft, watching for a flash of blood within the needle lumen. The side with the stronger flash is the arterial inflow limb. Often, when a newly inserted PTFE graft is used, the residual operative edema does not permit sufficient pressure to be applied to the graft, thereby preventing a noticeable difference in the

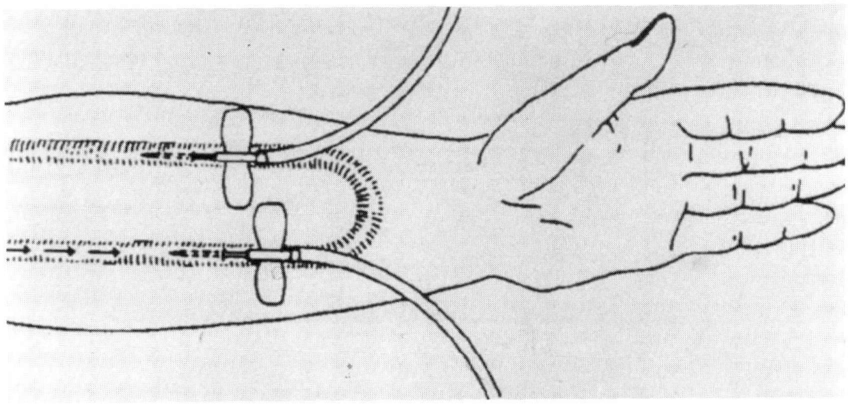

Figure 11-3. Direction of blood flow determines needle placement.

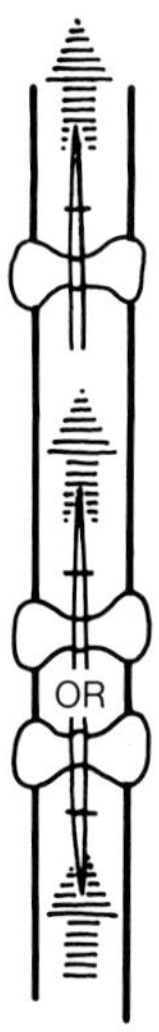

Figure 11-4. The arterial needle may be cannulated in either blood flow direction. The venous needle must always be cannulated with the bevel pointing in the direction of venous blood flow.

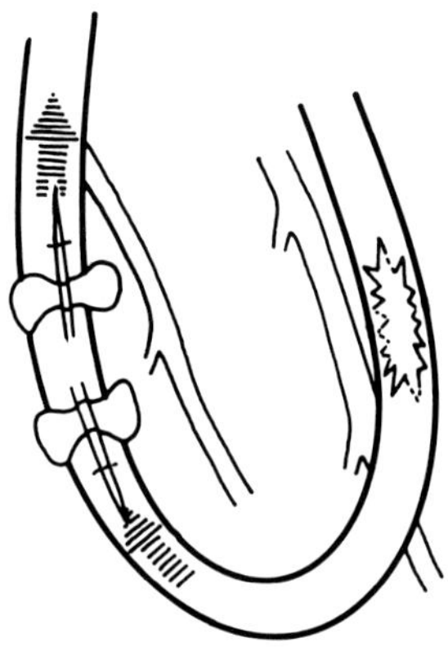

Figure 11-5. Needle placement if only one portion of the graft can be used for cannulation.

flash, bruit, or thrill. In that case, flow may be checked after the dialysis procedure has been initiated and the blood pump is running at 200 ml/ min. The midgraft is briefly compressed at a location between the two needles and the arterial pressure and venous pressure are monitored. In a regular graft, with the dialysis lines connected in the usual manner, the venous pressure will decrease when the midgraft is compressed. If the graft is reversed and the dialysis lines are connected in the usual manner, the arterial

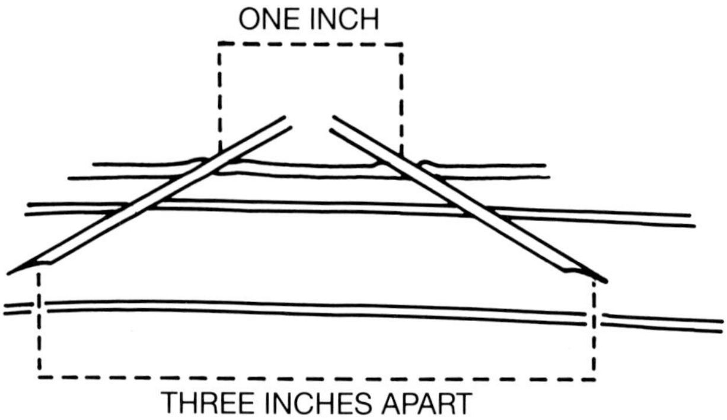

Figure 11-6. Correct minimum needle distances to prevent recirculation.

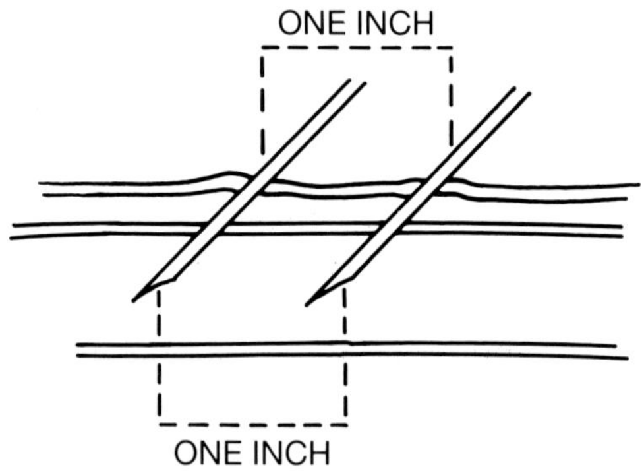

Figure 11-7. Incorrect needle distance, with the needles too close.

pressure will decrease to a more negative number and the venous pressure will increase. To confirm the clinical findings, recirculation studies can be performed with the dialysis lines connected both regular and reverse. The lower recirculation rate will indicate the correct direction of flow.

Needle placement and direction always depends on the direction of blood flow. The venous needle must always be cannulated with the bevel pointing in the direction of venous blood flow. The arterial needle placement may vary. In both PTFE grafts or A-V fistulas, the arterial needle may be cannulated in either flow direction (figures 11-3 and 11-4). The needles should be placed as far apart as possible to prevent recirculation. The minimum distance apart should be 1.5-2 inches[1]. If only one portion of the graft can be used for cannulation, needles placed in opposite directions permit the most effective use of limited space and decrease the risk of recirculation. This method places the needle bevels as far apart as possible. If both needles are placed toward each other, the possibility of the needle bevels touching, or lying less than an inch apart, is too great, and recirculation could be unnecessarily increased (figures 11-5, 11-6 and 11-7).

Cannulation procedures vary between units and even between nurses within the same unit. Familiarity with the basic principles of correct needle cannulation is necessary; these principles should be part of cannulation policies and procedures in

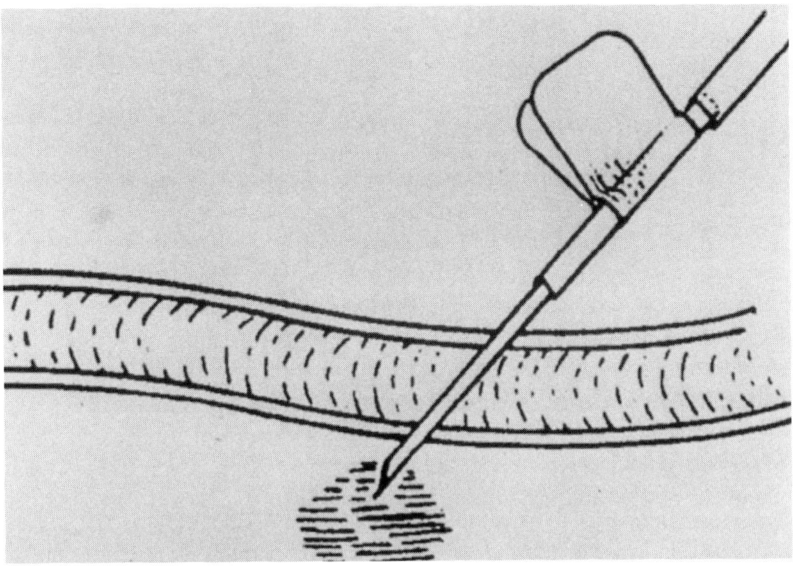

Figure 11-8. Needle advanced without 180-degree rotation, causing a back-wall infiltration.

every dialysis unit. The goal of correct needle cannulation is to prevent complications that can lead to graft infection, thrombosis, or failure. Before any dialysis access is cannulated, measures to control infection must be followed. Patients should be instructed in the importance of preventing infection and should actively participate in their own care. All patients should be taught to scrub the skin over their access site with antibacterial soap and water prior to dialysis. Patients unable to wash their own access limb should be assisted by the dialysis staff. Washing the area with a cloth using an antibacterial soap, or ready-to-use towel or prep, is mandatory.

Prior to cannulation, the sites should be assessed, palpated, selected, and prepped, using a topical antiseptic such as Betadine. It should be remembered that Betadine is truly effective only in the dry state, whereas alcohol is effective only in the liquid state.[2] The patient must be instructed not to touch the skin once it has been prepared for cannulation. Dialysis staff must strictly adhere to universal precautions, using gloves to protect both themselves and the patient from infection as well as from transmissible diseases.[1] As part of ongoing quality assurance monitoring, all infections occurring in dialysis patients should be tracked. Access-related infections can then be identified and common links found. Reeducation of patients and dialysis staff should be used to decrease the access infection rates if a break in the proper cannulation prep procedures is found to be linked to the infection[1,3]

Technique

Correct needle insertion into the access site will prevent a serious complication of back wall or posterior wall infiltration. All cannulation procedures should include the following principles:

45° Needle Insertion Angle. 1. Observation of a blood flashback. 2. 180° rotation of the needle bevel. 3. Leveling out of the angle and advancement of the needle up to the needle hub (figure 11-8).

The rotation of the needle bevel during cannulation reduces the risk of advancing the needle into the back wall; if the back wall is punctured, a hematoma readily forms. Should this occur prior to heparinization, the needle should be removed and digital pressure applied followed by the application of ice. It is extremely difficult to reach the back wall puncture by digital pressure, and bleeding into the surrounding tissue can be excessive, leading to a large hematoma. This hematoma formation can progress to compression of the graft lumen and thrombosis. A hematoma site can also lead to graft infection or abscess formation in the tissue surrounding the graft. Both thrombosis and infection can cause graft failure.

I once cared for a patient who had two separate episodes of back wall infiltration. During the first episode, the patient had an upper-arm graft. The back wall was punctured during the venous needle insertion. I was asked to assist the staff member cannulating the graft and found that bleeding from the puncture site was rapidly forming a large hematoma. The needle was removed, digital pressure held until the bleeding stopped, and ice applied. The hematoma was so large that no further cannulation could be attempted. The patient underwent hemodialysis that day via a temporary femoral catheter. When he returned for the next dialysis session, his graft was found to be thrombosed. He underwent a thrombectomy and revision with a patch repair of the back wall puncture. The revision was successful, and the graft continued to be used for dialysis. Six months later, this access failed and could not be salvaged. Another graft was placed in the neck and upper chest area between the brachial artery and internal jugular vein. The back wall of this graft was punctured with a needle during cannulation, and a massive hematoma formed. The patient was admitted to the hospital due to uncontrolled bleeding. During this admission, the patient suffered many other setbacks. I believe that these back wall punctures occurred because the needle was not rotated 180° during cannulation.

Needle Puncture-Site Rotation. Site rotation is essential to PTFE graft survival. Repeated needle punctures in the same site cause "one-site-itis" and lead to pseudoaneurysm formation. A bedside illustration of the patient's graft on which cannulation sites are tracked could help prevent "one-site-itis"[1,3] (figure 11-9).

Needle Removal. Postdialysis needle removal is very important in prevention of hematomas. The dialysis needle must be carefully removed from the needle track, following the angle used for insertion. Minimal digital pressure should be applied to the needle exit site during needle removal, thus preventing trauma to the graft lumen or surrounding tissues by the needle's cutting edge. After complete removal of the needle, adequate digital pressure must be applied to the needle skin exit site, as well as the graft lumen exit site[1] (figure 11-10). If the skin exit site clots but the graft wall has not, bleeding into the tissue between the graft and skin can occur. A hematoma can rapidly form, causing compression of the graft lumen. Caution must be taken when using topical clotting agents that may not reach the graft wall. The amount of digital pressure needed to achieve hemostasis varies from patient to patient, but should not occlude the graft lumen, or graft thrombosis can occur. Patient education is essential to ensure that patients are competent to hold "their own patches." If any patient is found to be unable to correctly hold his own needle site, family members may be asked to assist. The last possible solution should be the use of arm

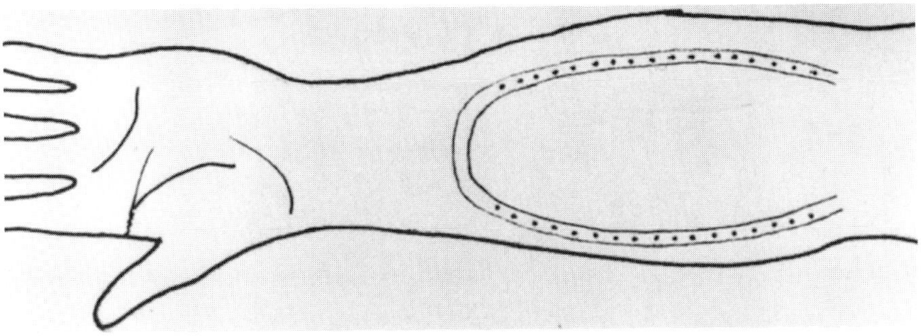

Figure 11-9. Bedside illustration to chart rotation of needle cannulation sites.

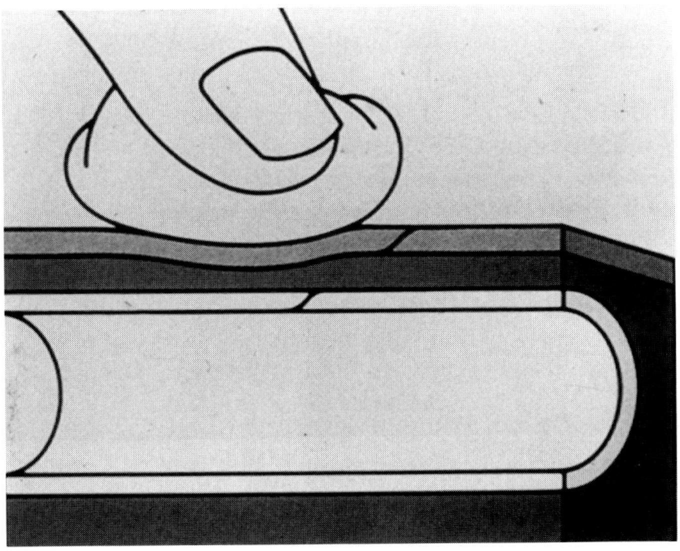

Figure 11-10. Proper digital pressure placement for post needle removal to ensure clotting of both the skin and graft needle exit site.

clamps. These are undesirable because they make it difficult to carefully adjust and monitor the pressure applied to the needle site, thus increasing the possibility of graft occlusion and thrombosis.[1]

Pressure should be held constant for 10 to 15 minutes before checking the needle site for bleeding. Bleeding should not be considered excessive until digital pressure has been applied for more than 20 minutes per needle site.

Patients should be informed of the time the needles are removed, and this time should be documented on the patient's chart to help monitor problems with prolonged bleeding. Hemostasis must be fully achieved before posttreatment dressings or adhesive bandages are applied to the access. The bandage must not occlude the access flow, and the presence of a bruit and thrill must be confirmed and documented before the patient leaves the dialysis unit. Patients and their care-givers must be instructed to check the patient's access for the presence of a bruit and thrill every morning and afternoon. Written instructions on whom to notify if there is a change or absence in the bruit or thrill must be included on all access education material. A patent access is every dialysis patient's life.

Adequate Blood Flow

The definition of adequate blood flow has greatly changed over the past 10 years. In the early 1980s, the standard practice was to slowly increase the patient's blood flow rate over the first 10 minutes of dialysis. Dialysis was initiated with the blood flow at 50-100 ml/min and increased to a maximum of 250 ml/min. Elderly or cardiac-compromised patients ran at 200 ml/min, because higher flow rates were believed to cause congestive heart failure. By the mid-1980s, high flux or high-efficiency dialysis meant blood flow rates were increased to 300 or 500 ml/min in order to achieve adequate clearances of the waste products across the larger dialyzer over a shorter time.[1] The vascular access blood flow must be able to support the 300-500 ml/min required by the dialysis blood pump. Low flow within the access is not usually seen in PTFE grafts, but is a common problem with catheters and poorly developed A-V fistulas. Hemodialysis machines equipped with a prepump arterial pressure gauge monitor the pressure in the dialysis blood circuit between the blood pump and the patient's fistula needle. Once the blood pump is started, the arterial pressure will be between 0 and −300. At arterial pressures of >-260, erythrocyte damage or hemolysis can occur. This is due to the excessive negative pressure or vacuum exerted on the blood cells by the blood pump when the access cannot meet the supply of blood demanded by the blood pump.[1,4]

If the hemodialysis machine is not equipped with a prepump arterial monitor, the only sign of excessive negative pressure will be arterial pillow or blood line collapse or "line sucking." If poor flow access continues at a high negative pressure without the nurse knowing, the line collapse may progress into secondary degassing, when visible air bubbles or segments will appear in the arterial line. The air is gas released from the patient's blood under excessive negative pressure. Prepump arterial monitoring can prevent excessive negative pressure. A limit of -200 should be used to prevent any risk of hemolysis. A dialysis access is considered nonfunctional if it cannot support a blood flow of 200 ml/min with an arterial pressure ≥ −200. The cause of the low flow must be investigated and corrected, or a new access must be established. Following is a sample of venous and prepump arterial pressures with the arterial pressure reflecting flows through various accesses. A one-day sample of first-hour dialysis pressures in 30 patients is reported below.

	Average Blood Flow ml/min	*Average Arterial Pressure mm Hg*	*Average Venous Pressure mm Hg*
Graft	321	188	223
Fistula	274	194	156
Permacath	263	203	141
Tesio catheter	230	197	122

Fistulas, Permacaths (Quinton, Seattle, Washington), and Tesio (Medcomp) catheters all reach maximum arterial pressure at a much lower blood flow rate than would be needed to reach the maximum venous pressure of 250 mm Hg. Without monitoring the prepump arterial pressure and relying only on venous pressure measurement, an excessive negative pressure within the arterial segment of the blood circuit could occur and potentially cause hemolysis. PTFE grafts usually hit the maximum venous pressure limit of 250 mm Hg before the arterial pressure limit is reached or exceeded. If a PTFE graft reaches maximum –200 arterial pressure at a low blood flow, such as 250 ml/min, an arterial inflow problem should be suspected.

Adequacy of Dialysis

Urea kinetic modeling is a tool used to determine the adequacy of the hemodialysis therapy. Kt/V is the mathematical calculation used to determine the removal of blood urea nitrogen (BUN). The Kt/V is based on the midweek, posthemodialysis BUN levels. The value can be calculated using different formulas and often is determined using a computerized program. The Kt/V value should be a minimum of 1.0. Any patient with a Kt/V of <1.0 must have all possible causes for poor urea clearance investigated, including the vascular access. Patients with Kt/V values of ≥ 1.2 have a lower morbidity and mortality rate than patients with Kt/V values of ≤ 1.0.[5]

Another tool commonly used to measure adequacy of dialysis is the urea reduction rate (URR). The percentage of urea reduction should be above 60%. URR value is easy to calculate using the following formula:

$$\frac{\text{pre BUN} - \text{post BUN}}{\text{pre BUN}} \text{ X } 100 = \text{URR}$$

ESRD networks are government-sponsored organizations that oversee the provision of end-stage renal disease therapy. The network develops and implements patient outcome guidelines and has chosen the adequacy of hemodialysis delivered to ESRD patients as a goal. The network can enforce criteria that facilities must follow. If a patient's Kt/V or URR values do not meet the network's set criteria, then a thorough investigation with corrective actions must be taken. Factors that affect measurement of adequacy of dialysis are related to length of dialysis time, blood flow or liters of blood processed during dialysis, and dialysis clearance. The role of vascular access in dialysis adequacy is related to blood flow rate. The higher the blood flow rate, the better the clearance due to the greater number of liters of blood that pass through the dialyzer. If the patient's access cannot support a blood flow rate of 200 ml/min, the patient will not achieve adequate clearance during a standard four-hour dialysis treatment. The percent of recirculation within the access also limits clearance. Any access with a high recirculation rate will reflect a poor clearance value. In the past, adequacy of dialysis was not monitored closely on all patients; therefore, a problem vascular access was not readily identified and aggressively treated. Changes in a patient's Kt/V or URR can be used as a marker for identifying a failing vascular access. Any patient with a Kt/V of <1.0 or URR of

<60% should be evaluated. If any corrective actions, such as a fistulogram with angioplasty are taken, the pre- and postintervention Kt/V or URR values can be compared. An improvement in the values should be achieved if the vascular access is the cause of the poor clearance values.

Catheters

The hemodialysis catheter is both a blessing and a curse for the patient and dialysis nurse. A properly functioning catheter allows for immediate access for acute hemodialysis and is a great lifesaver for the patient. If the catheter is functioning poorly, it creates discomfort and distress for both the patient and nurse. If access to the central circulation is difficult, several needle advancements before achieving vein cannulation can cause an increase in complications. Dialysis patients cannot afford trauma to the subclavian vein that may lead to stenosis and subsequent failure of a permanent access. To protect dialysis patients from the many possible complications of catheter insertion, only properly trained physicians should perform hemodialysis catheter insertion.[6]

One way to overcome the difficulty of subclavian catheter insertion is to employ the internal jugular approach using ultrasound-guided cannulation. One recent study by Denys et al. showed an ultrasound-guided cannulation success rate of 100% with an average of 1.4 insertions.[7] This technique has a success rate of 88% with an average of 2.5 attempts. The ultrasound-guided internal jugular approach can mean less discomfort for the patient, as well as fewer complications. Long-term complications such as vein stenosis are reported to be 10% for the internal jugular and 50% for the subclavian vein.[8,9] The purchase price of a portable ultrasound device would be recovered if only one patient was protected from an accidental pneumothorax requiring emergency treatment and transfer to a critical care unit.

The major problem with all catheters, temporary or permanent, is poor blood flow. To provide adequate dialysis, the catheter must be able to support blood flow of at least 200 ml/min, with a prepump arterial pressure of –200 or less. Blood flow rates of < 200 ml/min will not provide adequate clearances and will be reflected by poor Kt/V or URR values. Blood return with a syringe cannot determine if the catheter is able to support a blood flow rate of 200 ml/min. Research is needed to evaluate what occurs when attempts are made to use catheters at a higher blood flow rate than they can support. Perhaps damage to the vessel wall occurs when prolonged negative pressure from the blood pump causes the catheter to "suck" against the vessel wall. The trauma to the vessel wall may lead to the development of intimal hyperplasia and result in a stenosis. Dialysis units should monitor prepump arterial pressures to maintain catheters at blood flow rates that produce arterial pressures of ≤-200. Catheters used without arterial pressure monitoring must not be run at blood flow rates that produce prolonged periods of line collapse or line "sucking."

All catheters may be troubled by poor blood flow rates or thrombosis. One commonly used treatment is the infusion of a fibrinolytic activator. Urokinase (UK) is useful in clearing a clotted or poorly functioning catheter. If a catheter requires multiple injections of UK, i.e., every treatment or once a week, the catheter should be considered nonfunctional. For permanent catheters, investigations using contrast under fluoroscopy often show a fibrin sheath or tail formation that may have caused the malfunction.[10] The catheter may be successfully treated with UK to restore patency.

Correct catheter placement can prevent thrombosis or fibrin formation. Permanent catheters should be placed into the right atrium, not at the junction of the superior vena cava/right atrium. The lumen orientation should follow manufacturer recommendations to avoid the catheter tip from "sucking" against the arterial wall. Proper tip and lumen orientation also prevents the arterial and venous lumens from being reversed, thereby increasing the percentage of recirculation and decreasing the deficiency of the treatment.[11] Permanent catheters should be inserted under fluoroscopy to ensure proper placement. Many interventional radiologists are actively placing permanent hemodialysis catheters using percutaneous techniques under fluoroscopy. The interventional radiologist can play a key role in solving catheter access problems with imaging techniques. The catheter placement can be immediately verified and required corrections made before the procedure is completed.[12] Operating room timetables may not be as flexible due to their tight schedules and limited availability of fluoroscopy.

A correctly placed catheter that has frequent episodes of clotting should have the posthemodialysis flushing procedure reviewed. All catheters must be flushed adequately to ensure that the entire lumen has been cleared of blood. A normal saline flush should be rapid with the lumen clamps closed, ensuring that the entire lumen is flushed. Positive pressure created by the clamps prevents blood from backing up into the catheter. The heparinization flush must reach the entire lumen of the catheter and should follow the manufacturer's holding volumes (now printed on many catheters).

A permanent catheter option that has recently entered the market is a Silastic twin catheter. The Tesio catheter is two separate catheters that can be placed in different configurations to meet the patient's needs. The typical placement is a percutaneous method into the jugular vein with a subcutaneous tunnel to the clavicular region of the chest. The catheters are now available with a silver ion implantation process that results in a catheter surface that is thrombus and infection resistant. The Tesio catheter, as well as other catheter designs, must be considered to help provide more access options for the many dialysis patients rapidly exhausting all accesses.

Quality Assurance

The ESRD team currently consists of the nephrologist, dialysis nurse, renal dietician, renal social worker, transplant service representative, and the dialysis patient. The ESRD team must use a multidisciplinary approach to plan the care of each dialysis patient. The care plan must be outcome-based, with measurable short- and long-term goals. Each member of the ESRD team must address all identified goals and problems from their discipline's perspective. Vascular access creation and patency is a major issue for many dialysis patients. In one recent study, 20% of all inhospital days for hemodialysis patients were access-related.[13] Many access-related problems are dealt with on an outpatient basis and are not reflected by the percent of inhospital days. For many hemodialysis patients, the establishment and maintenance of a functional access is the main care plan goal. This is why the ESRD team should be expanded to include the vascular access surgeon and the interventional radiologist. The short- and long-term care plan goals must include interventions from all members of the ESRD team to help meet the goal of a functional hemodialysis vascular access. The following is an example of a patient care plan:

Patient

Thirty-five-year-old black, diabetic female on hemodialysis for six months with loss of first left forearm loop polytetrafluoroethylene (PTFE) graft due to repeated thrombosis. Patient currently is scheduled for outpatient surgery for creation of a left upper-arm PTFE graft and insertion of a temporary, left subclavian dual-lumen hemodialysis catheter.

SHORT-TERM GOALS

- Successful insertion of left temporary subclavian catheter and creation of left upper-arm PTFE graft.
- Prevent infection and maintain patency of the left temporary subclavian catheter for four to six weeks until new graft is ready for use.

LONG-TERM GOAL

- Maintain patency and function of the newly created left upper-arm graft.

Nephrologist

SHORT-TERM INTERVENTIONS

- Arrange for catheter and graft access placement.
- Monitor antihypertensive drug therapy and hemodialysis sessions to prevent posthemodialysis hypotension following new graft insertion.
- Monitor and evaluate blood sugar levels following surgical procedures; adjust insulin prescription as needed.
- Monitor and evaluate wound healing and catheter exit-site condition to detect any signs and symptoms of early infection; order antibiotic coverage as needed.
- Evaluate any signs and symptoms of uremia secondary to inadequate dialysis therapy via a temporary catheter.

LONG-TERM INTERVENTIONS

- Monitor and regulate anticoagulation therapy weekly.
- Evaluate any clinical findings that indicate malfunction of the graft, such as

ncrease in venous pressure, abnormal recirculation studies, or change in bruit or thrill.
- Evaluate any decreases in dialysis efficiency (Kt/V or urea reduction rate studies).
- Evaluate for any signs and symptoms of subclavian vein stenosis after the catheter has been discontinued.
- Order, guide, and oversee all interventions to maintain access patency.
- Pursue renal transplant as an option.

Dialysis Nurse

SHORT-TERM INTERVENTIONS

- Act as the patient's advocate to ensure that the patient's goals and wishes are followed.
- Document access procedure on patient's access history.
- Provide patient education regarding care of temporary catheter. Teach the patient to check the new graft for presence of bruit and thrill twice a day.
- Evaluate the access sites for any sign or symptom of infection. Report signs and symptoms promptly to other ESRD team members.
- Monitor patient's fluid removal and blood pressure response during hemodialysis. Support blood pressure with fluids as needed to prevent posttreatment hypotension.
- Administer or instruct patient to take medications as ordered, such as insulin, anticoagulants, antihypertensives, or antibiotics.
- Assess and report any signs or symptoms of uremia promptly to other ESRD team members.
- Coordinate the execution of physicians' orders to ensure that all tests and procedures (such as prothrombin times or blood sugars) are performed and results reported back in a timely manner.

LONG-TERM INTERVENTIONS

- Provide continuing patient education regarding care of the graft and interventions to maintain patency.
- Continue to act as the patient's advocate to ensure that patient wishes and goals are followed, including the pursuit of a kidney transplant.
- Monitor clinical signs and symptoms of access malfunction such as difficulty with needle cannulation, prolonged posttreatment bleeding, increasing venous pressure, and arm edema.
- Coordinate the execution of the access surveillance protocol tests and procedures, i.e., recirculation and adequacy studies. Report results to ESRD team members in a timely manner.

Renal Dietitian

SHORT-TERM INTERVENTIONS

- Evaluate dietary intake to promote good wound healing without developing uremic complications while the patient is being dialyzed via the temporary catheter.
- Evaluate blood sugars and determine if any dietary changes are needed to control the level.
- Evaluate changes in dialysis efficiency studies (Kt/V or urea reduction rates) and determine if any dietary intake changes account for the decreases in clearances.

LONG-TERM INTERVENTIONS

- Continue to evaluate dietary intake to control blood sugars as the patient's condition changes.
- Continue to evaluate dietary intake as it relates to dialysis efficiency studies. Identify any decrease in dialysis efficiency not related to increased protein intake.

Renal Social Worker

SHORT-TERM INTERVENTIONS

- Provide assistance in arranging transportation for access procedures.
- Provide support and encouragement to patients and family. Assist patients with venting frustrations with current access difficulties.
- Assist the patient in obtaining a stethoscope to assess the access for the presence of a bruit.

LONG-TERM INTERVENTIONS

- Assist with insurance coverage for tests and procedures.
- Provide ongoing support and encouragement, including the patient's pursuit of a renal transplant as an option.

Interventional Radiologist

SHORT-TERM INTERVENTIONS

- Assist with venous catheter placement, using fluoroscopy as needed.
- Evaluate chest x-ray after catheter line insertion to ensure correct line placement.

NAME ______________ DIAGNOSIS ______________________________

DATE	ACCESS LOCATION	PROCEDURE	M.D./ HOSPITAL	SURG/PROC. REMARKS	COMPLICATIONS
		PERITONEAL CATHETER			

Figure 11-11. This dialysis access history form is used to record all placement procedures and complications.

LONG-TERM INTERVENTIONS

- Perform fistulogram and angioplasty as needed under the access surveillance protocol.
- Perform UK thrombolysis of clotted hemodialysis access as needed.

Vascular Access Surgeon

SHORT-TERM INTERVENTIONS

- Surgical creation of access in nondominant arm and/or catheter line placement.
- Evaluate incision sites for normal healing and absence of infection.
- Monitor subclavian catheter function and absence of infection. Change line if needed.

LONG-TERM INTERVENTIONS

- Evaluate subclavian vein after catheter is discontinued for signs or symptoms of subclavian vein stenosis.
- Evaluate with other members of the ESRD team any clinical findings that indicate a change in function of the graft.
- Consult with the other team members regarding the treatment options and perform surgical interventions as needed.
- Continue to use the access surveillance protocol to monitor patients until renal transplant can be achieved.

The expanded ESRD team must work together to ensure that patient goals can be obtained. All dialysis facilities have active quality assurance (QA) or continuous quality improvement (CQI) programs. Currently, all members of the ESRD team participate in the QA or CQI programs. Various access surgeons and interventional radiologists should participate in these programs, which involve vascular access establishment and maintenance of patency. Vascular access can be easily monitored with a QA tracking tool. A dialysis access history must be obtained and updated on each patient; it should include all placement procedures and complications (figure 11-11). The dialysis staff must continuously update the access history for each patient. All access procedures, complications, and outcomes should be compiled monthly for review by the QA committee for trend identification.

Examples of a QA Trends

INFECTIONS: TWO GRAFTS

One infection was in a new graft in a 66-year-old female diabetic with poor wound healing who resides in a nursing home. The graft was never used for access. A culture and sensitivity test showed a methicillin-resistant *Staphylococcus aureus*

(MSRA) infection. The patient is still undergoing antibiotic therapy and MSRA precaution. Nasal culture remains negative. She is being dialyzed through a permanent dual-lumen catheter.

The second graft infection was with a four-month-old graft in a 25-year-old male. The patient had not washed his access arm with antibacterial soap prior to a needle cannulation. Culture and sensitivity showed a *S. aureus* infection. The graft continued to be used, with the patient washing his access arm prior to any needle cannulations. The infection cleared after antibiotic therapy. The patient was tested for nasal carriage and found negative.

MALFUNCTIONING PERMANENT DIALYSIS CATHETERS

All three clotted catheters were noted to be less than six months old. The same surgeon placed all catheters without the use of fluoroscopy. The catheters were found to be located in the superior vena cava, not the right atrium, and were treated with UK. Two catheters regained function with current blood flows of 250 ml/min. The third catheter was used for two treatments, rethrombosed, and was changed under fluoroscopy. The catheter is currently functioning at a 300 ml/min blood flow.

CLOTTED ARTERIOVENOUS ACCESS

The first patient, a 61-year-old female with a left forearm loop graft, had two episodes of clotting. The graft clotted initially after nine months. Venous pressures were slowly increasing to 150 mm Hg two weeks before the thrombosis. The patient was approached about the need for a fistulogram, but the graft clotted before the test. The graft was declotted and reclotted within 12 hours. The graft was then treated with UK and fistulogram with angioplasty. In addition, an upper-arm outflow vein stenosis of 70% was opened with balloon angioplasty. The graft remains patent after one week. The second failed access was an 18-month-old left upper-arm graft in a 52-year-old male. The patient experienced severe hypotension postdialysis on a Monday. When he presented for dialysis on Wednesday, the graft was found to be clotted. The patient underwent a declot procedure without complications. His dialysis dry weight was increased by 0.5 kg. The graft remains patent for two and one-half weeks with no further hypotension.

Monitoring Staff Techniques

Trends regarding issues with staff cannulation procedures can be identified by tracking all infiltrations. If the same staff member has multiple infiltrations with different patients, the staff member can be monitored during several cannulation procedures. Incorrect cannulation techniques should be corrected with the individual. If multiple staff members have difficulty cannulating the same patient, then the access should be evaluated for structural problems. The graft may be too deep to cannulate with a 1-in. fistula needle, and a 1¼-in. needle may be necessary. A fistula may be too underdeveloped and may need a surgical revision with a PTFE graft to correct the arterial inflow stenosis. Access complications can also be tracked according to surgical radiology group. Technical problems with access procedures by one member of a group can be identified and addressed. Monthly vascular access

NAME	ACCESS	ORIGINAL SURGERY DATE	REVISION DATE	KT/V	CREATININE REDUCTION	RECIR. PERCENT	VENOUS PRESSURE <200 @ 200 BFR	FISTULO-GRAM DATE/ RESULT	ANTICOAG. THERAPY	RESOLU-TION	COMMENTS

Figure 11-12. Each vascular access surgeon is provided a copy of this quarterly vascular access report.

QA results and identified trends should be reviewed by all surgical and radiology groups and quarterly reports should be compiled for their patients (figure 11-12). Input from the surgeons and interventional radiologists can help guide the QA committee with trend identification. QA goals must be changed to address identified trends and to monitor results. Long-term solutions to vascular access problems will be achieved only if the problems are addressed by a team approach, including the expanded ESRD team members.

Vascular Access Surveillance Protocol

The expanded ESRD team should use a vascular access surveillance protocol to detect and treat access complications. This protocol should be tailored to meet the needs of the individual unit. Wide implementation provides uniform access evaluation on all patients—not just those identified as problematic—and facilitates prompt intervention. Following is a sample vascular access surveillance protocol.

Clinical Problems

- Change in the quality of the thrill or pitch of the bruit.
- Difficulty with needle cannulation such as decreased blood flashback, clotted needles, clots in the tip of the needle, recurrent needle infiltration, or difficulty advancing the needle.
- Prolonged bleeding from access puncture sites postdialysis.
- Formation of access aneurysm or pseudoaneurysm formation.
- Unexplained, excessive fluid removal with ultrafiltration, controlled dialysis machine.
- High pressure with a closed system dialysis rinseback.

Venous Pressure Protocol and Other Procedures

Venous pressures (VP) should be monitored during each dialysis treatment or at least once a week. Within the first 60 minutes of therapy, during the vital sign check, decrease the blood flow to 200 ml/min until stable and then record the VP. A VP of > 150 mm Hg with a 16-gauge fistula needle is considered elevated. Any upward trend with venous pressure increases of 10% or more from one week to the next should be considered elevated.

Recirculation Studies. Obtain recirculation studies on all new vascular accesses and continue every three months. Repeat recirculation studies two weeks after any angioplasty or surgical revision. Repeat recirculation studies if the dialysis efficiency measurements are poor or change from acceptable to poor. A recirculation value of > 15% with three-needle technique or 10% with the two-needle technique is considered abnormal.

Dialysis Efficiency Measurements. Monitor monthly the dialysis efficiency by using kinetic modeling Kt/V or urea reduction rates of any decreases without changes in the dialysis prescription.

Color Flow Doppler Studies. Color flow Doppler allows noninvasive testing to evaluate access function. If the study is abnormal, or the subclavian vein is not visible or problems persist, proceed to the next step.

Fistulogram. This is the gold standard to evaluate access and subclavian vein.

Angioplasty. Percutaneous transluminal angioplasty is used as needed to open stenosis.

O.R. Surgical Intevention. Surgical revision of the new access is used as needed. Follow up with step one of the protocol and repeat steps as needed. This protocol helps guide the esrd team in maintaining a functional dialysis access for all patients under their care. The protocol can be adapted and updated as guided by the dialysis unit's ongoing QA or CQI goals.

Vascular access solutions will be found only if all members of the health care team work together, each respecting the talents and abilities of the others. The "political" walls that prevent interactions must be broken down. As we enter the era of health care reform, we must find solutions that will provide functional vascular accesses with long-term patency, and at an affordable cost for all. As a team, we can find the solutions to the current vascular access challenges and thus prolong the lives of our patients.

References

1. Lancaster LE. Core curriculum of nephrology nursing. New Jersey: Am Nephrol Nurses Assoc 1991; 203,291,235,263-268.
2. Perkins JJ. Principles and methods of sterilization in health services. Springfield, Ill.: Charles C Thomas; 337-338.
3. Fan PY, Schwab SJ. Vascular access: concepts of the 1990's. J Am Soc Neph 1992; 3(1):4,5,9.
4. Dhaene M, Gulbis B, Lietaer N, et al. Red blood cell destruction in single needle dialysis. Clin Nephrol 1989; 31(6);330.
5. Daugirdas JT, Ing TS. Handbook of dialysis. Boston: Little, Brown, 1994; 96.
6. Uldall PR. How should temporary vascular access for hemodialysis be achieved? Semin Dialysis 1993; 6(6):189.
7. Denys BG, Uretsky BF, Reddy PS. Ultrasound-assisted cannulation of the internal jugular vein. A prospective comparison to the external landmark-guided technique. Circulation 1993; 87(5):1560.
8. Schillinger F, Schillinger D, Montagnac R, et al. Post catherisation of vein stenosis in haemodialysis; comparative angiograph is study of 50 subclavian and 50 internal jugular accesses. Nephrol Dial Transplant 1991; 772-724.
9. Cimochowski GF. How should temporary vascular access for hemodialysis be achieved? Semin Dialysis 1993; 6(6):193-194.
10. Schneider TC, Krzywda E, Andris D, et al. The malfunctioning Silastic catheter-radiologic assessment and treatment. J Parenter & Enter Nutrition 1986; 10(1):70-73.

11. Whelchel JD. Central venous hemodialysis access catheters: a review of technical considerations and complications. In: Henry ML, Sommer BG, eds. Vascular access for hemodialysis—II. Chicago: W.L. Gore & Associates, Inc., and Precept Press, 131-132.
12. Mauro MA, Jaques PF. Radiologic placement of long-term central venous catheters: a review. Vasc Intervention; 4(1):136-137. QA tracking.
13. Besarab A, Dorrell S, Moritz M, et al. Preserving vascular access. Semin Dialysis 1991; 4(3):155.

DISCUSSION

Moderator:
Ronald M. Ferguson, M.D., Ph.D.
Panelists:
Deborah Joan Brouwer, R.N., C.N.N.
Ingemar J.A. Dawidson, M.D.
James R. DeBord, M.D.
Mitchell L. Henry, M.D.

Dr. Ferguson: I would like to begin by asking Dr. Dawidson to clarify a point. You said that if you stick a graft early, in less than 14 days, it has a greater probability of clotting, but you also said that was all due to patient or case mix. I would like you to follow up on that because it does not make sense to me.

Dr. Dawidson: In 1991-92 we were putting these grafts in and using them right away in acutely ill patients. If you know the Dallas patient population, these are sick patients. They come in with a creatinine of 25 and use up all of their veins, but still need dialysis. These were the patients who were accessed early in 1991-92. In 1993, these patients got an access earlier and, in 1993, there was no difference between the two groups. I am as puzzled as you are and we are obviously continuing to look at these results.

Discussant: Within that 14-day early cannulation period, how early are you willing to stick them?

Dr. Dawidson: Twenty-two percent of the 96 patients were accessed within 48 hours and 80% were stuck within seven days. I did not control this. The nephrologists controlled the timing. This is just something I found in retrospect. Several patients were stuck the same day. One patient went directly from the O.R. and was dialyzed with the graft within one hour and he had no problems. I do not think it is only the graft itself, but it also has to do with how you put it in. I use a very tight tunnel, a 6-mm dilator that is about 25 cm long. Second, I think it is crucial how you dialyze these patients. The dialysis nurse is perhaps even more important. You have to hold careful pressure for up to 20 minutes afterward.

Discussant: Do you have an early cannulation protocol? Do you use a smaller needle or lower pump speed, or do you use standard technique?

Dr. Dawidson: No, we use the same, standard technique.

Discussant: It seems clear to me, based upon the information presented and the literature, that flow is the best predictor of graft failure. I suspect that good vascular surgeons can put their hands on a graft, certainly if they have recent notes of their physical exam, and probably get within 20-30% of what the Doppler is going to tell you. I suspect there is a very high correlation between a good physical exam by an experienced examiner and what the Doppler is going to show. Assuming that is so, I wonder if just sending these patients more frequently to the vascular surgeon, or perhaps the vascular surgeon making rounds in the unit, should be the screening test. Perhaps teaching the dialysis nurses how to examine the patient and what to look for would be as effective.

Dr. Henry: I have absolutely no idea if that is true. If you follow a patient from point A to point B to point C and do serial physical exams, you probably can identify some aspects that may lead you to believe that the graft is failing or is otherwise okay. I do not think the doctors are the ones who are going to do that. If the nurses are very good, they may be able to do that because they see the patient three times a week. I would guess the physical exam does not correlate with Doppler or outcome. You have a great opportunity since you do access full time; you could design a study prospectively and do color flow Doppler versus physical exam. I would guess that the physical exam is not sensitive enough to identify those patients.

Dr. DeBord: Dr. Henry, what criteria did you use for the diagnosis of the significance of stenosis in these grafts? What do you consider significant in these grafts?

Dr. Henry: This was an observational study to identify if the stenoses are there, at what level the stenoses were, and how it correlated with flow.

Dr. DeBord: How can you diagnose your stenoses?

Dr. Henry: Simply with mapping both in the graft and in the outflow vein with the color flow Doppler.

Dr. DeBord: Can you make an estimation of the degree you stenosed?

Dr. Henry: Cross-sectional diameter was measured. Flow and flow reduction were then correlated with various degrees of stenosis.

Discussant: Ms. Brouwer, in terms of your patient control measures for patients with subclavian catheters, do you advise the use of masks and universal precautions?

Ms. Brouwer: Everywhere that I have worked, we mask the patient and we mask ourselves. We use strict precautions. You do not necessarily have to use sterile gloves with the catheters, but you need to use very strict precautions when touching the ends of the catheters. We use a povidone-iodine scrub before we take the catheters apart. We see more tunnel and exit site infections. That is usually from noncompliance on the part of the patients.

Discussant: Is that recommendation based upon data or is it just a common sense kind of thing? I asked the same question of Dr. Uldall yesterday, and he said they do not use masks in Canada.

Ms. Brouwer: We wear masks now as part of our OSHA policies. We have to have facial shields or masks, so the only additional masks are the ones we use on the patients.

Dr. Henry: There have been studies in the surgical literature looking at masks or no masks. In fact, the masks are totally worthless in preventing infections. I think that all of that garb we use these days is to prevent us from becoming contaminated rather than the other way around.

Discussant: Dr. Henry, I enjoyed your talk very much. Are there any data on flow rates in the A-V fistulas compared to bridge graft fistulas and thrombosis rate?

Dr. Henry: There are a lot of data. Both Barry Strauch and our data could not show any correlation in the A-V fistula, and I should have said that. It is really only very accurate in prosthetic grafts.

Discussant: Dr. DeBord, could you comment on your experience with arterial-to-arterial grafts? I have not had very good success with these and I would like to know what the experience of others has been.

Dr. DeBord: I have had no experience with arterial-to-arterial grafts for dialysis. You have to have some obstruction between your two arterial beds in order to have a gradient for flow, so I guess it would be accomplishing two things, the dialysis access and a vascular bypass in one graft. I do not know if I would want to be sticking it three times a week.

Dr. Ferguson: Ms. Brouwer, have you ever stuck one?

Ms. Brouwer: No. I cannot imagine what the venous pressures on that would be and how you would even get the blood pump to return the blood. I would not want to do it.

Discussant: The venous pressures are very high, and it is a very bad thing to do, but there are nephrologists who keep pushing to do that. They have said that it has been done in other places. I have done only a couple and they have been terrible.

Discussant: Dr. Henry, regarding the color flow Doppler, how does the color imaging help in your examination? Is it really necessary?

Dr. Henry: The color itself does not, but the relative flow rates do. It is a nice, pretty picture, and you can look at it and tell very quickly visually where the stenoses or flow abnormalities are. The color itself does not help you, but the technology does.

Discussant: Could a good ultrasound technician do the same thing in gray scale?

Dr. Henry: Yes. The newer machines will calculate the flows directly; therefore, you do not need to go through velocities, and you get flow rates rather than velocities.

Discussant: Do you have any studies that show the relationship with flow on hyperplasia on venous site down the road relatively?

Dr. Henry: The vast majority of these failures were due to venous hyperplasia in the outflow tract. The decreased flow in these grafts did predict those that thrombose more frequently and those that had good flow. Did I misunderstand your question?

Discussant: No. The only thing I was concerned about was how your flow caused more hyperplasia.

Dr. Henry: This study has not addressed that at all.

Dr. Ferguson: Dr. Henry, if flows are so important, with all of those zeroes in front of the p-value, it looked as if it were far and away the most significant thing. What should we be doing in the O.R. for an end point? Should we be shooting for an end point of flow as opposed to anatomic correction?

Dr. Henry: I think it makes perfect sense. We have all been trained in the O.R. to use various clues that make us think we have increased the flow. It goes back to the question of whether we can identify changes in flow by putting our hands on the graft. I think if this type of examination is available and you can use it cost-effectively, it might be able to help significantly. If you have done your best operation, there is probably no reason to measure flow at that time, because it is not going to help you make any decisions unless you look more centrally for an abnormality.

Dr. Ferguson: What if you do a thrombectomy on a graft that previously had 300 cc of flow, and you think you fixed it and at that time in the O.R. you have 280 cc of flow? What is the fate of that graft?

Dr. Henry: You should look for another abnormality that you have not addressed.

Dr. Ferguson: So what you are saying is, maybe we should be measuring flows with similar kinds of instruments in the O.R.?

Dr. Henry: Perhaps for routine activity it is going to be very expensive and you will not be reimbursed for those activities as far as your patients are concerned. You or your patient will have to pay those bills.

Discussant: My comment is that the arterial jump graft is in the access literature. It enjoyed a brief period of popularity. I would like to ask Ms. Brouwer if she has recommendations for routine inservice training by the access surgeons in the dialysis unit.

Ms. Brouwer: Inservice training is very important. The big problems are with the dialysis staff turnover rate in many of the units, the lack of ongoing education, and the fact that there are really very few references that can be used to train the nurses. One of the best available materials is a booklet that the Gore company distributes on how to correctly cannulate grafts. Even the nursing literature is lacking in that, and that is something the nurses need to fix.

Discussant: Dr. Henry, does anybody try to map the natural history of the graft from the beginning in time right after the graft is inserted and then every three to six months?

Dr. Henry: That is the problem with all of these studies. Some of the patients who have come onto this study have been followed over time from the beginning of the graft, but the average age of those grafts was two and a half years. Those are the studies that need to be ongoing.

Dr. Ferguson: But I think you pointed out that if we use the databases that are now available, and if we all were to prospectively start to follow these parameters longitudinally, we would have some very interesting prospectively collected data in a couple of years. We would not have to depend on these cross-sectional studies that are really very difficult to interpret.

Dr. Henry: There is no question about that. These studies have been designed to identify if it is cost-efficient to identify the failing access and to intervene before the access fails. I think we can show this in the near future, so that third-party payers will recognize that it is an important modality to pay for and that in fact money can be saved. But at this time, capital outlays, as well as the technician's time and professional fees, are being reimbursed poorly or not at all.

Discussant: Dr. DeBord, you said that in thigh grafts one of the problems was infection because the groin was dirty. Do you have data supporting that there are more infections in thigh grafts?

Dr. DeBord: I do not have any personal data showing this. The groin has a higher number of infections in those incisions in vascular surgery and has an associated incidence of infection in the vascular graft.

Discussant: I have tried to tunnel the graft laterally on the thigh. You put the graft in a position so it is accessible for nurses with the patient in a chair. We purposefully tunnel the graft out laterally on the thigh, and it is anecdotal, but we really have not seen many thigh graft infections.

Dr. DeBord: That is an excellent point in terms of anatomy and practicality of the graft.

Dr. Henry: I am aware of no prospective trials, that have looked at arm versus groin in a prospective fashion to see which one is more prone to infection. In most studies that have looked at vascular access and reported both arm and groin grafts, the evidence of infection is higher in the groin access patients. You have to remember that those patients are more likely to get an infection overall because they do not have any other access sites.

Discussant: To my knowledge, there are three techniques for doing recirculation studies. It seems that any technique that would use the opposite arm for recirculation studies on a routine basis would be counterproductive. Does anyone have any thoughts about the stop-flow or low-flow techniques?

Ms. Brouwer: That is the reason the stop-flow was designed. The problem with the stop-flow is that the recirculation rates are very low. The studies will often show up as zero or below 5% recirculation. If you are still using a traditional 10% or 15% recirculation, it is unacceptable. A 5% recirculation may be unacceptable. You need to individualize those levels that you are using. That is why stop-flow was developed—to save the other arm.

Dr. Ferguson: Ms. Brouwer, I would like to ask one last question. Yesterday Dr. Uldall presented some very interesting data on a new catheter, not a temporary catheter, but a long-term catheter with a very low complication rate. What do you think of catheters like that as a primary, long-term access for hemodialysis? You are the one who is going to have to use them and dialyze a patient successfully.

Ms. Brouwer: Well, if they work, great! They are wonderful. The problem is that often the long-term catheters do not function well. A lot of that has to do with how they are inserted. We have used the Tesio catheters, which are the softer catheters with the blunt end. They work very well, and we get good flow rates out of them. We have not seen a lot of infections with the two tunnels. I have nightmares over the Permacaths. They do not function well in my experience.

Discussant: Is there any indication in your dialysis unit for capping catheters with urokinase versus capping off those catheters with heparin?

Ms. Brouwer: I have done that. I think we overuse urokinase. The catheter that needs to have urokinase put in it that regularly needs to be investigated as to why. Urokinase became a very easy way to treat these catheters so that nobody has to bother with them. It is not cost-effective. We have one patient we have used it on because she is allergic to heparin, but urokinase should not be used routinely.

SECTION V

12

15-YEAR EXPERIENCE WITH TAPERED (4–7-mm) AND STRAIGHT (6-mm) PTFE ANGIO-ACCESS IN THE ESRD PATIENT

P. Sabanayagam, M.D., F.R.C.S. (C)., F.A.C.S.

THE EXPONENTIAL INCREASE AND PREVALENCE OF END-STAGE RENAL DISEASE (ESRD) is well documented. Hypertension and glomerulonephritis were the prevailing causes during the initial decade (1973-83). This has been superseded by diabetes during the second decade (1983-93). In addition, elderly patients with multisystem disease have entered the renal program during the past decade. At present, more than 157,000 patients receive hemodialysis as their primary mode of renal replacement therapy. The projected population of patients that will receive hemodialysis in 2000 is estimated at 240,000.

The provision of an adequate reliable angio-access is essential for hemodialytic renal replacement therapy. This continues to challenge the ingenuity of the vascular surgeon in the long-term survivors and in the changing population of patients. The autologous arteriovenous (A-V) fistula still remains the ideal angio-access. This can be created in only 15% of all patients as a primary adequate angio-access. In patients in whom the primary angio-access has failed and in those in whom this cannot be created, a prosthetic bridged graft is created. During the past two decades, a variety of biologic and synthetic prosthetic conduits have been used to create the bridged A-V graft. The early failure rate and the increased incidence of complications with the biologic angio-access are well documented.[5-7] This has led to the use of synthetic conduits in the creation of the bridged A-V graft.

The desirable characteristics of an ideal conduit for the creation of angio-access should be nonantigenic and carry a nonthrombogenic inner surface.[1-5] It should resist infection and maintain its structural integrity in an infected human milieu. In the event of an infection, it should localize to the affected area. It should seal and heal puncture sites with autologous tissue following cannulation. It should possess desirable mechanical handling properties, with a low implantation porosity and high healing porosity. In the event of thrombosis, it should offer easy thrombectomy leaving a smooth inner surface. It should conduct a fixed volume of blood without any incremental increase with maturation. Ideally, the conduit should be free of neointimal fibroplasia along the body of the graft and anastomotic sites.

Evaluation of Patient

The reported five-year survival of patients with ESRD is 60%, whereas the 10-year survival is 40%. An occasional survivor over 25 years is reported. The provision and maintenance of angio-access in the long-term candidate is a challenging problem, thus careful planning of the primary and subsequent angio-access is essential for the survival of these patients. The following guidelines help achieve this goal and allow long-term patency of the bridged arteriovenous graft:

- The upper extremities are the preferred site over the lower extremities.
- Whenever feasible, the angio-access should be created in the distal upper extremity to preserve proximal sites for subsequent procedures.
- Gentle handling of tissue and incisions placed along the long axis of the extremity are essential to prevent excessive swelling partly due to interruption of the lymphatics.
- Avoid using anticoagulation during the initial creation of the angio-access, as this will render the graft a wettable surface allowing seepage of serum into surrounding tissue. This leads to excessive swelling and/or seroma.
- Anticoagulation is indicated with declotting and revision of well-healed grafts.
- Antiplatelet therapy and Coumadin anticoagulation are indicated in patients with recurrent thrombosis.
- Avoid atherosclerotic arteries, especially in the distal extremity, as this will lead to poor inflow with a high incidence of ischemia to hand and digits.
- Avoid skeletonizing the artery and vein circumferentially. The dissection should be limited to allow control and to carry out the anastomosis.
- Avoid placing the venous anastomosis at or near joints, allowing sufficient length of vein for future revisions in the event of thrombosis.
- Whenever possible, the venous anastomosis should be placed over the junction of a venous branch, as this creates less turbulence, reducing neointimal hyperplasia at the anastomosis.
- Excise valves at the anastomotic site. The anastomosis is preferably placed distal to this excision site.
- The prosthetic graft should be placed in an adequate subdermal tunnel. The best healing occurs in this layer of skin.

Table 12-1. Site of Graft

Site	Straight grafts	Tapered grafts	Total	%
Forearm	168	599	767	50
Upper arm	109	620	729	48
Axil-axil	11	10	21	2
Leg	3	6	9	—
Total	291	1,235	1,256	100

- The angio-access should be anatomically placed to allow easy access for cannulation and patient comfort during hemodialysis.
- Prophylactic antibiotics are indicated during the placement of the initial angio-access, during revisions and in the event of posterior puncture of the graft.

Materials and Methods

All patients receiving the bridged A-V fistula during the study period between 1978-93 are included. A total of 1,229 patients received 1,526 polytetrafluoroethylene (PTFE) bridged A-V grafts. The straight (6-mm) and tapered (4–7-mm) PTFE grafts were used during the period 1978-81 in a prospective random study. Since 1981, the tapered PTFE graft was used exclusively to create the bridged A-V graft. There were 53% males and 47% females, with an average age of 58 years; 73% were over 50 and 16% were younger than 40. Seventy-eight percent were hypertensive and 348 were diabetic.

Bridged grafts created in the upper extremity totaled 1,496 (98%). There were 767 forearm grafts and 729 upper-arm grafts. The remaining 30 grafts were placed as biaxillary and leg grafts (table 12-1). The creation of an angio-access invariably shunts arterial blood from the extremity distal to the angio-access. As almost all angio-access is created in the upper extremity, it is essential to investigate the arterial perfusion to the hand and digits prior to and following the creation of the graft. The Allen's test is an objective form of this evaluation. The measurement of digital pressures and wave form is an accurate, noninvasive evaluation of the perfusion to the hand and digits (Doppler model 1052, Parks Electronics) (figure 12-1). Because blood pressures in these patients are variable, a more accurate interpretation of digital perfusion is the digital index:

$$\text{Digital index} = \frac{\text{distal systolic pressure}}{\text{systemic systolic pressure}}$$

Patients receiving the forearm straight or loop graft, upper-arm straight graft, the biaxillary graft, and the autologous A-V fistula were the subject of this study. The distal forearm angio-access had the most impairment of perfusion to digits, with the exception of the autologous A-V fistula. The more proximal biaxillary graft manifests the least impairment to the perfusion of the hand and digits. The upper-arm graft occupies an intermediate position. This information is essential in deciding the site of the angio-access in a vascularly impaired patient.

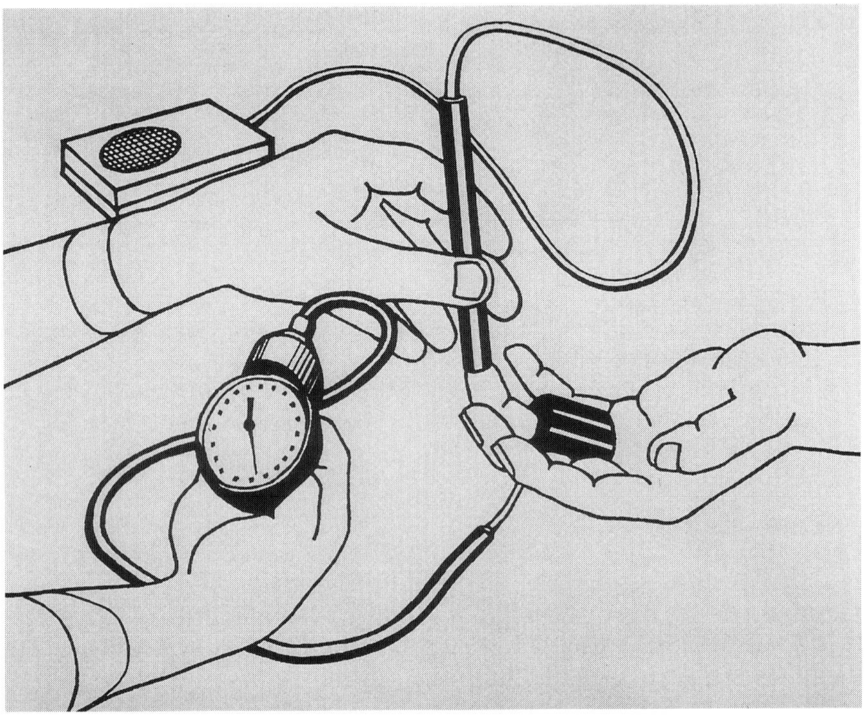

Figure 12-1. Measurement of digital pressures and wave form is an accurate, noninvasive evaluation of the perfusion to the hand and digits.

Digital pressures were measured and digital indexes calculated in all patients prior to the placement of the angio-access, during the first postoperative day and at monthly intervals for a period of six months. The greatest drop in perfusion is seen during the immediate postoperative day. However, during the ensuing period, there is an increase in perfusion due to collateral blood flow. This collateralization occurs during the initial three months, stabilizing the perfusion to the hand and digits. This finding allows one to monitor patients with mild symptoms of ischemia during this period before subjecting them to banding of the graft.

The perfusion of the hand and digits is increased when tapered (4–7-mm) grafts are used in the creation of bridged A-V grafts, compared to the straight 6-mm grafts. This is uniformly seen at all sites with prosthetic angio-access. The type of prosthetic, tapered (4–7-mm) or straight (6-mm), the site, and the configuration are presented in figure 12-2.

Surgical Technique

All procedures were performed under regional anesthesia or local infiltration anesthesia in the upper extremity and lower extremity. General anesthesia was used in patients receiving a biaxillary graft. The vessel size, atherosclerosis in

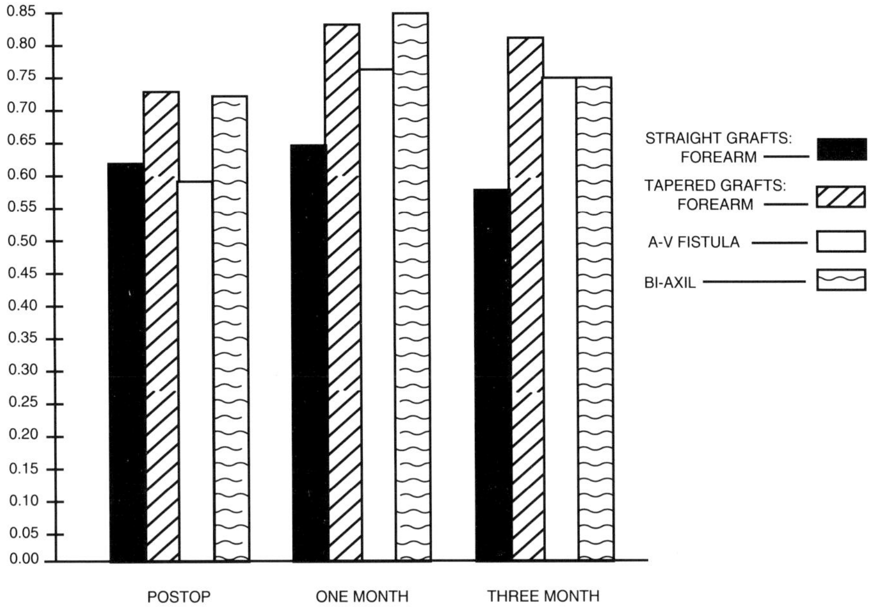

Figure 12-2. Mean digital perfusion index (mean of five digits).

the artery, and sclerosis of the vein determine the site and type of angio-access. An artery with an internal diameter of 2.5 mm and vein with an internal diameter of 3 mm is suitable for the creation of the prosthetic angio-access. All vessels should be handled gently, avoiding excessive forcible dilatation. A smooth transition of the luminal surface of the prosthetic to the intimal lining of the vein is essential to prevent platelet deposition with ensuing neointimal hyperplasia. The largest available vein, preferably opposite the branch, is selected as outflow. This improves energy dissipation, delaying the arterialization and neointimal hyperplasia at the venous anastomosis. A sharp entry of the prosthetic into the outflow vein is also avoided.

The subdermal tunnel for the prosthetic is created overlying the muscle. The tunnel should be calibrated with a metal sizer, 10 mm in diameter, to avoid constriction of the body of the prosthetic graft. The use of heparin anticoagulation and/or forcible irrigation with heparinized saline solution during the creation of the angio-access causes seepage of serum into the adjacent tissue. This leads to the inevitable swelling along the graft insertion site and seroma formation.

Results and Complications

The data were analyzed using life table analysis, and life tables were compared using log rank test of significance. The incidence of complications was computed and presented as a proportion of 100 graft months of follow-up. There were 1,393

Table 12-2. Type and Incidence of Complications

Type of complication	No. observed	Incidence/100 graft-months of follow-up
Thrombosis	1230	3.22
Infection	73	0.188
Aneurysm	60	0.16
Ischemia	16	0.05
Venous hypertension	9	0.023
Seroma	5	0.13
Total	1,393	3.64

complications during 38,242 graft months of follow-up. These complications in order of frequency are shown in table 12-2.

Thrombosis

Thrombosis is the most frequent cause of angio-access failure. There were 1,230 angio-access thromboses during the study period, which extended over 38,242 months. An incidence of 3.22 occurrence of thrombosis in 100 graft months follow-up was seen in this study. Thrombosis during the early follow-up period is usually secondary to hypotension, dehydration, hypercoagulability, and (rarely) from external pressure. In most cases, patency of the angio-access can be established with a simple thrombectomy. The most common cause of thrombosis is fibrous intimal hyperplasia at the venous anastomosis involving a short segment of the vein and graft. This localized area of mechanical obstruction is corrected with a patch angioplasty using prosthetic material. Occasionally, thrombolysis using urokinase with transluminal angioplasty restores patency of the angio-access.

In selected cases, when the graft and vein can be mobilized, the area of stenosis can be resected. An end-to-end anastomosis between the graft and the outflow vein can be done to reestablish patency. In instances where the area of stenosis along the venous outflow is long, a segmental replacement using a 6-mm graft as an interposition graft reestablishes patency.

Central Vein. The stenosis or thrombosis of the central subclavian vein, innominate vein, and superior vena cava is seen with increasing frequency in these patients. This central venous stenosis can be corrected with transluminal dilatation of the stenosis with stenting.

Body of Graft. Repeated cannulation of the graft for hemodialysis leads to accumulation of organized thrombus. This causes fibroplasia and associated stenosis of the body of the graft. These areas of stenosis can be successfully dilated using metal dilators and/or Fogarty thrombectomy catheters to reestablish patency. In the long-term patient, arteriosclerotic changes, including calcification, can occur in the graft. This is treated by resection of the affected segment with an interposition graft.

Arterial Inflow. Thrombosis secondary to poor arterial inflow is rare. This often signifies progression of the arteriosclerotic process in the inflow artery. The arterial inflow is augmented by bypassing a more proximal artery to the arterial end of the graft, converting a straight graft into a loop graft.

Table 12-3. Summary of Clinical Results of All Grafts

Type	No. used	No. patients	% of patients experience	Avg. months weighted experience	Months maximum
Forearm	767	579	75	28.9	154
Upper arm	729	626	86	21.1	171
Leg	9	8	89	29.2	121
Axil-axil	21	16	76	19.3	70
Total	1,526	1,229	81	25.1	171

Infection

Infection is the second most common complication encountered with angio-access. An incidence of 0.188 occurrences in 100 graft months follow-up was seen. Localized infection over the needle puncture site without bacteremia is treated with systemic antibiotics and local drainage. However, if this is associated with bacteremia, the graft is resected with angioplasty of the artery and vein. Infections of the anastomotic area are always treated with the excision of the graft and ligation of vessels.

Aneurysms

The evolution of the pseudoaneurysm is secondary to repeated needle punctures at the same site. The pseudoaneurysm may be solitary or multiple. Solitary aneurysms are treated by resection with angioplasty or interposition graft. Multiple aneurysms of the graft are treated with resection of the graft and placement of a parallel graft. An incidence of 0.16 occurrences per 100 graft months was seen in this series.

Ischemia

A relative ischemia of the distal extremity is an inevitable sequela of the creation of an angio-access. In most patients, this manifests as coldness of the extremity with mild paresthesia. This mild manifestation of ischemia disappears with increased collateral blood flow. The most severe manifestation of ischemia presents as pain during exercise or rest and/or motor dysfunction of the hand and digits. This requires urgent correction with banding of the graft and in the rare case, termination of the flow through the graft.

Results

The upper extremity is the preferred site in 98% of all patients. Forearm grafts were placed in 50% of these patients as compared to 48% placed in the upper arm

Table 12-4. Life Table Analysis of Patency of PTFE Angio-access

	Primary (%)	Secondary (%)
0–1 yr.	92	98
1–2 yr.	69	92
2–3 yr.	56	83
3–4 yr.	45	77
4–5 yr.	39	70
5–6 yr.	33	67
6–7 yr.	28	59
7–8 yr.	25	48
8–9 yr.	22	43
9–10 yr.	20	35

Table 12-5. Incidence of Ischemia

Straight (6-mm) versus tapered (4–7-mm) angio-access		
	Straight	**Tapered**
Number in study	294	1,232
Graft-months of follow-up	9.347	28,636
Grafts with ischemia	9	6
% of grafts affected	3.10	0.50

(table 12-3). The remaining 2% of grafts were placed over the anterior chest wall and lower extremity. Life table analysis shows that one-third of the grafts are patent at five years and one-fifth are patent at 10 years without intervention (table 12-4). Intervention procedures, such as thrombectomy, patch angioplasty, and interposition graft, have a doubling effect on the patency rate. Life table analysis following the first intervention procedure shows an extension of the graft patency by three years in 50% of the patients.

Summary

No statistically significant difference was noted when the cumulative patency rate is compared between tapered (4–7-mm) and straight (6-mm) bridged A-V graft (table 12-5). The tapered graft A-V fistula shows a significant reduction in the steal syndrome ($p < 0.005$). There was no statistically significant difference seen when the cumulative patency rate of the upper-arm graft was compared with the forearm graft. The cumulative patency rate of bridged A-V graft in the diabetic ESRD patient is significantly reduced compared to the nondiabetics ($p < 0.002$). However, no significant difference in primary patency rate is seen when the juvenile diabetics are compared with adult-onset diabetics.

The secondary patency rate of PTFE graft A-V grafts[8-10] is slightly lower than the best reported series of autologous A-V fistulas by Zerbino et al.,[12] but better than the series reported by Higgins et al.,[11] and also the median patency rates of the autologous A-V fistula (figure 12-3).

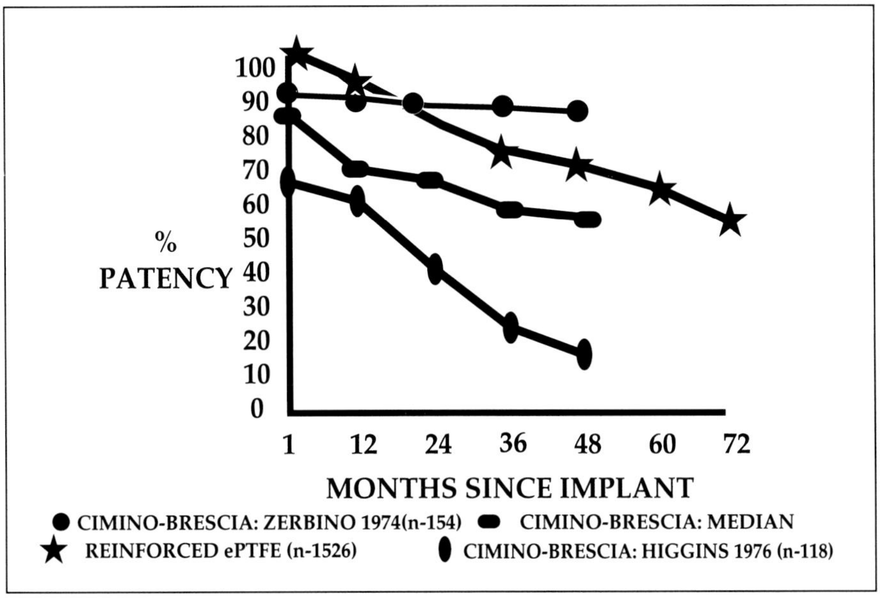

Figure 12-3. Vascular access for hemodialysis: comparative secondary patencies for Cimino-Brescia fistula ePTFE vascular grafts.

The incidence of complications requiring secondary procedures is definitely higher when compared to the complication rate of the autologous A-V fistula. The PTFE graft remains the prosthesis of choice for the creation of an A-V graft.

References

1. Sabanayagam P et al. Experience with two hundred and twenty five expanded PTFE fistulae for chronic maintenance hemodialysis. Proc Soc Artif Organs 1970; 6:126.
2. Campbell CD et al. Expanded microporous polytetrafluoroethylene (Gore-Tex) as a vascular conduit. In: Vascular grafts. New York:Appleton-Century-Crofts, 1978; 335.
3. Rosenberg N. The bovine arterial graft and its several applications. Surg Gynecol Obstet 1976; 142:104.
4. Sabanayagam P et al. Experience with one hundred reinforced expanded PTFE grafts for angioaccess in hemodialysis. Trans Am Soc Artif Intern Organs 1979; 26:126.
5. Sabanayagam P et al. A prospective random study comparing Gore-Tex graft and bovine graft as fistulae for maintenance hemodialysis. Proc Eur Soc Artif Organs 1982; 9:8.
6. Shack R et al. Expanded polytetrafluoroethylene as dialysis access grafts; serial study of histology and fibrinolytic activity. Am Surg 1977; 43:817.
7. Abbott WM et al. The role of mechanical properties in graft design. In: Dardik H, ed. Materials in vascular surgery. Miami:Symposia Specialists, 1978;59.
8. Sabanayagam P et al. A comparative study of 402 bovine heterografts and 225 reinforced PTFE grafts as AVF in the ESRD patient. Trans Am Soc Artif Intern Organs 1980; 26:88-92.
9. Sabanayagam P et al. IV. Prosthetic bridged AV fistulae, PTFE (Gore-Tex) versus bovine grafts; 13 years of experience with over 1300 fistulae. Trans Am Soc Artif Intern Organs 1983; 29:791.

10. Sicard GA, Allen BT, Anderson CB. Polytetrafluorethylene grafts for vascular access. In: Sommer BG, Henry ML, eds. Vascular access for hemodialysis. Chicago: W.L. Gore & Associates, Inc., and Pluribus Press, 1989.
11. Higgins MR et al. Blood access in hemodialysis. Clin Nephrol 1976; 6(5):473-77.
12. Zerbino VR et al. A 6 year clinical experience with arteriovenous fistula bypasses for hemodialysis. Surgery 1974; 76(6):1018-23.

13

STENOTIC LESIONS ASSOCIATED WITH A-V GRAFTS FOR HEMODIALYSIS: EXPERIENCE WITH INTRAOPERATIVE BALLOON ANGIOPLASTY AND POSTOPERATIVE ENDOVASCULAR STENT PLACEMENT

E. Steve Woodle, M.D., Mary Pat Knoerzer, R.N., M.S.N., Kenneth A. Newell, M.D., Craig Hackworth, M.D., Jordan Rosenbloom, M.D., and Jeff Leef, M.D.

POLYTETRAFLUOROETHYLENE (PTFE) ARTERIOVENOUS (A-V) grafts remain the most common type of vascular access for patients on hemodialysis. Stenotic lesions, located within the A-V graft (intragraft), at the level of the venous anastomosis, or in the distal vein, remain the primary cause of A-V graft loss and failure. Initial approaches for correction or salvage consisted of surgical approaches (patch angioplasty or PTFE bypass grafts). Over the past decade, percutaneous balloon angioplasty has proved to be an acceptable alternative to surgical correction of stenotic lesions.[1-4] Percutaneous balloon angioplasty, however, is often complicated by significant rates of recurrent stenosis.[1-4] More recently, metallic endovascular stents have been developed as a means for maintaining vascular patency following balloon angioplasty of arterial and venous lesions and in creation of transhepatic internal portosystemic shunts.[5,6] We have recently employed a combined surgical and radiologic approach for the management of A-V graft stenoses consisting of intraoperative balloon angioplasty (IBA) and postoperative endovascular stent (EVS) placement. Here we report our initial experience with this approach in patients with stenotic lesions associated with PTFE A-V grafts.

Materials and Methods

Intraoperative Balloon Angioplasty. A-V graft thrombectomy procedures were performed using two incisions, one in the arterial limb of the A-V graft and another near the venous anastomosis. A-V graft thrombectomy was performed using Fogarty embolectomy catheters, and the A-V graft was probed with coronary dilators. The caliber of individual stenoses was defined by the size of the smallest coronary dilator that offered resistance during passage. Mechanical dilatation of individual stenoses was performed with coronary dilators to a caliber of 3.5 mm. Balloon angioplasty was performed by introducing a balloon angioplasty catheter (Meditech, Watertown, Massachusetts) advanced via the graftotomy. Each stenosis was treated by three inflation procedures, after which a 5-mm coronary dilator was passed to assess the success of the angioplasty. Success of IBA was defined as an absence of (1) resistance to passage of a 5-mm coronary dilator and (2) evidence of stenosis on postoperative angiography. Following the IBA procedure, a heparin bolus was given (30 U/kg) and a constant infusion initiated (7 U/kg/hour).

Postoperative Angiography, Balloon Angioplasty, and Endovascular Stent Placement. Postoperative angiographic evaluation was performed in each patient. The goal of these studies was to evaluate the entire A-V graft, and distal and central venous anatomy. Treatment of residual stenoses consisted of repeat balloon angioplasty and EVS placement. EVSs were placed via a percutaneous approach using the Seldinger technique; they were premounted on balloon angioplasty catheters, advanced into position under fluoroscopic guidance, and secured into position by balloon inflation. The stents consisted of the Wallstent (Schneider, Minneapolis, Minnesota) and the Palmaz stent. (Johnson & Johnson Interventional Systems, Warren, New Jersey).

Follow-up Studies. Following IBA, A-V grafts were reassessed at one and three months post-IBA by angiography. Additional studies were performed when patients demonstrated increasing venous pressures on hemodialysis or decreasing dialysis efficiency (increased recirculation times).

Results

IBA was performed in 20 patients, including 12 females and 8 males. As with our dialysis patient population in general, most were elderly, with an average age of 57.9 ± 14.7 years. Median follow-up post-IBA was nine months.

Most A-V grafts were forearm loop grafts. In addition, six upper-arm loop grafts and two upper-arm straight grafts were treated by IBA (figure 13-1). Venous outflow in forearm loop grafts was relatively equally divided among the basilic vein above and below the elbow and the cephalic vein below the elbow. At the time of IBA, 36 stenoses were identified. Of these, half were intragraft stenoses, 15 were venous anastomotic stenoses, and three were located in the distal vein (figure 13-2). IBA successfully treated each intragraft stenosis, as postoperative angiography revealed no

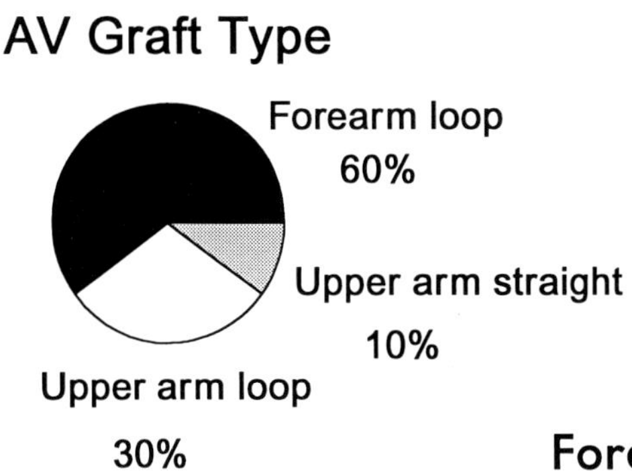

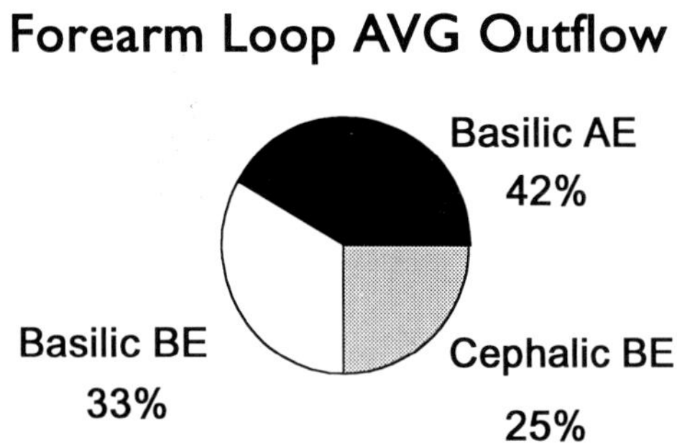

Figure 13-1. A-V graft configuration and venous outflow distribution of forearm loop A-V grafts. AE = above elbow, BE = below elbow.

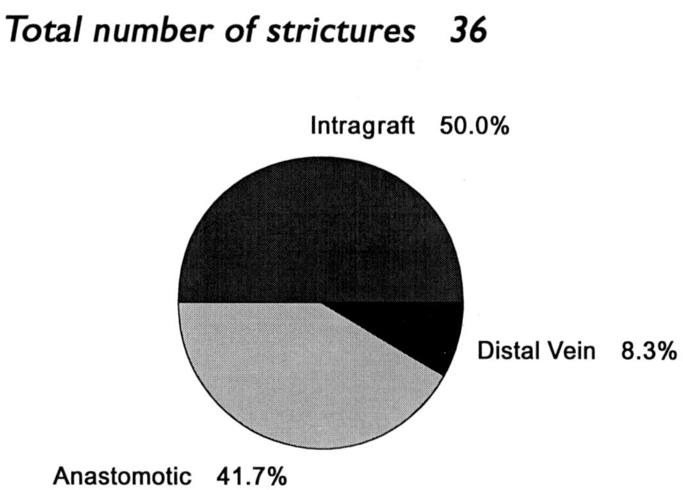

Figure 13-2. Distribution of stenoses identified at the time of intraoperative balloon angioplasty.

intragraft stenoses (figure 13-3). However, postoperative angiography revealed residual stenosis in 46% of venous anastomotic lesions, providing an overall success rate of 77%. EVS placement was performed in 35% of patients in the immediate postoperative period. An additional 30% of patients required EVS placement at a later point.

A-V graft thrombosis occurred at a rate of one per 6.9 patient months. Analysis of current A-V graft status revealed that 80% of A-V grafts are patent (figure 13-4). Of the four A-V grafts that were lost, two were lost to recurrent stenosis and A-V graft thrombosis, and one each was lost to inflow stenosis and to infection.

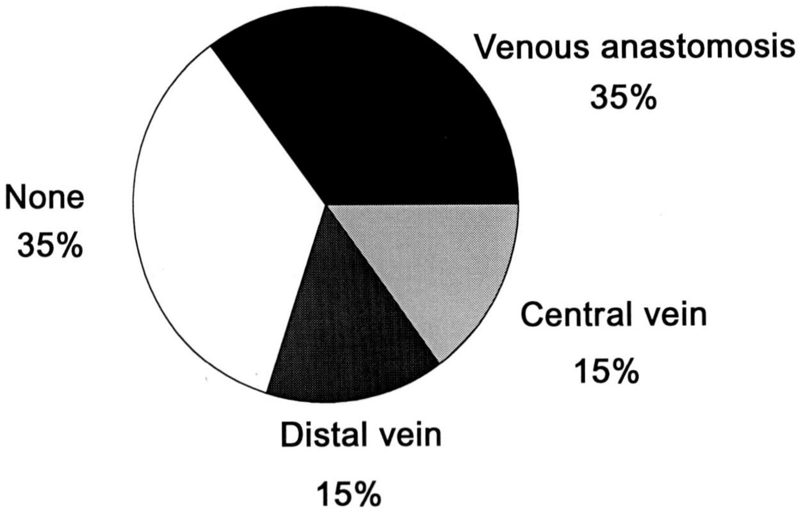

Figure 13-3. Distribution of venous stenoses identified at the time of immediate postoperative balloon angioplasty.

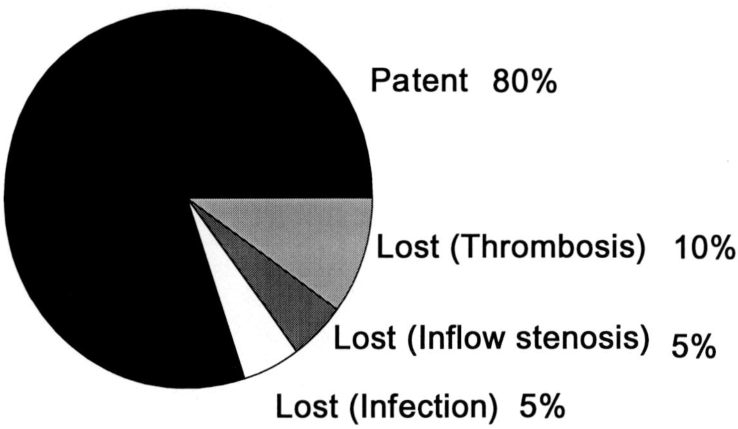

Figure 13-4. Current status of A-V grafts following intraoperative balloon angioplasty ± EVS placement.

Discussion

Our experience with IBA revealed significant differences between intragraft and venous anastomotic stenoses. Intragraft stenoses were successfully treated in all patients and did not recur, suggesting that IBA may be the therapeutic modality of choice for these lesions. Venous anastomotic stenoses, however, were successfully treated by intraoperative angioplasty alone in only 56% of patients, thus requiring additional intervention in about half of the patients. These observations indicate that fundamental differences exist between intragraft stenoses and venous anastomotic stenoses with respect to recurrence following balloon angioplasty.

Table 13-1. A-V Graft Thrombosis Following Intraoperative Balloon Angioplasty

	No. patients
No A-V graft thrombosis episodes	7
One A-V graft thrombosis episode	7
Two A-V graft thrombosis episodes	2
Three A-V graft thrombosis episodes	3
Four A-V graft thrombosis episodes	1

The patency rate following IBA was comparable to that previously reported following surgical revision and/or percutaneous balloon angioplasty procedures.[1-4,7] As with other approaches, maintenance of A-V graft patency required subsequent interventions, (table 13-1), as the A-V graft thrombosis rate following intraoperative balloon angioplasty was one episode per 6.9 patient-months. Of the 20 A-V grafts, only two were lost to recurrent stenosis and thrombosis. The observation that long-term patency is comparable to other approaches indicates that EVSs may perform in the peripheral venous circulation with an efficiency that approaches that observed in more central veins.

Complications observed with IBA and postoperative endovascular stenting were low. Vascular perforations were low, and EVS migration was not observed. Although all patients were treated with heparin to avoid perioperative A-V graft thrombosis, perioperative bleeding from the wound or other sites was not observed. It is likely that the low incidence of bleeding complications may be related to the relatively low doses of heparin that were administered. Currently, heparinization is continued for a total of only 12 hours following IBA or postoperative EVS placement. Indeed, heparin therapy may prove to be unnecessary with future experience.

The patency rates observed in this study may have been achieved in part due to the assiduous monitoring by routine postoperative angiography that was performed not only in the immediate postoperative period but also during the first three months after IBA. Similarly, the thorough evaluation of each A-V graft (including assessment of both the arterial and venous limbs in addition to the venous anastomosis) and the distal venous circulation (including the distal arm veins and the central veins) may have contributed to the observed success rates.

IBA may offer several advantages over standard surgical approaches for the correction of stenotic lesions. One advantage may be a reduction in operating time. Although data were not presented regarding operating time, each IBA procedure took less than 15 minutes to perform, and most took less than 10 minutes. In contrast, surgical revision may take 45 minutes or more for completion. IBA may also provide the additional advantage of avoidance of additional incisions and/or dissection, thus may decrease patient morbidity. Finally, IBA may provide the additional advantage of salvage of vein length by avoidance of PTFE bypass procedures for surgical correction.

This experience indicates that intraoperative balloon angioplasty provides a viable alternative to surgical correction of stenoses associated with PTFE A-V grafts for hemodialysis access. Further study is warranted, and should include comparison with established surgical approaches.

References

1. Rodriguez-Perez JC, Maynar M, Rams A, et al. Percutaneous transluminal angioplasty as best treatment in stenosis of vascular access for hemodialysis. Nephron 1989; 51:192-196.
2. Glanz S, Gordon DH, Butt KM, Hong J, Lipkowitz GS. The role of percutaneous angioplasty in the management of chronic hemodialysis fistulas. Ann Surg 1987; 206(6):777-781.
3. Smith TP, Cragg AH, Castaneda F, Hunter DW. Thrombosed polytetrafluorethylene hemodialysis fistulas: salvage with combined thrombectomy and angioplasty. Radiol 1989; 171:507-508.
4. Dapunt O, Feurstein M, Rendl KH, Prenner K. Transluminal angioplasty versus conventional operation in the treatment of haemodialysis fistula stenosis: results from a 5-year study. Br J Surg 1987; 74(11):1004-1005.
5. Zollikofer CL, Largiader I, Bruhlmann WF, Uhlschmid GK, Marty AH. Endovascular stenting of veins and grafts: preliminary clinical experience. Radiol 1988; 167(3):707-712.
6. Woodle ES, Darcy M, White HM, et al. Intrahepatic portosystemic vascular stents: a bridge to hepatic transplantation. Surgery 1993; 113:344-351.
7. Palder SB, Kirkman RL, Whittemore AD, Hakim RM, Lazarus JM, Tilney NL. Vascular access for hemodialysis. Ann Surg 1985; 202(2):235-239.

14

PROXIMAL ARTERIAL WAVEFORM AS AN INDICATOR OF FUNCTIONAL SIGNIFICANCE IN COLOR DOPPLER IMAGING OF THE A-V FISTULA FOR HEMODIALYSIS

William W. Harkrider, M.D., R.V.T.,
and Michel E. Comeaux, R.N., B.S.N., R.D.M.S.

PREDICTION OF VASCULAR ACCESS THROMBOSIS appears to be important in the prolongation of vascular access survival. Anatomic variation and stenosis of the prosthetic arteriovenous (A-V) fistula for hemodialysis is readily discernible with color Doppler imaging. The functional significance of these findings has yet to be defined.[1,2]

Materials and Methods

Retrospective analysis of color Doppler studies, both hard copy and real-time video tapes, were made of two selected groups of patients with A-V fistulas. The first, or "normal" group, was defined as patients without significant abnormalities in Doppler studies who had maintained a patent A-V fistula for longer than six months from the time of the Doppler study. The second, or "abnormal" A-V fistula group, was defined as those with significant abnormalities as shown by Doppler, thrombosed, and/or those who had surgically proven high-grade stenoses of the fistula within one month of the study.

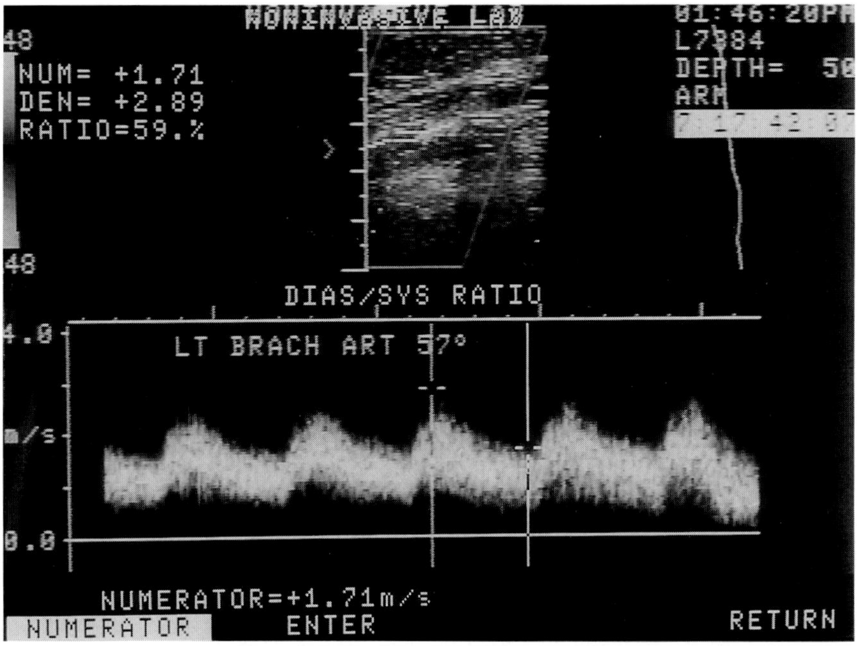

Figure 14-1. "Normal" A-V fistula with increased diastolic flow and a ratio > 0.4.

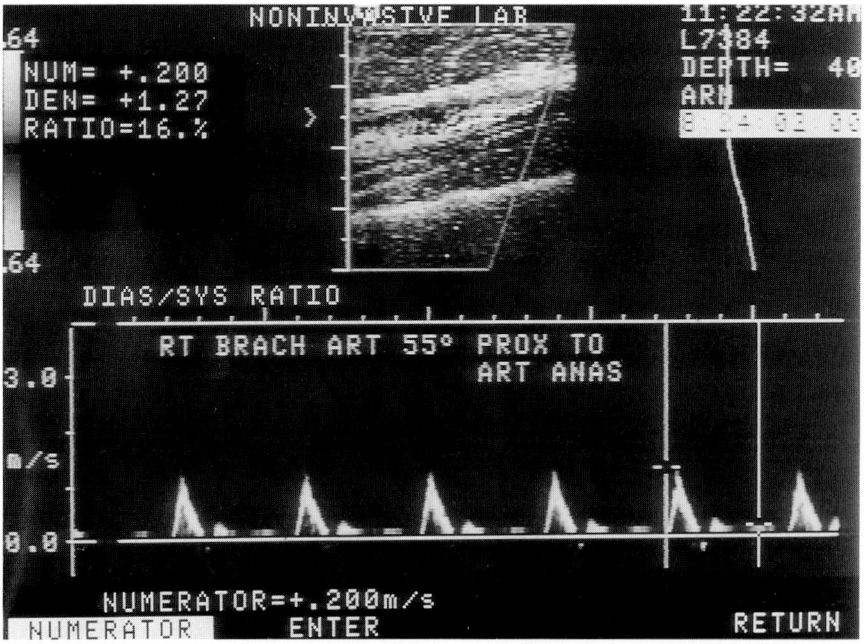

Figure 14-2. "Abnormal" A-V fistula with decreased diastolic flow and a ratio < 0.2.

Doppler imaging was performed in the supine position beginning with the subclavian vein, bilaterally, using a 5-MHz transducer equipped with a pulsed Doppler. A 7.5 MHz transducer equipped with a pulsed Doppler was used for evaluation of the upper extremity to include documentation of the proximal artery, the arterial anastomosis, the arterial and venous limb of the graft, the venous anastomosis, and the distal vein (proximal arm). Longitudinal and transverse planes were used with gray scale and color. The color pattern proximal to the graft, within the graft, and distal to the graft was scrutinized. Color patterns were divided into categories of solid (red or blue), mixed (combination of red and blue), or mosaic (turbulent with all colors of the spectrum). Doppler waveform samples were obtained at the sites mentioned, as well as of the contralateral brachial artery, in an attempt to determine whether a specific Doppler waveform pattern existed. The velocity waveform was obtained using an angle of ≤60º. The peak-diastolic-to-peak-systolic ratios were calculated and recorded. The diameter measurement of the arterial and venous limb about 1 cm from the anastomosis was recorded.

The group of 26 patients studied between August 1990 and August 1992 consisted of 16 females and 10 males with an age range of 28 to 80 and a mean age of 64. Twenty (77%) patients had a history of hypertension. Twelve (46%) were diabetics. The age of the graft at the time of the study varied from one month to three years. The patency from the time of the scan of the normal group of patients ranged from six months to two years and four months. The graft material was polytetrafluoroethylene (PTFE) and the configuration was forearm loop in all but two patients. Of these two patients, one had a Brescia-Cimino fistula and one had an upper-arm straight graft.

Results

Color pattern was inconsistent within the graft itself of each patient as well as between the two groups. Velocity measurements were nonspecific except with isolated increases in or near obvious obstructions when compared to the velocity proximal or distal to this area. The proximal arterial waveform 1 cm from the arterial anastomosis was that of a low-resistant artery (high diastolic flow) for all of those patients in the "normal" group (figure 14-1). In contrast, the "abnormal A-V fistula" group had a proximal arterial waveform of a high-resistant vascular bed approaching that of the contralateral brachial artery. The peak-diastolic-to-peak-systolic ratio in the "normal" group was ≥0.4. In contrast, the "abnormal" peak-diastolic-to-peak-systolic ratio was ≤0.3 (figure 14-2).

Discussion and Conclusion

Much has been written about the noninvasive evaluation of A-V grafts in hemodialysis access. However, consistent findings and concrete criteria that predict thrombosis have yet to be defined.

The A-V fistula for hemodialysis is an abnormal communication of a high-resistant peripheral artery to a low-resistant peripheral vein. The expected change in the proximal artery waveform is from a low diastolic flow to that of a high diastolic flow.[3,4] This can be readily documented with color Doppler imaging of the proximal artery. The peak systolic velocity and the peak diastolic velocity are easily measured with modern technology.

As the "normal" fistula progresses to the "abnormal" fistula as demonstrated by increased resistance and decreased flow within the fistula, the proximal artery reflects this with a decrease in the diastolic flow. Occlusion of the A-V fistula returns the arterial waveform to the presurgery high-resistant peripheral artery.

This observation was apparent in this limited retrospective study. The peak-diastolic-to-peak-systolic ratio is a simplistic number that is easily obtained and repeatable; it appears to have some value in predicting A-V fistula thrombosis. Further studies using this ratio in addition to other parameters (i.e., percent of stenosis, volume of flow, etc.) should demonstrate increased accuracy in predicting graft thrombosis.

Isolated stenosis of the A-V fistula graft can adequately be defined by color Doppler imaging. The functional significance of this stenosis or stenoses should be guided by the proximal arterial reflector of the distal vascular bed.

References

1. Strauch BS, O'Connell RS, Geoly KL, Grundelhuner M, Yakub N, Tietjen DP. Forecasting thrombosis of vascular access with Doppler color flow imaging. Am J Kidney Dis 1992; 19(6):554-57.
2. Tordoir JH, de Bruin HG, Hoeneveld H, Eikelboom BC, Kitslarr PJ. Duplex ultrasound scanning in the assessment of arteriovenous fistulas created for hemodialysis access: comparison with digital subtraction angiography. J Vasc Surg 1989; 10:122-28.
3. Nonnast-Daniel B, Martin RP, Lindert O, et al. Colour Doppler assessment of arteriovenous haemodialysis fistulas. Lancet 1992; 339:143-45.
4. Riedhammer HH, Weise A. Die dopplersonographicische Beurteilung der Thrombosegefahrdung bei artriovenosen Fieteln. Nieren Hockdrukkrank 1988; 17:85-92.

15

THE EFFICACY OF DISCHARGING RENAL PATIENTS WITH A VENOUS CATHETER IN PLACE FOR HEMODIALYSIS TREATMENTS

Clive O. Callender, M.D., Bert Williams, M.D., Charles Murigande, Ph.D., Roger Wilmer Jr., Joel Stevens, M.D., and Oswald Warner, M.D.

CATHETERIZATION OF THE SUBCLAVIAN VEIN was introduced in the late 1970s to provide temporary vascular access for acute hemodialysis. Although it has proven to be a relatively safe and effective procedure, long-term complications can result from human error, causing stenosis or thrombosis of the subclavian vein and pneumothorax.

Femoral vein catheterization is also a popular choice for venous access in patients requiring hemodialysis, because it is easier to control complications. In addition, femoral catheterization avoids the complication of pneumothorax. Like subclavian vein catheterization, this method has its share of complications. Such complications include puncture site hematoma, arteriovenous (A-V) fistulas, and femoral nerve damage. Because of the associated complications, few, if any, patients were discharged from the Howard University Hospital dialysis/transplant center (Washington, D.C.) with subclavian or femoral catheters in place until 1988.

In the interest of meeting the patient's health care needs and decreasing health care costs, the unit modified its management of patients requiring venous catheters for dialysis. In this report, we demonstrate that there is no difference in complications requiring hospitalization (morbidity) or mortality between patients discharged with venous catheters in place and those hospitalized until the venous catheter is no longer needed. We also show that discharging patients with the venous catheter in place decreases the length of hospital stay, thus lowering health care costs. Our data

Table 15.1. Increasing Outpatient Dialysis Sessions from Era 1 to Era 3

Era	No. patients	No. dialysis sessions	No. inpatient sessions	No. outpatient sessions	% outpatient sessions
1	94	950	758	192	20.21%
2	94	906	632	274	30.24%
3	123	883	484	399	45.00%

Table 15-2. Table of Era by Type of Dialysis

Frequency expected cell chi-square row %	Inpatient	Outpatient	Total
86-88	758	192	950
88-90	632	274	906
90-92	484	399	883
Total	1,874	865	2,739

p1/i = the probability of an inpatient dialysis given the era i (i=1 for 86-88, i=2 for 88-90 and i=3 for 90-92). We are testing homogeneity hypothesis given by:
Ho : p1/1 = p1/2 = p1/3 = p
p1/1 = 0.798
p1/2 = 0.697
p1/3 = 0.548
This test was carried out by chi-square, and we rejected the hypothesis of homogeneity with p value < 0.0001 (chi-square = 133.245 df = 2).

clearly indicate that there is no difference in complications between subclavian vein and femoral vein catheterization in patients who are discharged early.

Materials and Methods

A retrospective analysis was performed on 311 patients who were identified from a list of 700 patients as having end-stage renal disease (ESRD) and having Shiley catheter (Vas-Cath, Quinton) placement at the transplant/dialysis center. This study excluded patients whose database on the Shiley catheter was incomplete or absent. The 311 patients were chosen from three two-year periods—1986-88, 1988-90, 1990-92. Each patient's database was analyzed for the following information: (1) number of days catheterized, (2) number of days the patients was discharged or hospitalized with the catheter in place, (3) number of dialyses performed using the Shiley catheter in hospitalized versus discharged patients, and (4) total dialysis time in hospitalized versus discharged patients. The data were then used to compare the three two-year periods, allowing us to evaluate the overall efficacy of discharging patients with Shiley catheter in place. Statistical significance was identified by chi-square test.

Table 15-3. Table of Era by Complications

Frequency expected cell chi-square Row %	Inpatient	Outpatient	Total
86-88	11	4	15
88-90	5	4	9
90-92	7	4	11
Total	23	12	35

We could not reject the hypothesis of homogeneity (p value = 0.664). Therefore, there is no evidence that the probability of complications requiring patients to be hospitalized differs between inpatients and outpatients from era to era.

Table 15-4. Complications, Subclavian versus Femoral Catheterization

Era	Subclavian catheterization (%)	Femoral catheterization (%)
1	54	46
2	45	55
3	45	55

Table 15-5. Complication Rate per Era, Inpatient versus Outpatient

Era	Inpatient rate (%)	Outpatient rate (%)
1	12	4
2	5	4
3	6	3

Results and Discussion

The results of our examination are shown in the accompanying tables and figures. Table 15-1 shows how the percentage of dialysis treatments given on an outpatient basis grew from era 1 to era 3.

In reviewing the literature, we found that the subject of discharging patients with venous catheters in place had not been addressed. Because this was being done at our institution, we decided to present the results seen with our patients and in turn show that it is an efficacious practice. From the results in table 15-2 it can be seen that the probability of an inpatient dialysis via venous catheter decreased from era 1 to era 2. This confirms the fact that more patients were being discharged with venous catheters in place and dialyzed as outpatients. Table 15-3 shows that there was no difference in complications requiring hospitalization from era to era. We also show that the percentage of patients being dialyzed as outpatients increased from era 1 to era 3 (table 15-4 and figure 15-1). In terms of health care cost (figure 15-2), there is a $75,000 decrease in hospital bed cost (for dialysis days only) from era 1 to era 3.

Our study also demonstrates that subclavian and femoral catheterization did not differ in terms of complications requiring hospitalization (table 15-4). In addition, the overall complication rate decreased from era 1 to era 2 (table 15-5). The most

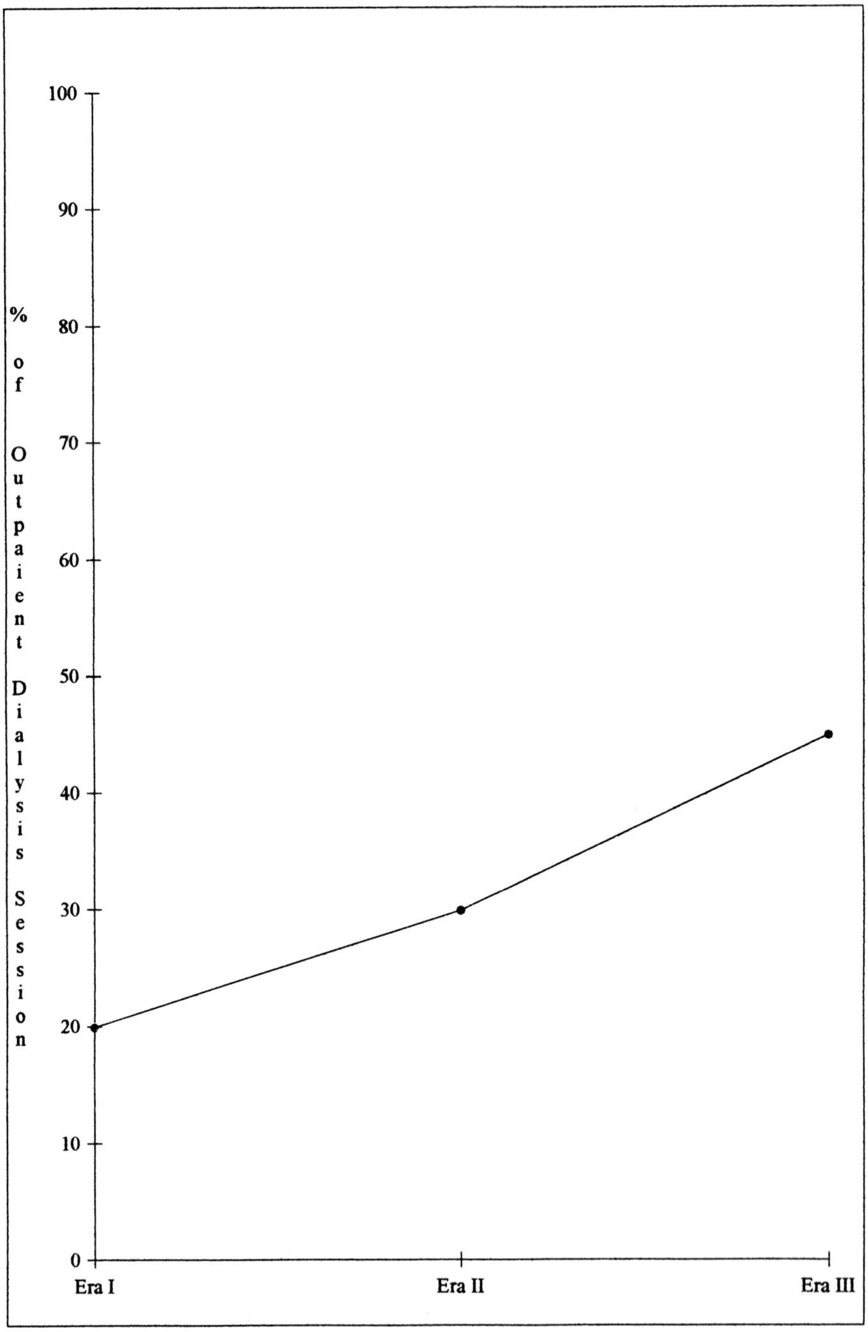

Figure 15-1. Increase in percentage of patients dialyzed as outpatients, era 1 to era 3.

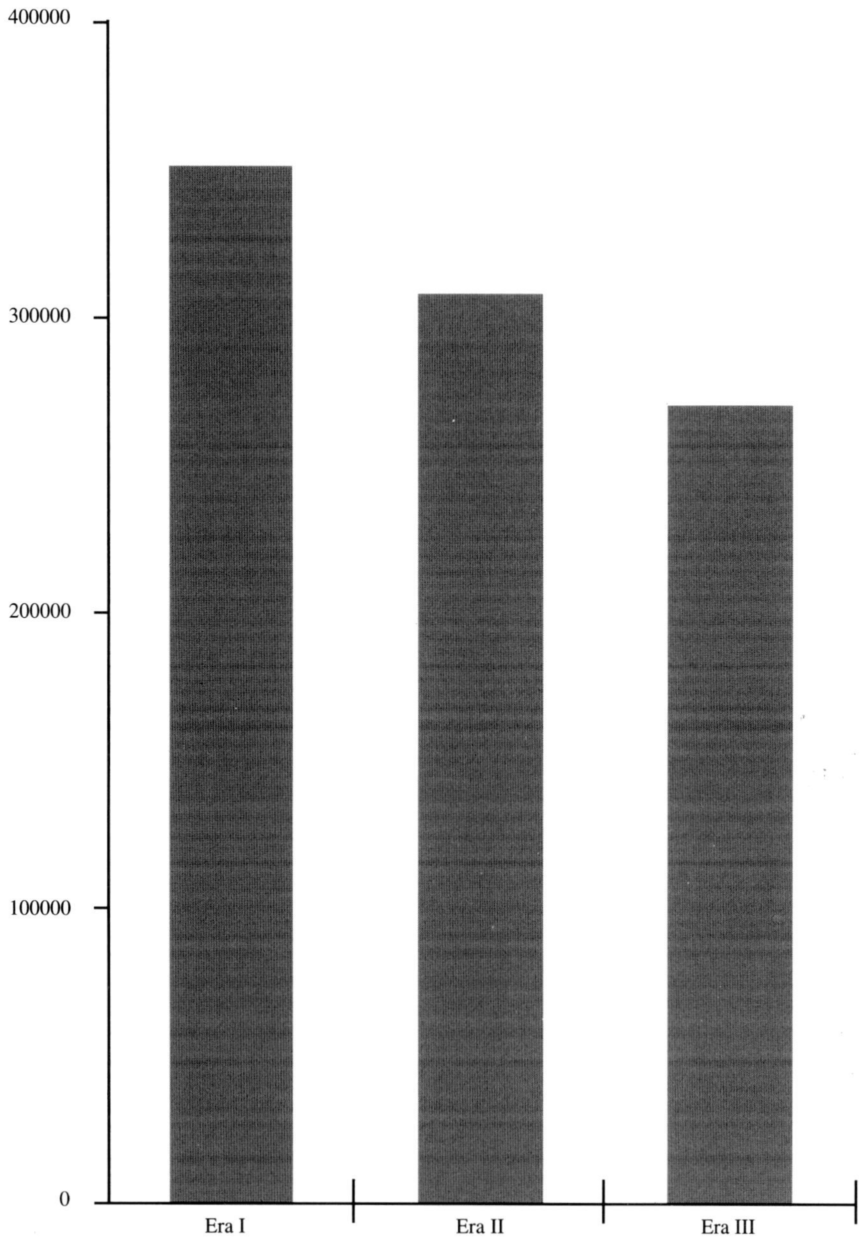

Figure 15-2. Decrease in hospital bed cost (dialysis days only) was $75,000 from era 1 to era 3.

Table 15-6. Complications Requiring Hospitalization

Complication	No.	% of Total
Thrombosis	16	46
Infection	11	31
Accidental removal of catheter	8	23
Total	35	

common complication requiring hospitalization was thrombosis followed by infection (table15-6). The least common complication requiring hospitalization was accidental removal of the catheter.

We conclude that there is no statistically significant difference in complications requiring hospitalization between inpatients and outpatients from era 1 to era 3. The results also show that discharging patients with a catheter for dialysis decreases hospitalization time and thus health care cost. In addition, there was no significant difference between complications seen in subclavian versus femoral venous catheters. We further conclude that discharging patients with venous catheters in place is a safe, efficacious practice.

References

1. Fant GF, Dennis VW, Quarles LD. Late vascular complications of the subclavian dialysis catheter. Am J Kid Dis 1986; VII(3):225-228.
2. Nand N, Scott SJ, Main J. Successful hemodialysis via an unusually sited subclavian catheter. Int J Artif Organs 1991; 14:97-98.
3. Alarabi A, Eklund T, Claesson K, Wikstrom B, Danielson BG. Experience with vascular access for acute renal failure: using Buselmeier shunt and femoral vessel catheter. Nephron 1991; 58:192-195.
4. Palmisano BW, Clifford PS, Coon RL. Chronic vascular catheters in growing piglets. J Dev Physiol 1989; 12:363-367.
5. de Los Angeles A, Lerner A, Goldstein SJ, Kramer MS, Raja RM. Comparison of coaxial and side by side double lumen subclavian catheters with single lumen catheter. Am J Kidney & Kidney Dis 1986; VII(3):221-224.
6. Gibson SP, Mosquera DA, O'Donnell MJ, Odurny A. Streptokinase in the treatment of innominate-vein thrombosis association with hemodialysis catheter. Preservation of a precious arteriovenous fistula. Nephrol Dialysis Transplant 1991; 6:206-208.
7. Carlisle EJF, Blake P, McCarthy F, Vas S, Uldall R. Septicemia in long-term jugular hemodialysis catheters: eradicating infection by changing the catheter over a guidewire. Int J Artif Organs 1991; 14(3):150-153.
8. Yerdel MA, Karayalcin K, Naras, Bozathi L, Idirm EY, Anadol E. Mechanical complications of subclavian vein catheterization. A prospective study. Int Surg 1991; 76:18-22.

16

THE USE OF UROKINASE IN PERMANENT DOUBLE-LUMEN JUGULAR HEMODIALYSIS CATHETERS

Alan G. Wasserstein, M.D., Kenneth L. Brayman, M.D., Sidney M. Kobrin, M.D., Mark Phalen, M.D., and Charlotte Thomas-Hawkins, R.N.

DACRON-CUFFED SILASTIC CATHETERS inserted into jugular or subclavian veins have come into widespread use for intermediate and long-term hemodialysis.[1-4] In a survey of hemodialysis patients with permanent double-lumen catheters (PDLCS), recurrent thrombosis occurred in 24%. Urokinase (UK) was required in 14% of patients one to two times per month, in 9% once to twice a week, and in 4% at every treatment.[2] In another study, UK was required for clotting or poor flow in 46% of patients, but no catheter was lost because of thrombosis.[5] In a third series, 30% of catheters were removed because of thrombosis or poor flow.[3] Uldall et al. have recommended aspirin in all patients with PDLCS, with the addition of warfarin when thrombosis occurs, and I.V. high-dose UK (250,000 U) for acute thrombosis.[5] In the previously noted survey, only 10% of patients with such catheters were receiving some form of anticoagulation agent.[2]

We report here our experience with UK in maintaining patency of PDLCS. Because we have been reluctant to employ anticoagulation in dialysis patients because of their propensity to bleed, we have relied on UK in large amounts to maintain patency. We have had no bleeding complications, but extensive use of UK has been expensive.

Materials and Methods

We examined the use of UK in PDLCS in the outpatient dialysis unit of the Hospital of the University of Pennsylvania for the period of October 1 through

Table 16-1. Patient Characteristics

	Required urokinase	No urokinase
Number	28	21
Age	58.0	57.6
M:F	9:19	11:10
Diabetes+/–	9:19	3:18
Hct (%)	30.6	29.3
Blood flow (ml/min) prescribed	404	426
Blood flow (ml/min) delivered	311*	357

*p <0.01 compared with patients who did not receive UK

Table 16-2. Total Urokinase Administration

	Low-dose	High-dose
Treatments given (%)	116 (6)	43 (2)
No. same-day low-dose UK	—	11
Same-day low-dose UK	—	32
No. doses	343	43
Doses per treatment (U)	2.95 (22.1K)	1 (250K)
Elapsed time to next UK (days)	12.2	12.8
Total UK (U)	2,572,500	10,750,000

December 31, 1993. Catheters (Permacath, Quinton, Seattle, Washington) were inserted because of failure of peripheral access in most cases and in some cases because of impaired cardiac output, advanced age, or patient preference. Catheters were inserted in the internal or external jugular vein by the surgical or interventional radiology service. Tip placement was in the right atrium or at its junction with the superior vena cava. Target blood flow rate was 300 ml/min or more. Kt/V was targeted at 1.3 for patients whose dialysis lasted three and one-half hours or more and 1.5 for patients with shorter dialysis times. Catheters were instilled with heparin (1,000 U/ml) at the end of dialysis in an amount sufficient to fill each lumen to its tip (1.5 ml). Catheter dressings were changed under sterile conditions at each treatment.

UK was administered in either low or high dose for absence of flow or poor flow (250 ml/min). UK was instilled in low dose (5,000 U/ml) in one or both lumens in a volume (1.5 ml) sufficient to fill the lumen to the tip. After 20 minutes the catheter was used. If adequate flow was not restored, low-dose UK was instilled repeatedly in one or both lumens to a maximum of three instillations per lumen. If low-dose UK did not restore flow, high-dose urokinase was administered. High-dose UK consisted of 12,500 U to each lumen by infusion over 30 minutes, followed by immediate use of the catheter. High-dose UK was given initially (without prior low-dose UK) if the patient had received low-dose UK during recent dialysis treatments or if blood flow rate had been unsatisfactory after low-dose UK at previous treatment. The choice of low- or high-dose UK was at the discretion of the nursing staff. If flow was not restored, the need for dialysis on that day was assessed and, if dialysis could be postponed, the patient was told to return on the following day for treatment.

Table 16-3. Distribution of Urokinase Administration

No. treatments (%)	No. patients Low-dose	No. patients High-dose	Total UK (U)
1–2(2.5–5.0)	10	11	4,344,000
3–4(7.5–10)	5	6	5,650,000
5–6(12.5–15)	8	1	2,368,000
7–8(17.5–20)	2	0	332,000
9–10(22.5–25)	3	0	631,000
Totals	28	18	13,325,000

Table 16-4. Frequency of Urokinase Administration

	Frequency (%) Never	0.3–2x/mo	2.1–3.3x/mo
Low-dose	43	47	10
High-dose	63	37	0

Table 16-5. Urokinase Cost and Reimbursement

	Cost*
Low-dose	$11,456.08
High-dose	12,726.29
Total	24,182.37
Reimbursement	23,261.26
Profit (loss)	($ 1,896.11)

*Does not include staff time and materials

Results

Forty-nine patients in the period of study had PDLCs for maintenance dialysis (32% of the hemodialysis population), and 28 (70%) received UK on at least one occasion. Characteristics of patients with PDLCs are given in table 16-1. Patients with catheters were older than those with peripheral vascular access (58 versus 54 years, respectively). There was no difference in age, sex, hematocrit, or presence of diabetes mellitus between patients who did or did not receive UK. Lower blood flow rate was prescribed (NS) and delivered ($p < 0.01$) in patients who received UK.

Total UK administration is summarized in table 16-2. Low-dose UK was administered at 116 treatments (6% of all treatments of patients with PDLCs). High-dose UK was administered at 43 treatments (2%), following low-dose UK at 11 treatments and without prior (same day) low-dose UK in 32 treatments. Elapsed time to the next use of UK was 12.2 days following low-dose UK and 12.8 days following high-dose UK. Low-dose UK was given in a dose of 7,500-37,500 U per treatment in which low-dose UK was used (mean 22,125 U, or 2.95 doses/treatment). Although low-dose UK was used more frequently than high-dose UK, the latter accounted for the bulk of UK administered.

The distribution of UK administrations is shown in tables 16-3 and 16-4. Seventy percent and 45% of patients required low-dose and high-dose UK, respectively, at least once in the period of study. Surprisingly, the group of patients with the highest rate of UK administration did not account for the bulk of UK usage (table 16-3).

Cost and reimbursement for UK are given in table 16-5. Despite the disparity of use of low-dose and high-dose UK, total expenditures for each dosage level were comparable. Reimbursement did not cover cost of UK, and this shortfall would be greater if staff time and materials were included.

In all but four instances, dialysis was given on the day that UK was administered. In these four cases, dialysis was performed via PDLC on the following day, presumably because UK had resulted in clot lysis overnight. Dialysis time was lost on the day that UK was used. In patients who required UK, duration of dialysis was 3.21 hours on days when UK was administered and 3.63 hours on days when UK was not needed (difference: 25 minutes or 11%, p=0.025).

Twelve patients received warfarin 1.0 - 7.5 mg daily, beginning in one patient prior to and in 11 during the period of study. Target prothrombin time was 13-14 seconds. Four patients received aspirin, beginning in two patients prior to and in two during the period of study. Two patients of the 12 who received warfarin did not require UK. When warfarin or aspirin was started during the period of study, no effect on frequency of administration of UK was observed (data not shown), but the period of observation was too brief to have shown a significant change. No bleeding complications were encountered.

Discussion

Use of UK in this study was successful in that catheter patency was maintained and catheter life was prolonged. However, the frequency of use of UK was higher than has been reported previously.[2,5] Presumably, this increased requirement is due at least in part to minimal use of anticoagulants. Even in the few cases in which warfarin was prescribed, the prothrombin time was only minimally increased. The use of anticoagulants is often contraindicated in dialysis patients because of the potential bleeding diathesis. On the other hand, the bleeding diathesis of dialysis patients is probably less than in former years because of widespread use of recombinant erythropoietin. The current study suggests that PDLCs are associated with high UK utilization and increased costs but with minimal loss of dialysis time. Assuming the frequency of PDLCs in the hemodialysis population is 15%[2] and the size of the hemodialysis population to be 150,000, the annual cost of UK in the United States at our rate of use would be $66 million. This figure does not include use of UK in declotting peripheral vascular access or temporary central venous catheters. Even if the use of UK can be reduced by oral anticoagulants, UK is a significant expense of hemodialysis.

Our study shows that it is possible to use UK on the day of dialysis to achieve adequate blood flow rate with only moderate loss of dialysis time. As compared with the study of Uldall et al., we did not use high-dose UK exclusively and did not wait three to four hours for effect. We were able to use low-dose UK on many occasions, with savings in the total dose of UK administered. If UK had been administered at high dose levels at every treatment where required, total UK administration would have been 39,750,000 U (159 treatments x 250,000 U/treatment), a threefold increase. Cost would have been $46,905 (159 treatments x $295/treatment), a twofold increase. Since the use of high-dose (rather than low-dose) UK did not prolong the time until UK was again required, low-dose UK apparently reduced cost. However, it is possible that we used high-dose UK only when clot had become more extensive, and that more liberal use of high dose UK would have reduced the total number of UK uses. An optimal algorithm of UK administration would require direct comparison of alternative protocols.

Delivered dialysis was less in patients with PDLCs who required UK. Both blood flow rate and duration of dialysis were reduced. Thirty percent of treatments were shortened by 11%, an overall reduction of 3.3%. Missed dialysis time and erratic blood flow could increase dialysis morbidity and mortality in the long term. Patients with PDLCs, especially those who require UK, are at risk for underdialysis. We recommend vigilance for this complication and a safety margin in dialysis prescription.

Anticoagulants would, if effective, reduce the inconvenience and expense of UK administration. Our data do not permit any assessment of the efficacy of oral anticoagulation in maintaining catheter patency.

Summary and Conclusions

Thirty-two percent of hemodialysis patients used PDLCs for vascular access, and 57% of them required UK at least once in a three-month period.

Repeated use of low-dose UK (7,500 U/lumen, 2.95 doses/treatment) restored catheter patency and function at most dialysis treatments on the day of dialysis. Time to next UK administration was similar with low-dose and high-dose UK. Repeated administration of low-dose UK allowed substantially less total UK use than did less frequent use of high-dose UK.

Patients with PDLCs have a shortfall of delivered dialysis. As a result of decreased dialysis duration and blood flow rate, this shortfall is magnified in those who require UK.

Patients with PDLCs require repeated UK administration to restore catheter function and patency on the day of dialysis without increased risk of bleeding.

Underdialysis is a hazard of PDLCs, especially in patients who require UK.

Urokinase is a significant expense of hemodialysis. Repeated administration of low-dose UK, supplemented by high-dose UK when necessary, may be as efficacious and more economical than reliance on high-dose UK only.

References

1. Shusterman NH, Kloss K, Mullen JL. Successful use of double lumen, silicone rubber catheters for permanent hemodialysis access. Kidney Int 1989; 35:887-890.
2. Dunea G, Domenico L, Gunnerson P, Winston-Willis F. A survey of permanent double lumen catheters in hemodialysis patients. ASAIO Trans, 1991; 37:M276-M277.

3. Shaffer D, Madras PN, Wiliams ME, D'Elia JA, Kaldany A, Monaco AP. Use of Dacron cuffed silicone catheters as long-term hemodialysis access. ASAIO J 1992; 38:55-58.
4. McDowell DC, Moss AH, Vasilakis C, Ball R, Pillai L. Percutaneously placed dual lumen silicone catheters for long-term hemodialysis. Am Surg1993; 59:569-573.
5. Uldall R, Besley ME, Thomas A, Slater S, Nuezca LA, Vas M. Maintaining the patency of double-lumen silastic jugular catheters for hemodialysis. Int J Artif Organs 1993; 16:37-40.

DISCUSSION

Moderator:
Mitchell L. Henry, M.D.
Panelists:
William W. Harkrider, M.D., R.V.T.
P. Sabanayagam, M.D.
Alan G. Wasserstein, M.D.
Bert Williams, M.D.
E. Steve Woodle, M.D.

Discussant: I would like to thank Dr. Harkrider for his presentation, because it seems as though he has finally given us something that seems objective and reproducible to follow our grafts with the noninvasive lab. We have been just as disappointed with following velocities because of the turbulence. My question is to Dr. Woodle. Do you use any imaging when you do your intraoperative balloon angioplasty? If not, it seems as if we have now taken something that can be done in one setting with only one set-up fee and moved it into the O.R. with one set-up fee and then over to the angiography suite for a second set-up fee.

Dr. Woodle: No, we do not do any imaging. The only time we would do any imaging in the O.R. is when we re-perfuse a graft and are not happy with how the graft feels. We are concerned as to whether or not it will remain patent until we get down to the angiography suite. Then we will do an on-table angiogram to level the axilla. The reason that we went to doing balloon angioplasty in the O.R. was because we wanted to get away from the extra time that it required and the extra incision necessary to revise these grafts. Routinely, when we do a balloon angioplasty, we are out of the room in 30 to 45 minutes. The time we are in the O.R. is shorter than our turnover.

Discussant: We have started taking it out of the angiography suite entirely and moving it into the O.R. The turnover time is just as long, and we have found that we can thrombectomize a graft quickly on-table and then do our angiogram. If there is an anastomotic stenosis, we do not use balloon angioplasty; we either patch or revise them. If there is a more proximal venous stenosis, depending on the surgeon we either do our own balloon angioplasty or call the interventional radiologist to the O.R. to do it. Part of the key to that is we have a digital C-arm in the operating room that has imaging capability.

Dr. Woodle: We have stayed away from distal lesions, for the reason that we think that if you are going to address those in the operating room, that is where you must have imaging equipment. The perforation rate would be higher. The lesions in the graft or at the anastomoses are fairly fixed, encased in scar, but the ones that are distal have fairly tenuous support. We get the balloon across by dialating with coronary dilators up to about 3.5 mm. Then we can manually and semiblindly put the catheter across. As long as you are at the venous anastomoses, that is fine. However, I am not comfortable blindly putting a catheter across the distal venous lesion without a very high rate of perforation. The level of expertise that it takes to do an angioplasty on anintragraft lesion is minimal, but you have to have your catheter positioned properly and advanced accurately for a distal venous lesion. As a surgeon, I do not have extensive training in that and I do not do it. I would ask a radiologist do it.

Discussant: We have started doing our own, only because it seems that it is at an inconvenient time of the night and we cannot get an interventional radiologist. It is based upon having good imaging in the O.R.

Discussant: Dr. Williams, in your presentation you had some data on femoral vein catheters. Did you send home a significant number of patients with femoral vein catheters? If so, was their outcome the same?

Dr. Williams: We found that there was really no difference in the complications occurring in the femoral versus the subclavian.

Discussant: In your population, about what percentage of patients went home with femoral catheters?

Dr. Williams: I do not remember the exact numbers on my slide. When you look at the complications that occur, the percentage per catheter is equal. Almost 50% of our patients went home with femoral catheters.

Discussant: How long were they left in there without changing, and were the patients ambulatory?

Dr. Williams: On average, close to two weeks, the time it took for the graft to mature. Yes, they were ambulatory.

Discussant: One of the things that prompted this trial was that we had heard that patients cannot be discharged with femoral catheters, and many of the institutions in our area told us not to do it. But we had been doing it. Our institution is one in which most patients are dialyzed in house under constant watch, as opposed to a system under which they go to multiple community centers, so that made a difference.

Discussant: We have some six patients with the Cook catheter tunneled to exit from the anterior surface of the thigh 10 cm below and lateral to the insertion site in the ligament. These patients have been at home with catheters for two years at a stretch with very few problems. The thrombus obstruction rate we see with long-term femoral catheters is somewhat higher than that with jugular catheters. I do not think the femoral site is ideal for long-term catheters, but it is an alternative if you cannot use the jugular site. I have a question for Dr. Sabanayagam. I am not sure I fully understood some of the results of your very interesting work with the tapered graft. It seems to me that there are potential advantages to tapered grafts. I assume that if you are reducing the arterial blood flow into the graft because the tapering is at the arterial end, there should be a reduction in the incidence of steal syndromes and ischemia of the hand. Do you have any comparisons between standard grafts and tapered grafts in terms of reducing steal complications?

Dr. Sabanayagam: I showed a slide that compared the standard 6-mm graft with the tapered graft. There were nine instances in which we recorded steal syndrome that required some kind of surgical intervention with the standard straight, 6-mm graft. Six patients developed steal syndrome with the 4–7-mm tapered graft. The incidence was about 3.5% with the straight grafts (about 294 of them), while with the tapered graft it was about .5%.

Dr. Henry: Let me clarify that a bit. Where do you base your arterial takeoff with either the loop or straight grafts? Are they at the brachial artery or the branch of the brachial artery?

Dr. Sabanayagam: Virtually all of my grafts are straight grafts, so I have to use the radial artery or the brachial artery.

Dr. Henry: We take great care to take it off a branch of the brachial artery, and we rarely see steal with a standard 6-mm graft. I think that is probably a more important consideration when you look at steal rather than what graft you use.

Discussant: Dr. Sabanayagam, is your incidence of venous stenosis substantially less with the tapered graft than with the 6-mm graft?

Dr. Sabanayagam: The Reynold's number for the tapered graft is less compared to that of the straight graft. So, in theory, we should have less venous stenosis with the tapered graft compared with the straight graft. However, when I look at this large series followed over 15 years, the patency rates between these two look pretty much identical.

Dr. Henry: There is some compelling information in the lab that did in fact say you had less stenosis with the tapered graft, but I am not aware of any good clinical data published to demonstrate that there is a difference.

Discussant: Dr. Wasserstein, although you are using less urokinase per treatment, it did not seem to me that your total usage was costing less.

Dr. Wasserstein: Part of that is a function of the pricing structure. The large, 250,000-U vial costs $295, and the smaller vial, 5,000 U, is $34. You are getting 50 times more urokinase for only nine times the price. That is part of the reason for the difference in cost. It is very difficult to make cost comparisons. I am assuming that if we used high-dose urokinase every time it might have cost us more. On the other hand, we probably would not have needed repeated low doses of urokinase, and that would have lowered the cost. It is possible that if we used high-dose urokinase more frequently, we would have had better resolution of clot each time we used it. That would have had a cumulative effect of giving us better long-term results. So I am not going to argue that the low-dose was in fact more economical. I think you need a direct comparison.

Discussant: So your prime motive for using the low-dose was that it was safer?

Dr. Wasserstein: Yes, although it was also the economical aspect of it as well.

Discussant: One of the points you stressed was that the obstructed catheters waste dialysis time and patients get shortchanged in their dialysis time. If you have a patient who arrives for dialysis with an obstructed catheter, why don't you just sit them in a room somewhere with urokinase and put them on the next shift, then bring somebody else into the first shift?

Dr. Wasserstein: It is not always that easy. Transportation is a major issue in an inner-city dialysis unit. Also, we are often full, and scheduling other treatments on the same day is not always possible. I must say, I think our patients on urokinase are well dialyzed. We try to leave a generous and substantial margin in our dialysis prescription.

Discussant: From a nursing perspective, a catheter that needs to be treated with urokinase on such a regular basis is not a functional access. Did you look at the catheters with a contrast study to verify what the tip location is? Are they "sucking up" against the wall and causing obstruction?

Dr. Wasserstein: We did have that problem in some cases. I agree with you. It is not a good thing, but I think in any series you look at there are patients who have a high urokinase requirement. Even in Dr. Uldall's series, there is a fair urokinase requirement even in patients who are taking anticoagulants in reasonable doses. It is not an easy problem to eliminate.

Discussant: That is a very good point. If you are having to use urokinase very frequently, one should question the position of the tip and question anatomical items such as superior vena cava stenosis. We have simply moved the catheter from somewhat above the entrance to the right atrium down into the right atrium. This has solved the problem.

SECTION VI

17

PROLONGATION OF HEMODIALYSIS ACCESS SURVIVAL WITH ELECTIVE REVISION

Jeffrey J. Sands, M.D., and Carol L. Miranda, R.V.T.

FAILURE OF HEMODIALYSIS VASCULAR ACCESS remains a major source of morbidity and hospitalization for patients with end-stage renal disease. (ESRD). Hemodialysis access failure, the most frequent cause of hospitalization for dialysis patients, is also the single largest cause of hospitalized days.[1] Many modalities, including recirculation studies,[2-4] venous pressure indices,[5,6] duplex ultrasonography,[4,7-9] and angiography,[4,9] have been used to evaluate hemodialysis accesses in an attempt to predict and localize the source of access problems. Several groups have previously reported the ability to select patients at high risk of future access failure using duplex ultrasonography.[10,11] We also reported the ability to decrease thrombosis in a subset of polytetrafluoroethylene (PTFE) grafts with the use of elective revision of areas of graft stenosis.[12] The present study was undertaken to see whether a program of electively repairing areas of stenosis either surgically or with angioplasty would prolong the survival of hemodialysis access sites when compared to repairing the access only after clotting.

Methodology

In this study, 153 dialysis accesses (56 arteriovenous [A-V] fistulas and 97 PTFE-grafts) were followed from placement of the vascular access until the end of the study

Table 17-1. All Accesses

	No.	Flow volume (cc/min)	Maximum % stenoses	% of patients still dialyzing
Fistulas	56	1,263	21.86	67.9
Grafts	97	1,168	39.92	59.8
p value		NS	0.002	NS

NS = not significant

period. Excluded were patients who died, were transplanted, or were transferred to a different dialysis unit. The dialysis accesses were grouped by their access type (A-V fistulas or PTFE grafts) and compared. Each access type was subdivided into three groups. Group 1 patients had no interventions (no episodes of clotting, surgical revisions, thrombectomies, or angioplasties) from the time of placement until the end of the study. Group 2 patients had an episode of thrombosis as their first event or intervention occurring after placement of the access. Group 3 patients had an elective revision of an area of stenosis within the access or the runoff as their first intervention subsequent to the placement of the access. The total survival of the access site was measured from access placement until the access was abandoned or until the end of the study period. Accesses were abandoned due to the inability to maintain patency or maintain flows adequate to administer dialysis. The number of clotting episodes and the number of elective revisions were recorded throughout the life of the access. Each hospitalization and its attendant surgeries was accounted as one event, defined by its initial finding (either clotting or elective revision). Efforts were made to declot all clotted accesses within 48 hours of presentation. Screening duplex ultrasonography was performed on patients at six-month intervals. Data regarding flow volumes and maximal percent stenosis in the access and runoff were obtained as previously described.[12] Statistical analysis was performed on all groups and subgroups using the Student's t-test and chi-square analyses provided in the computer program GB Stat 4.0.

Results

As noted previously, the 153 accesses were followed from the initial placement of the access until the end of the study period. The mean follow-up was 772 days (minimum 14 days, maximum 2,755 days). The ultrasound characteristics of all accesses are described in table 17-1. Mean flow volumes were similar in A-V fistulas and grafts—1,263 cc/min and 1,168 cc/min, respectively (NS). Maximal percent stenosis averaged 21.86% in fistulas and 39.92% in PTFE grafts (p=.002). The majority (67.9%) of the fistulas and 59.8% of the grafts continue to function (NS). As noted in table 17-2, PTFE grafts had more clotting episodes per patient-year than fistulas (2.28 versus 0.99, p=.029). Elective revisions were similar in PTFE grafts and fistulas (table 17-2). The number of interventions per patient-year (clotting episodes and revisions combined) was higher in PTFE grafts than in fistulas (2.57 versus 1.20, p=.019). Total survival of the access averaged 644.49 days in fistulas and 840.36 days in PTFE grafts, approaching statistical significance (p=.068).

Table 17-2. All Access

	No.	Clotting per patient-year	Revisions per patient-year	Interventions per patient-year	Access survival (days)
Fistulas	56	0.99	0.21	1.2	645
Grafts	97	2.28	0.36	2.57	840
p value		0.029	0.126, NS	0.019	0.068, NS

NS = not significant

Table 17-3. Fistulas

	No. patients	Flow volume (cc/min)	Maximum % stenosis*
Group 1 (no events)	34	1,379	11.24
Group 2 (initial clotting)	11	1,056	40.22
Group 3 (initial revision)	11	1,065	40.4
p value		NS	0.038

*p=0.038 for group 1 v. 3

Table 17-4. Fistulas

	Revision per patient-year	Clot per patient-year	Intervention per patient-year
Group 2 (initial clotting)	0.408	4.84	5.29
Group 3 (initial revision)	0.655	0.543	1.2
p value	NS	0.063 (NS)	0.060 (NS)

NS = not significant

The groups of A-V fistulas and PTFE grafts were subdivided into three groups: Group 1 had no episodes of clotting or revisions, group 2 had an episode of clotting as the initial event after placement of the access, and group 3 had an elective revision or angioplasty as the initial event.

In fistulas (table 17-3), there were no significant differences in flow volumes in all three groups. The maximum percent stenosis in the access was significantly higher in groups 2 and 3 patients than in those with no events. Total revisions per patient-year were similar in groups 2 and 3 patients (0.408 in group 2 versus 0.655 in group 3, NS—table 17-4). Clotting episodes per patient-year were higher in group 2 (primary clotting) than in group 3 (4.84 versus 0.543, p=.063). Total events per patient-year averaged 5.289 in those with primary clotting (group 2) versus 1.19 in those with primary elective revision (group 3) (p=.061). Fistulas with elective revisions (group 3) had a significantly prolonged survival when compared to fistulas in patients who originally clotted (group 2) (998 days versus 357 days, p=.004—table 17-5). This difference persisted when fistulas still in use were excluded (group 3, 772.5 days versus group 2, 212.2 days, p=.03).

In PTFE grafts, flow volumes were similar in all three groups (table 17-6). Maximum percent stenosis was significantly higher in group 3 compared to the group of patients in group 1 and group 2 (table 17-6). Clotting episodes per patient-year were higher in group 2 than in group 3 (3.57 versus 1.07 episodes, p=.003—

Table 17-5. Fistulas

	Total access survival (days)	% of fistulas still dialyzing	Abandoned accesses survival (days)
Group 2 (initial clotting)	357	54.50	212
Group 3 (initial revision)	998	63.60	772
p value 0.004	NS	0.033	

NS = not significant

Table 17-6. PTFE Grafts

	No. Patients	Flow volume (cc/min)	Maximum % stenosis*
Group 1 (no events)	18	1,292	27.41
Group 2 (initial clotting)	54	1,141	35.02
Group 3 (initial revision)	26	1,137	58.58

*p=0.385 group 1 v. 2; p=0.001 group 1 v. 3; p <0.001 group 2 v. 3

table 17-7). Group 3 patients had more elective revisions per patient-year (.745) than group 2 patients (.284) (p=.003). The total number of interventions per patient-year was, however, significantly higher in group 2 patients than in group 3 patients (3.74 versus 1.82 interventions, p=.016).

In PTFE grafts (table 17-8), survival of the access was markedly prolonged in those with elective revision (group 3) compared to those with primary clotting (group 2) (1,022.7 days versus 689.23 days, p =.013). These differences were also present when the patients who continue to be dialyzed were excluded (987.37 days in group 3 versus 495.1 days in group 2, p=.014).

Discussion

The failure of dialysis vascular accesses (A-V fistulas and PTFE grafts) has remained problematic throughout the history of the ESRD program. In the most recent U.S. Renal Data System report, dialysis access failure remained the most frequent cause of hospitalization for patients with ESRD and the leading cause of hospital days.[1] As noted earlier, various screening methods have been used to predict which accesses will fail, in the hope that elective intervention will prevent future episodes of clotting. Our group and others have described the ability of duplex ultrasonography to predict accesses at high risk of failure[10-12] and the ability to decrease clotting episodes in a subset of PTFE grafts over the subsequent six months.[12] To be effective, a screening technique must influence subsequent outcome, preferably on both a short- and long-term basis. Screening is based on the assumption that elective repair of accesses will improve long-term access outcome. Our current study proves the premise that screening duplex ultrasonography, coupled with elective repair of accesses, effectively improves both short- and long-term outcome.

In fistulas, elective revision resulted in a 640-day (1.8-year) increase in access longevity when compared to repair after the fistula had clotted. Clotting episodes

Table 17-7. PTFE Grafts

	Clotting per patient-year	Revision per patient-year	Intervention per patient-year
Group 2 (initial clotting)	3.56	0.284	3.74
Group 3 (initial revision)	1.07	0.745	1.82
p value	0.003	0.003	0.016

Table 17-8. PTFE Grafts

	Total access survival (days)	% of grafts still dialyzing	Abandoned accesses survival (days)
Group 2 (initial clotting)	689	48.10	495
Group 3 (initial revision)	1,023	69.20	987
p value	0.013	0.076	0.014

per patient-year and total interventions were also decreased, but only approached statistical significance. This appears to be due to the small numbers in these groups. We believe that the short total life of fistulas in our series was due to a relatively short follow-up and the large percentage of fistulas in continued use. This is in part due to recent efforts to increase the number of patients with native A-V fistulas in our dialysis facility. Of interest, patients who died with functioning fistulas had an average fistula life of 1,679 days, or 4.6 years.

A comparison between the groups of PTFE grafts is more revealing. PTFE grafts with initial elective revision had nearly a full year increase in survival compared to grafts that first clotted (1,022.8 days versus 689.2 days total increase in longevity of 333.6 days). Electively revised PTFE grafts had significantly fewer episodes of thrombosis per patient-year (1.08 versus 3.57) and fewer interventions per patient-year (1.82 versus 3.74 episodes). On an individual basis, patients who had initial elective revisions required about two fewer surgeries or angioplasties per year and had 2.5 less episodes of clotting per year. The limited number of PTFE grafts with prolonged survival without any incident emphasizes the difficulty of maintaining adequate access and the limitations of PTFE grafts.

In summary, in both A-V fistulas and PTFE grafts, patients who underwent an initial elective revision to correct anatomic abnormalities of their access had fewer subsequent clotting and interventions than those who clotted initially. Patients undergoing an initial elective revision had fewer operations, about a one-year increase in the total survival of PTFE grafts, and a 1.8-year increase in survival in A-V fistulas.

This study confirms the ability of elective procedures to significantly improve access outcome on a long-term basis and proves that screening ultrasonography, combined with elective revision, improves access outcome. We propose that duplex ultrasonography and elective revisions will decrease hospitalization as well as the total cost of maintaining accesses. Future prospective trials are indicated to further delineate these matters and to compare the efficacy of different methods of screening.

References

1. U.S. Renal Data System. 1992 annual data report. Bethesda: National Institutes of Health, National Institute of Diabetes and Digestive and Kidney Diseases, 1992.
2. Nardi L, Bosch J. Recirculation: review, techniques for measurement and ability to predict hemoaccess stenosis before and after angioplasty. Blood Purif 1988; 6:85-89.
3. Kobrin SM, Kriger FL, Raja RM. Measurement of hemodialysis access recirculation: a two-needle method at the start of dialysis. Trans Am Soc Artif Intern Organs 1989; 35:508-10.
4. Schleifer CR, Jones K, Blakenbiller A, Snyder S. Access surveillance methods to prevent clotting in hemodialysis patients (abstr). Am J Kidney Dis, ASN Prog & Abst, 1993; 4:102.
5. Besarab A, Dorrell S, Moritz M, Michael H, Sullivan K. Determinants of measured dialysis venous pressure and its relation ship to true intra-access venous pressure. Trans Am Soc Artif Internal Organs 1991; 37(3):270-71.
6. Besarab A, Moritz M, Sullivan K, Dorrell S, Price JJ. Venous access pressures and the detection of intra-access stenosis. Trans Am Soc Artif Intern Organs 1992; 38:519-23.
7. Tordoir JH, Hoeneveld H, Eikelboom BC, Kitslarr P. The correlation between clinical and duplex ultrasound parameters and the development of complications in arteriovenous fistulae for haemodialysis. Eur J Vasc Surg 1990; 4:179-84.
8. Kottie SP, Gonzalez AC, Macon EJ, Fellner SK. Ultrasonographic evaluation of vascular access complications. Radiology 1978; 129:751-54.
9. Middleton WD, Picus DD, Marx MV, Melson GL. Color Doppler sonography of hemodialysis vascular access: comparison with angiography. AJR 1989; 152:633-39.
10. Shackleton CR, Taylor DC, Buckley AR, Rowley VA, Coopersberg PL, Fry PD. Predicting failure in polytetrafluoroethylene vascular access grafts for hemodialysis: a pilot study. Can J Surg 1987; 30 (6):442-44.
11. Strauch BS, O'Connell RS, Geoly KL, Grundlehner M, Yakub YN, Tietjen DP. Forecasting thrombosis of vascular access with Doppler color flow imaging. Am J Kidney Dis 1992; 19(6):554-57.
12. Sands J, Young S, Miranda C. The effect of Doppler flow screening studies and elective revisions on dialysis access failure. Trans Am Soc Artif Intern Organs 1992; 38(3):524-27.
13. Mehta S. Statistical summary of clinical results of vascular access procedures for hemodialysis. In: Sommer BG, Henry ML, eds. Vascular access for hemodialysis—II. Chicago:W.L. Gore & Associates, Inc., and Precept Press, 1991: 145-57.

18

BRACHIAL-JUGULAR EXPANDED PTFE GRAFTS FOR DIALYSIS

José R. Polo, M.D., Juan Sanabia, M.D., and Javier Calleja, M.D.

SOME PATIENTS IN WHOM A CENTRAL VEIN CATHETER has been used for dialysis may develop stenosis in the intrathoracic veins, especially if the subclavian route was used.[1] On the other hand, intimal hyperplasia affecting the axillary vein in upper-arm grafts may produce a long stenosis precluding a proximal vein bypass to treat graft dysfunction or thrombosis. In these cases, either the external or the internal jugular vein can be used to perform or to maintain an upper-arm graft. Isolated case reports on the use of jugular veins in vascular access for dialysis have been published previously.[2-5] We have previously published a preliminary experience with brachial-jugular grafts for dialysis.[6] In this report, the long-term outcome of 40 patients with brachial-jugular grafts is analyzed.

Materials and Methods

All patients in whom a vascular access using the jugular vein was performed in the Hospital Universitario Gregorio Marañón, Madrid, Spain, were studied. Age, presence of diabetic nephropathy, complications of the angio-access, and therapeutic methods to treat complications were analyzed.

Expanded, standard wall polytetrafluoroethylene (ePTFE) (GORE-TEX, W.L. Gore & Associates, Flagstaff, Arizona) was used in all cases; 6-mm grafts were used in children and in patients with previous 6-mm brachioaxillary grafts. Grafts used in remaining patients were 6–8-mm manually tapered grafts.

All surgical procedures were performed under local anesthesia using alkalinized 0.25% bupivacaine. A 2-g dose of cephazolin was administered preoperatively. If the patient was on dialysis through a temporary venous catheter, cloxacillin was

Table 18-1. Complications Treated in 40 Brachial-Jugular ePTFE grafts (5.8 revisions per 100 graft-months)

Complication	No.	Patients
Thrombosis	39	18
Late infection	9	8
Graft dysfunction	5	2
Venous hypertension*	2	2
Pseudoaneurysm	2	2
Totals	57	32

*Facial edema in external jugular vein graft

Table 18-2. Surgical Treatment of Occlusive Complications

Procedure	Thrombosis	Dysfunction
Thrombectomy	15	
Surgical angioplasty	10	
ePTFE graft bypass	8	3
Bypass to internal jugular vein	1	2
Contralateral brachioaxillary ePTFE graft	5	

administered orally for one week. Whenever the patient was not hospitalized for other reasons, the operation was performed in an ambulatory surgical setting.

Graft dysfunction was defined in the following cases: patients with dialysis pressure of >200 mm Hg with dialysis flow of 300 ml/m; recirculation of >20%; or Kt/V <0.8. Fistulography was obtained in all cases of dysfunction.

The duration of angio-access was analyzed using the life table method. Event-free patency was defined as the interval between graft construction and the occurrence of any complication requiring surgical therapy. Overall patency was defined as the interval between graft placement and definitive loss of function due to a non-recoverable complication. Comparison between curves was obtained using the Haenzel-Mantel method (log rank).

Results

Between September 1986 and October 1993, 1,068 surgical procedures were performed in our center to create a vascular access for dialysis: 766 (71.5%) were autologous fistulas (radiocephalic, n=543; brachiocephalic, n=137; and brachiobasilic, n=83); 305 were ePTFE grafts (straight forearm, n=48; loop forearm, n=18; brachioaxillary, n=191; brachial-jugular, n=40, femoro-femoral, n=8).

Brachial-jugular grafts (13% of all grafts) were performed in two groups of patients. In 14 cases, the graft was placed to salvage a brachioaxillary graft threatened by a central vein stenosis. In the other 26 cases, the graft was used to create an upper-arm conduit in patients with subclavian or axillary vein stenosis previously documented by phlebography. Eight of these patients had subclavian dialysis

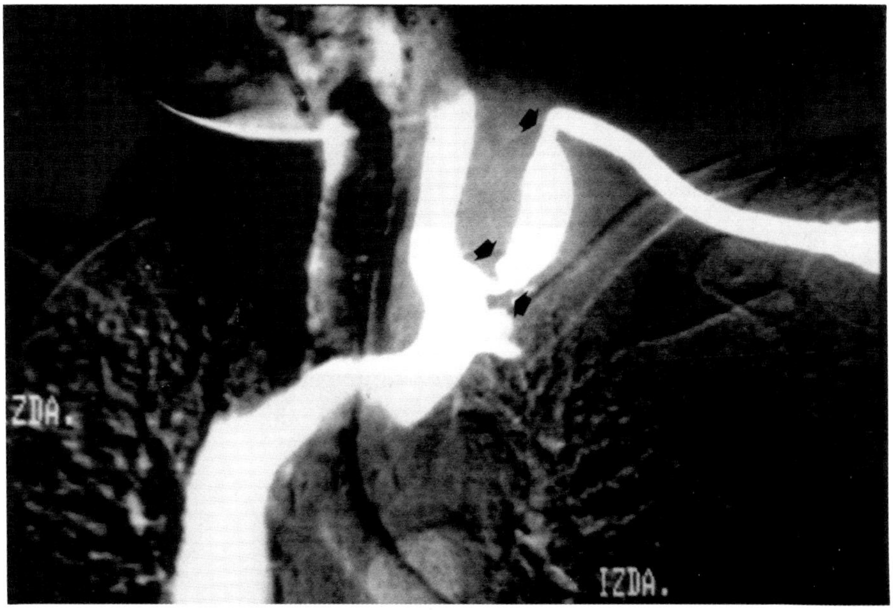

Figure 18-1. Fistulography in a patient with brachial-jugular graft showing stenosis in the proximal external jugular vein (arrows). Patient was treated with bypass to the internal jugular vein.

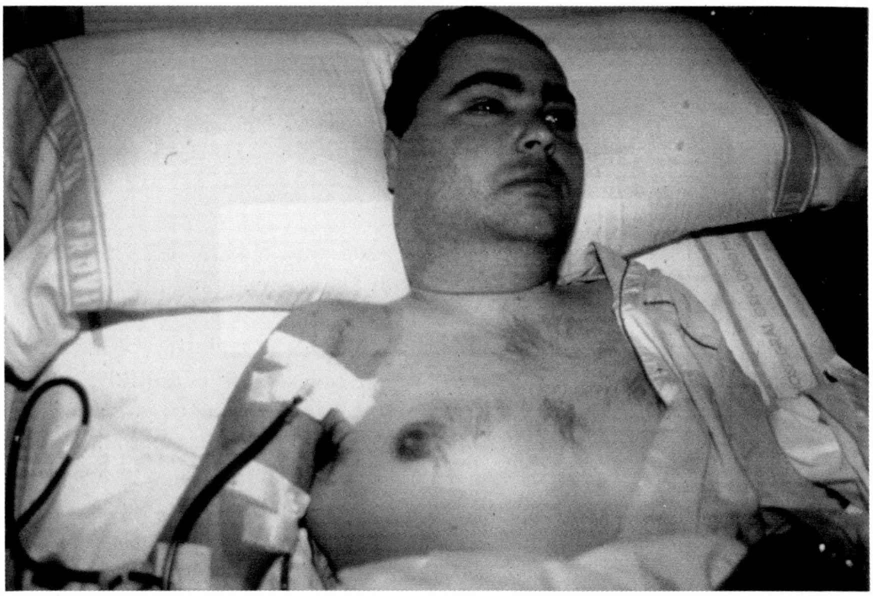

Figure 18-2. Facial edema due to venous hypertension in a patient with a brachial-jugular graft placed in the external jugular vein.

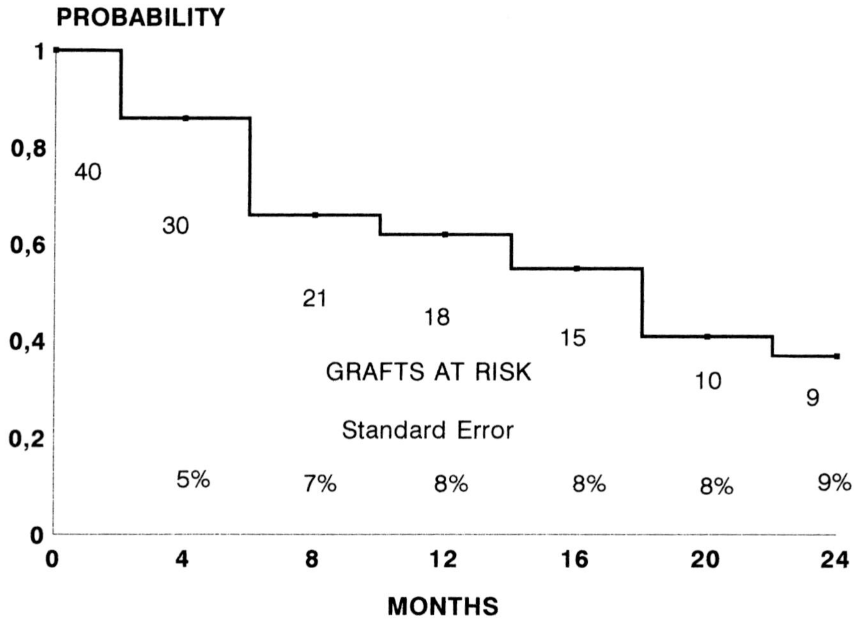

Figure 18-3. Actuarial analysis of event-free patency (primary patency) in 40 brachial-jugular grafts for dialysis.

catheters placed in the past. An axillary vein occlusion due to a previously failed brachioaxillary graft was found in the other 18 patients.

Age of the patients ranged from 8 to 72 years (mean: 49, C.I.: 44, 55). Diabetic nephropathy was observed in 22% of the patients. The external jugular vein was used in 20 cases and the graft was anastomosed to the internal jugular vein in another 20 patients. In 18 accesses, 6-mm grafts were used; 6-8-mm tapered grafts were placed in another 22 patients. Ambulatory surgery was done on 75% of patients.

Early failure was not observed. Late complications are shown in table 18-1. The complication rate was 5.8 episodes per 100 graft-months (0.7 episodes per graft-year). Venous stenosis was diagnosed by fistulography in all cases of graft dysfunction, and associated distal graft stenosis was observed in two of them. The surgical treatment of occlusive complications is given in table 18-2. Either a venous or a graft stenosis was detected during the operation in 61% of the patients with graft thrombosis. Proximal external jugular vein stenosis (figure 18-1) was treated with a bypass to the internal jugular vein in two patients. Proximal internal jugular vein stenosis, observed in a patient with contralateral subclavian vein occlusion, was treated with a bypass to the contralateral internal jugular vein. A new form of distal venous hypertension causing facial edema is described in two patients each with an external jugular vein graft (figure 18-2). Venous stenosis was excluded by fistulography. This syndrome was successfully treated with proximal vein ligation.

Event-free patency and overall patency are shown in figures 18-3 and 18-4. Comparison between event-free and overall patency curves was statistically significant (log rank, p=0.0011). Five grafts are still being used for dialysis more

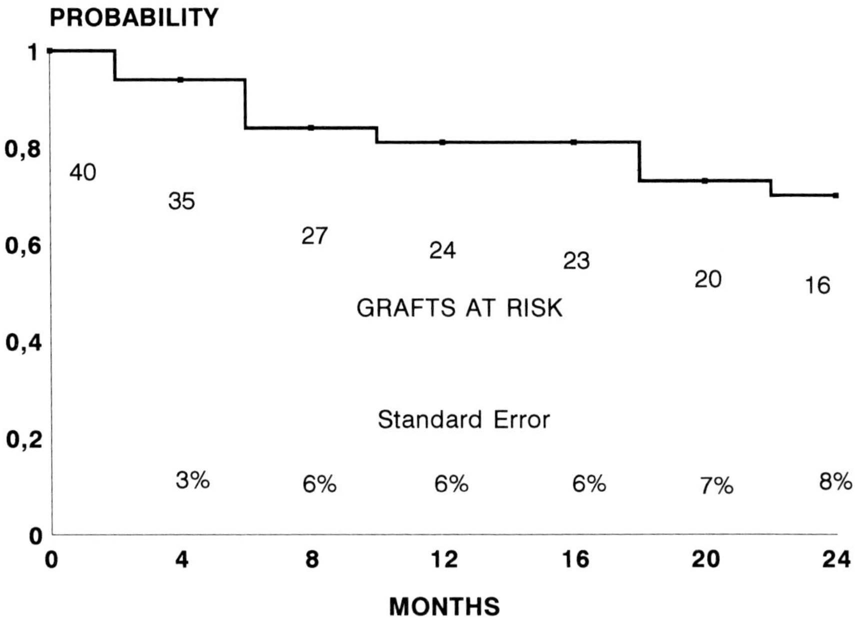

Figure 18-4. Actuarial analysis of overall patency (secondary patency) in 40 brachial-jugular grafts for dialysis.

than four years after their construction. An external jugular vein graft remains functioning for 70 months after eight surgical salvage procedures.

Discussion

A subclavian vein stenosis in patients with a vascular access in the same limb can be treated by means of percutaneous transluminal angioplasty or endoluminal stenting.[7,8] However, re-stenosis occurring after angioplasty frequently requires repeated dilatations,[9] and the placement of an endoluminal stent does not necessarily prevent restenosis.[10] Moreover, long or multiple stenosis, and complete venous obstructions in some cases preclude treatment of this pathology by means of interventional radiology.

Brachial-jugular grafts can be done under local anesthesia as ambulatory surgery. This procedure can be an alternative to other, more complex operations such as axillofemoral graft or intrathoracic vein bypass graft, in patients with nondilatable axillary or subclavian vein stenosis.[11,12] As with other dialysis grafts, the most common complication observed in the brachial-jugular graft was intimal hyperplasia affecting the vein in the area of the graft outflow.

Early diagnosis of graft dysfunction and intraoperative detection of venous stenosis during thrombectomy was observed in 61.5% of the cases in our series. This early diagnosis allowed surgical correction of this complication and increased the life of the graft. This fact has been shown by several authors in other series of dialysis grafts.[13-15] The difference between event-free and overall patency shows the efficacy of surgical salvage procedures. In our small series of patients with brachial-jugular grafts, this difference was statistically significant (log rank, p=0.0011). However, due to the different graft size and different venous outflow (external or internal jugular vein), statistical studies must be cautiously considered. The small number of patients precludes a separate analysis of the different groups of grafts.

A new form of venous hypertension has been found in patients in whom the graft was placed in the external jugular vein. Two out of 20 cases with external jugular vein grafts had facial edema, which was resolved with distal vein ligation. A fistulogram excluded proximal vein stenosis in these patients. Currently, we ligate the distal vein in every graft placed in the external jugular vein.

Due to the large number of patients in which thrombosis was associated with venous stenosis in our series, we believe that the hemodynamics and biochemical parameters defining graft dysfunction in our protocol were inadequate to detect all of the vascular stenoses. Perhaps routine color flow Doppler studies, along with hemodynamic parameters and biochemical analysis of dialysis efficiency, could better detect stenosis due to intimal hyperplasia and allow early treatment of this kind of pathology. Because jugular veins can be the last resort to maintain an upper-arm graft, a warning must be given against the use of dialysis catheters through the jugular vein route. We believe that brachial-jugular grafts can be an alternative to complex intrathoracic procedures, Dacron cuff catheters, or lower limb grafts, in cases of nondilatable central vein stenosis. Patency of the jugular vein axis up to the right atrium must be confirmed by radiologic studies when this surgical procedure is considered.

References

1. Shilinger F, Shillinger D, Montagnac R, Milcent T. Post catheterisation vein stenosis in hemodialysis: comparative angiographic study of subclavian and internal jugular access. Nephrol Dial Transplant 1991; 6:722-724.
2. Haimov M. Vascular access for hemodialysis. New modification for the difficult patient. Surgery 1982; 92:109-110.
3. Thomsen MB. A grafted arteriovenous fistula between the subclavian artery and ipsilateral internal jugular vein. Acta Chir Scand 1983; 149:637-638.
4. Posner MP, McNeil P, Lee HM et al. Salvage of hemoaccess in the presence of symptomatic subclavian vein stenosis/ occlusion. Transplant Proc 1987; 19:137-145.
5. Campistol JM, Abad C, Torras A, Revert L. Salvage of upper arm access graft in the presence of symptomatic subclavian vein thrombosis. Nephron 1989; 51:551-552.
6. Polo JR, Sanabia J, Garcia-Sabrido JL, Luño J, Menarguez C, Echenagusia A. Brachial-jugular polytetra-fluoroethylene fistulas for hemodialysis. Am J Kidney Dis 1990; 16:465-468.
7. Beathard GA. Percutaneous transvenous angioplasty in the treatment of vascular access stenosis. Kidney Int. 1992; 42:1390-1397.
8. Turmel-Rodrigues L, Pengloan J, Blanchier D, et al. Insufficient dialysis shunts: improved long-term patency rates with close hemodynamic monitoring, repeated percutaneous balloon angioplasty, and stent placement. Radiology 1993; 187:273-278.
9. Kumpe DA, Cohen MAH. Angioplasty/thrombolytic treatment of failing and failed hemodialysis access sites: comparison with surgical treatment. Prog Cardiovasc Dis 1992; 34:263-278.

10. Vorwerk D, Günter RW, Bohndorf K, Kistler D, Gladziwa U, Siebert HG. Follow-up results after stent placement in failing arteriovenous shunts: A three-year experience. Cardiovasc Intervent Radiol 1991; 14:285-289.
11. Rueckmann I, Ouriel K, Berry C, Hoffart N. The synthetic axillofemoral graft for hemodialysis access. ANNA J 1991; 18:567-571.
12. Duncan JM, Baldwin RT, Caralis JP, Cooley DA. Subclavian vein-to-right atrial bypass for symptomatic venous hypertension. Ann Thorac Surg 1991; 52:1342-1343.
13. Etheredge EE, Haid SD, Maeser MN, Sicard GA, Anderson CB. Salvage operations for malfunctioning polytetrafluoroethylene hemodialysis access grafts. Surgery 1983; 94:464-470.
14. Rizzuti RP, Hale JC, Burkart TE. Extended patency of expanded polytetrafluoroethylene grafts for vascular access using optimal configuration and revisions. Surg Gynecol Obstet 1988, 166:23-27.
15. Leapman SB, Pescovitz MD, Thomalla JV, Milgrom M, Filo RS. Salvage surgery for arteriovenous conduits: does it make sense? In: Henry ML, Ferguson RM, eds. Vascular access for hemodialysis—III. Chicago:WL Gore & Associates, Inc., and Precept Press, 1993; 169-174.

19

ILIOFEMORAL VENOUS STENOSIS ASSOCIATED WITH THIGH FISTULAS

Richard C. Dillihunt, M.D.

Chronic hemodialysis is generally accomplished using Brescia-Cimino or polytetrafluoroethylene (PTFE) A-V shunts surgically placed in the upper extremities. Such accesses can be used for a considerable time before they fail and require revision or reconstruction. Early failures are usually due to venous stenosis caused by intimal fibromuscular hyperplasia at or near the venous anastomosis.[1] Other causes of failure include infection, laminated clot in PTFE grafts, and pseudoaneurysms.

Intimal hyperplasia at the venous anastomosis is generally repaired by excision of hyperplastic tissue with patch angioplasty. This commonly results in further long-term patency of the salvaged fistula. A more difficult problem causing failure of upper extremity fistulas is stenosis due to venous intimal hyperplasia considerably distant from the venous anastomosis. Such stenoses require balloon catheter dilation, various revisions, jump grafts, or stents. More central stenoses in the subclavian veins may be attributed to prior multiple subclavian vein catheterizations and will often respond to balloon angioplasties, at least temporarily. Additionally, internal jugular catheters may be used for chronic hemodialysis, but eventually these fail due to thrombosis or infection.

Once one upper extremity or the internal jugular veins are no longer suited for chronic hemodialysis, the other may usually be used. Despite imaginative variations and techniques, however, in a small percent of patients, it is necessary to abandon the upper extremity and seek other routes for continued hemodialysis. Assuming peritoneal dialysis is not a better option and renal transplantation is not available, it therefore becomes necessary to consider placement of an A-V fistula in the lower extremity.

In experience with lower extremity accesses for hemodialysis at Maine Medical Center (Portland) over the past several years, we have concluded that a tapered 4–7-mm loop PTFE fistula from the common femoral artery (CFA) to the common femoral vein (CFV) is the most suitable conduit when an upper extremity or neck source is no

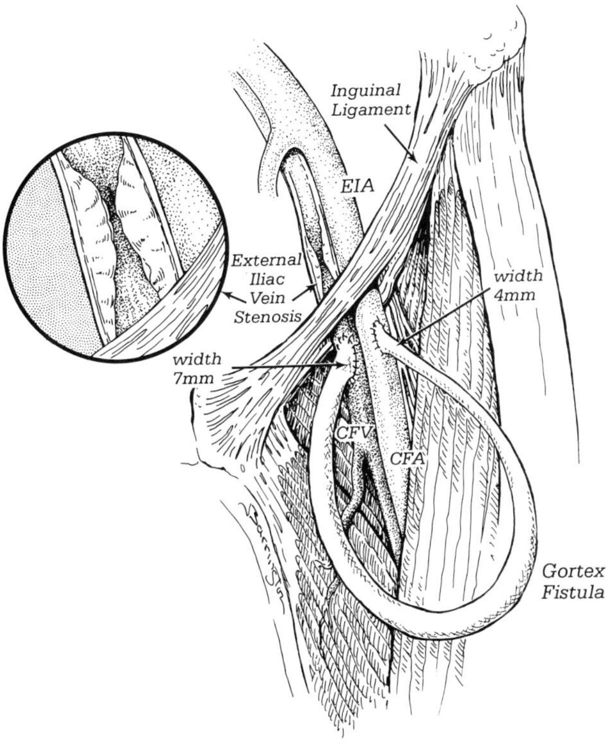

Figure 19-1. Tapered 4-7-mm loop PTFE from common femoral artery to common femoral vein.

longer available (figure 19-1). Concerns regarding potential groin wound sepsis and arterial steals for the most part have been unfounded.[2] Although we place PTFE accesses in the upper extremity preferentially, we have not hesitated to place such a shunt in the thigh when necessary.

During the past few years, we have encountered a troublesome complication in four patients who had placement of A-V fistulas from CFA to CFV. This complication is venous stenosis of the common femoral and/or external iliac vein above, and some distance from, the venous anastomosis of the loop graft. This stenosis is very similar to those seen in the upper extremity and is assumed to be due to intimal fibromuscular hyperplasia. Our experience with four patients we have identified with this complication are briefly summarized in the following section:

Case Summaries

1. Insulin-Dependent Juvenile Diabetic Male

This 42-year-old insulin-dependent juvenile diabetic male developed end-stage renal disease (ESRD) in 1978. From that time, until December 1992, he was dialyzed

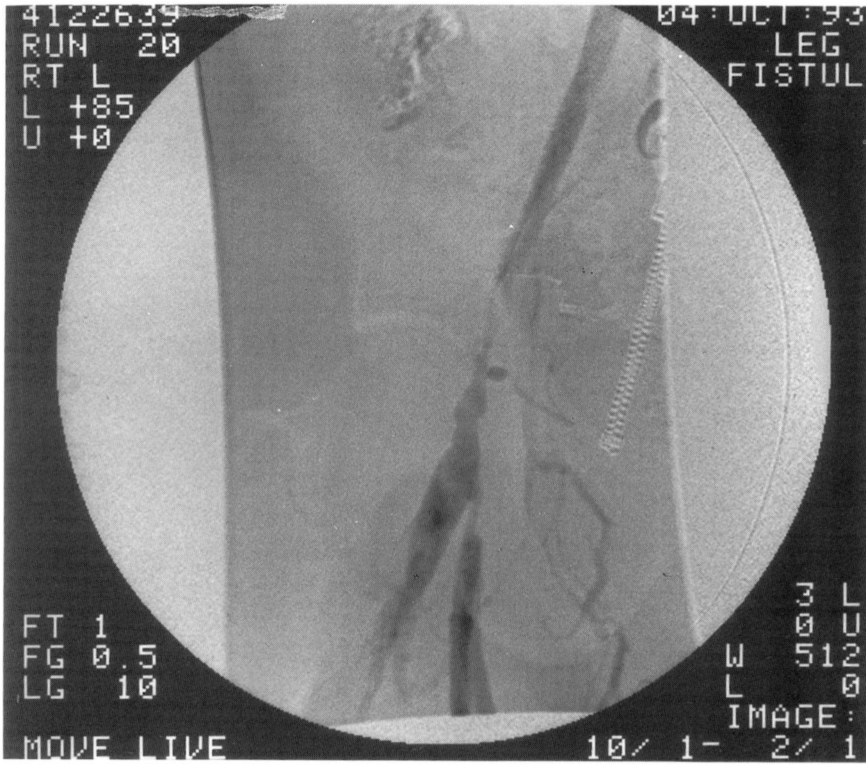

Figure 19-2. Fistulogram demonstrating external iliac vein stenosis above the venous end of the thigh fistula.

via various venous neck catheters and upper extremity fistulas. Eventual failure of all catheters and shunts required placement of a right thigh fistula, utilizing a 4–7-mm tapered PTFE graft from CFA to CFV in December 1992.

By October 1993, evidence of venous obstruction prompted a fistulogram disclosing external iliac vein stenosis above the venous end of the thigh fistula (figure 19-2). This was successfully treated with a PTFE jump graft for the venous end of the fistula to the external iliac vein above the stenosis. No further problems have developed in the ensuing brief follow up.

2. *Noninsulin-dependent Diabetic*

This 71-year-old noninsulin-dependent diabetic developed ESRD, requiring dialysis in July 1992. Hemodialysis was maintained thereafter with neck and subclavian catheters and with upper extremity accesses. Multiple complications, including venous thrombosis and steal syndromes, eventually required placement of 4–7-mm tapered loop PTFE graft from the right CFA to CFV in March 1993.

By January 1994, increased fistula venous pressures prompted a fistulogram demonstrating stenosis of the CFV and external iliac vein above the venous anastomosis (figure 19-3). The patient has continued on hemodialysis using this fistula without progression of obstruction to date.

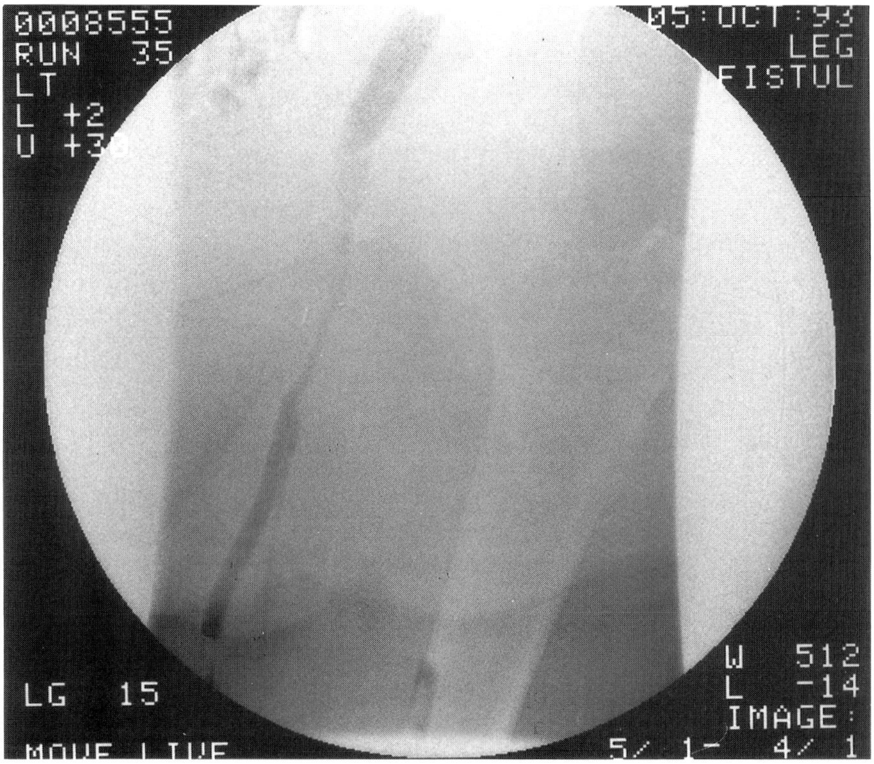

Figure 19-3. Fistulogram demonstrating stenosis of the CFV and external iliac vein above the venous anastomosis.

3. Nondiabetic Female

This 31-year-old nondiabetic female developed ESRD due to glomerulonephritis in 1972 at age 10. Following this, she was on hemodialysis for three years, after which she received a living related donor renal transplant. This failed, requiring transplant nephrectomy and resumption of dialysis shortly thereafter.

After years on hemodialysis via neck catheters, subclavian catheters, and upper extremity accesses, she required placement of a left thigh 4–7-mm tapered loop PTFE graft from CFA to CFV in July 1991. This fistula functioned well until January 1992, when she developed swelling of the left lower extremity and elevated venous pressures with recirculation on dialysis. A fistulogram disclosed stenosis (figure 19-4), which was treated and improved with balloon angioplasty (figure 19-5).

This condition recurred, requiring repeated balloon angioplasties at decreasing intervals until October 1993. At this time she underwent bypass of the stenosis, using an 8-mm PTFE jump graft from the venous end of the fistula to the external iliac vein above the stenosis, relieving the obstruction.

Hemodialysis continued without difficulty for four months until February 1994, when she developed recurrent left lower extremity swelling. This was associated with elevated venous pressures and recirculation in her shunt, prompting

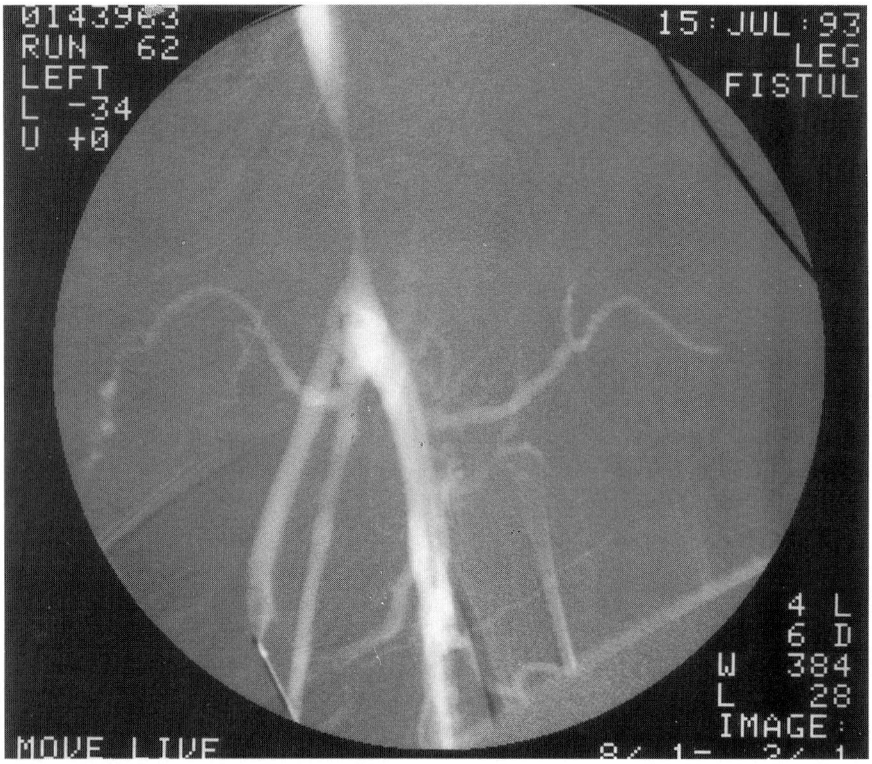

Figure 19-4. Iliac vein stenosis to be dilated.

repeat fistulogram revealing stenosis in the iliac system central to the jump graft. Following this, she required venous balloon angioplasty on two occasions, with temporary relief.

On April 20, 1994, she underwent cadaveric renal transplantation with excellent early function and discontinuation of dialysis.

4. Nondiabetic White Female

This 40-year-old nondiabetic white female developed chronic renal failure of undetermined etiology in 1983 at age 30 and has since been on hemodialysis. Over the ensuing nine years, she required various neck catheters, subclavian catheters, and upper-arm shunts to maintain access for hemodialysis.

In February 1992, she required placement of a 4-7-mm tapered PTFE loop fistula in the left thigh for continued hemodialysis due to failure of all other accesses. This thigh fistula functioned well until August 1992, when increased venous pressure, recirculation, and leg swelling prompted a fistulogram that disclosed iliac venous stenosis above the venous anastomosis (figure 19-6). Angioplasty afforded temporary relief, with recurrences requiring repeat angioplasties.

In August 1993, marked edema of the left lower extremity prompted another fistulogram, revealing left iliac vein occlusion that was treated with a left-

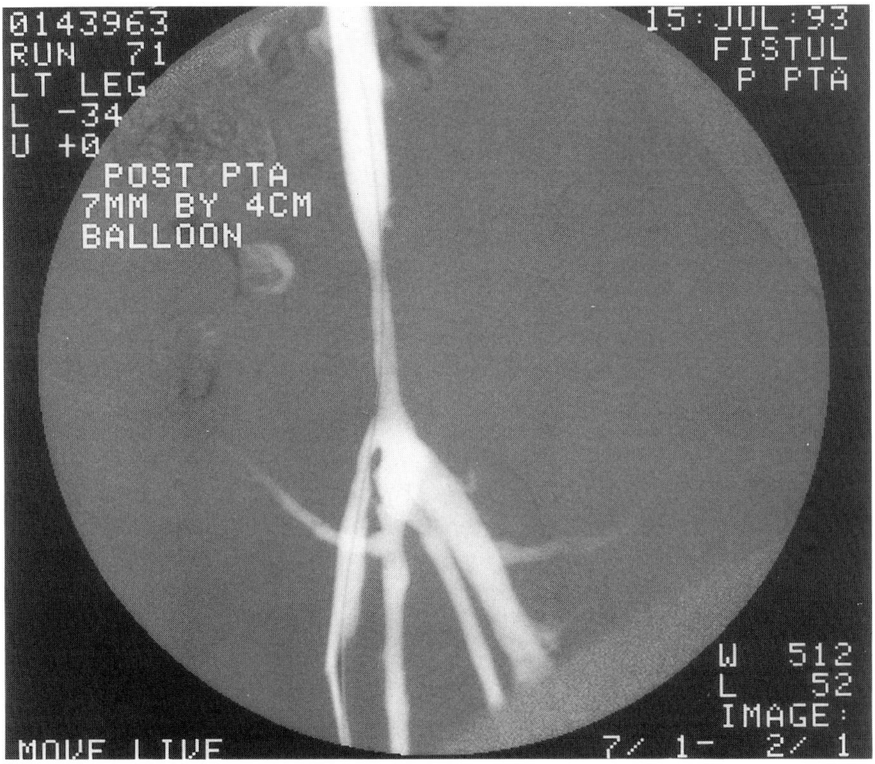

Figure 19-5. Balloon angioplasty treatment of stenosis.

femoral-vein-to-right-femoral-vein 10-mm PTFE bypass with resolution of swelling and return of normal fistula function. In April 1994, marked left thigh swelling with increased venous pressures recurred, and a fistulogram disclosed occlusion of the femorofemoral venous crossover graft (figure 19-7). The left thigh fistula continues to function with runoff via common femoral collaterals.

Discussion

All of the above cases previously had multiple accesses in the upper extremities, with revisions and eventual failure. None of the patients was suitable for peritoneal dialysis, and only one was suitable for renal transplantation (she has recently received a transplant). We have not reviewed all of our thigh fistulas over the years to see if other such patients exist; consequently, we do not know the incidence of this complication. Given the small number of thigh fistulas we do, it must be high. Such a review is currently being done.

The appearance of symptomatic venous stenosis in our patients has occurred in a relatively brief time after placement of the shunts (average: 7.5 months). The development of this complication is generally signaled by the appearance of edema of the

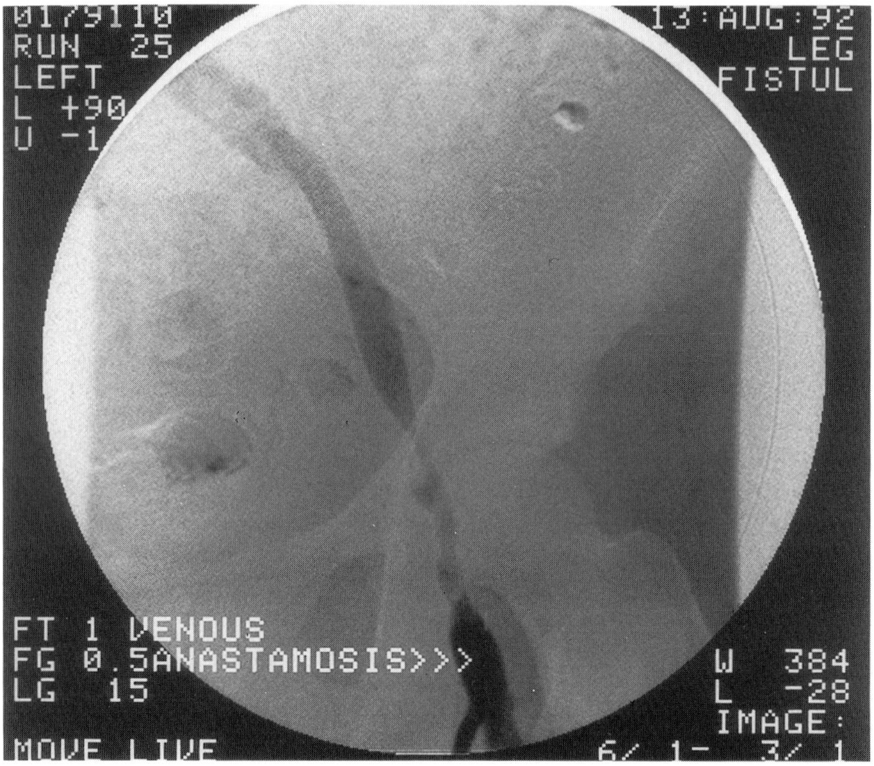

Figure 19-6. Fistulogram demonstrating iliac venous stenosis above the venous anastomosis.

entire lower extremity, often with blue discoloration and increased venous pattern mimicking deep vein thrombosis. Concomitant increases in venous pressures on dialysis with recirculation as the condition worsens have been observed. The pathophysiology of this complication is unclear. None of our patients had previous catheters or fistulas in the affected veins.

The diagnosis of venous stenosis can be made by duplex imaging.[3] Following this, a fistulogram is confirmatory, and treatment by balloon angioplasty is appropriate at that time. Our experience is that balloon angioplasty results in reversal of symptoms with radiographic improvement of the stenosis, but unfortunately, recurrences developed early. Repeated angioplasties were needed, with decreasing duration of success.

Because of the limitations of angioplasty, we elected to bypass the stenosis in two patients (cases 1 and 3), using a PTFE jump graft. Success of this technique is questionable, however, as one developed a new venous stenosis above the bypass (case 3), and the other has been followed for only six months (case 1).

Our last patient (case 4) appears to demonstrate the natural history of this condition. The stenosis was treated periodically by angioplasty. Venous thrombosis occurred, prompting a crossover venous bypass to enhance runoff, and now she has recently presented with thrombosis of her crossover graft. Most likely, this occurred because of venous stenosis in the contralateral iliac vein above the distal end of the crossover graft.

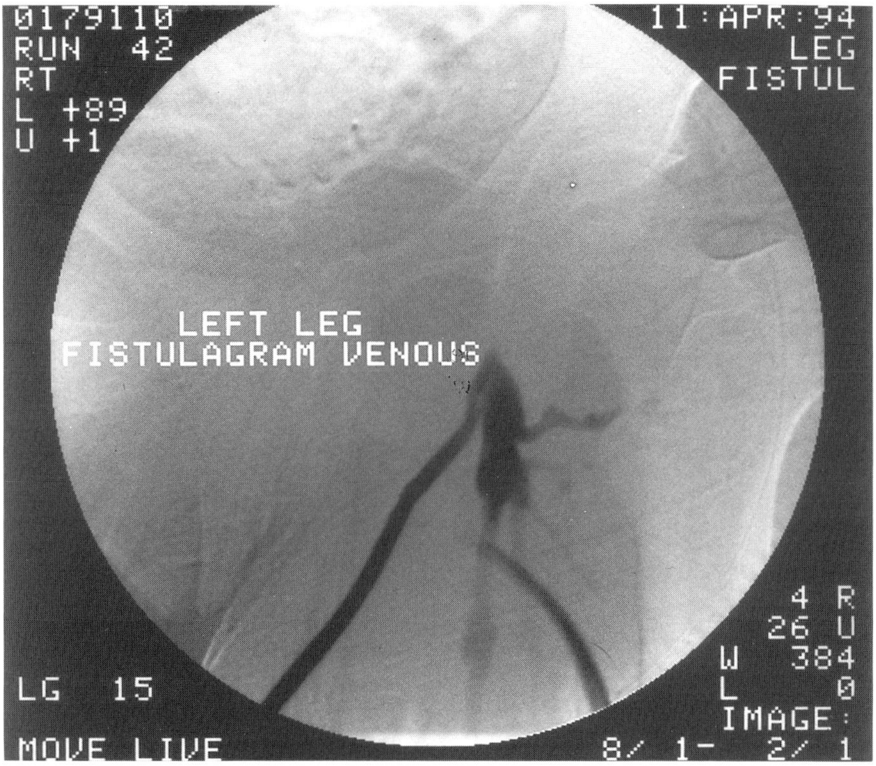

Figure 19-7. Fistulogram demonstrating occlusion of the femorofemoral venous crossover graft.

The development of venous stenosis above the venous anastomosis in thigh fistulas appears to be a serious problem in patients requiring this form of hemodialysis. As more patients are placed on dialysis for longer and longer periods of time, it seems likely that we can expect to see this complication more frequently. With fewer kidneys available for transplantation, we can expect this situation to worsen. We suspect that venous obstruction complications in lower extremity fistulas cause much more morbidity than similar complications in upper arm shunts. These anatomic lesions may also preclude placement of a renal transplant in the ipsilateral iliac fossa.

Continued study of this problem is therefore needed. The cause of stenosis is assumed to be fibromuscular hyperplasia, and this needs pathological documentation. New techniques are needed to deal with these patients. Long-term anticoagulation is untried. Stenting of venous stenosis in the iliac venous system would appear to offer some promise, but long-term follow-up of this mode of treatment will be necessary to determine its efficacy. The possibility of stent placement at the time of construction of thigh fistulas may be worth consideration.

References

1. Swedberg SH, Brown BG, Sigley R, Wight T, Gordon D, Nicholls SC. Intimal fibromuscular hyperplasia at the venous anastomosis of PTFE grafts in hemodialysis patients. Circulation, 1989; 80(6):1726-1735.
2. Kumpe DA, Cohen MAH. Angioplasty thrombolytic treatment of failing and failed hemodialysis access sites: Comparison with surgical treatment. Prog Cardiovasc Dis, 1992; 34(4): 263-278.
3. Miranda CL. Importance of imaging the venous run-off system during duplex evaluation of hemodialysis access grafts. J Vasc Tech 1993; 17(6):303-306.

20

USE OF WECK CLIPS TO ADJUST FLOW IN AN A-V PTFE BRIDGE GRAFT

Arthur L. Humphries Jr., M.D., Robert R. Nesbit Jr., M.D., B. Carter Rogers, M.D., Charles H. Wray Jr., M.D., and James J. Wynn, M.D.

AN A-V FISTULA AT THE WRIST is the first choice for hemodialysis access. More frequently, we have used the larger antecubital cephalic vein to the brachial artery. If the upper-arm basilic vein is large, we have elevated it for creation of a fistula, as we have pioneered.[1] But frequently a polytetrafluoroethylene (PTFE) graft is more practical. A large vein is also very desirable for a graft, to minimize stenosis from intimal hyperplasia. From 1980 through October 1990, we placed 350 8-mm PTFE grafts from the brachial artery to the axillary vein or from the femoral artery to the femoral vein. At least three grafts have remained patent for 10 years. Only one patient suffered a severe nerve palsy (ischemic monomelic neuropathy).

From October 1990 until March 1993, we created 49 grafts; 84% of 32 upper-arm grafts and 92% of 17 thigh grafts were patent up to two and a half years. Eleven percent required at least one declotting operation, however.

The size of the arterial anastomosis is by far the most critical factor determining graft flow, as the flow increases proportionally to the fourth power of the radius. It is also the easiest factor to modify. Other important factors that may affect flow are the size and length of the graft; whether it is flattened, curved or kinked; the diameter of the artery and vein; blood pressure; cardiac output; and the coagulability of the blood. As time goes by, the characteristics of the shunt may change. The artery, the anastomosis itself, and the vein may dilate. On the other hand, either the anastomosis or vein may become smaller from platelet deposition or intimal hyperplasia. Blood might flow faster (though total flow may not be greater) through a 6-mm graft, but since 1976 we have used the 8-mm graft because the inner surface of the graft may soon become narrowed by pseudointima and thrombotic excrescences.

Table 20-1. Poiseuille's Law

$$\text{Flow} = \frac{(P_1 - P_2)\pi r^4}{8L\eta}$$

Diameter (mm)	D x D x D x D
8	4,096
6	1,296
5	625
4	256
3	81

If the diameter is 3, then 3 to the fourth power is 81. By chance, 81 ml/min would be roughly the flow through a graft with a 3-mm arterial anastomosis. Thus, if the diameter is 4 mm, flow could be up to 256 ml/min theoretically; if 5 mm, up to 625, etc.[8]

Thus, to choose the optimal flow for a given patient is nearly impossible. Even if one could calculate the appropriate diameter for the anastomosis, making the precise anastomosis would be difficult. The critical problem of anastomotic size is best illustrated by the following calculations based on Poiseuille's law (see table 20-1). If the anastomosis is 3 mm, then 3 to the fourth power is 81. By chance, this is a reasonable estimate of flow in ml/min. A 4-mm diameter theoretically could increase flow up to 256 ml/min; a 5-mm diameter up to 625, a 6-mm to 1,296; and an 8-mm to 4,096 ml/min flow. Even if a 5-mm diameter were known to be ideal and it was sutured precisely so, the anastomosis might still turn out to be a slit or oval rather than a circle.

Because of our fear of creating a steal, we had always narrowed the end of the PTFE graft to 4 or 5 mm with a "one size fits all" philosophy. But vascular surgeons routinely make an anastomosis to the femoral or more distal artery two to three times as long as the artery. Taylor et al., when using PTFE, have added a vein patch to its end to allow an even longer anastomosis.[2]

Since August 1992, we have made the arterial anastomosis 8 to 15 mm long. Then, if necessary to prevent steal of blood from the hand or foot, we narrowed the graft with a clip. The concept is not new. Braunwald and Castanedo used a doubly tapered graft (W.L. Gore & Associates, Inc., Flagstaff, Arizona) for the creation of a systemic-pulmonary arterial shunt.[3] Each end of the graft was 5 or 6 mm and the waist 3 or 4 mm in diameter.

Materials and Methods

We reviewed the records of the 36 patients operated upon from August 1, 1992, through March 31, 1994. Telephone follow-ups were required in a few instances. The patients ranged from 22 to 77 years of age. A majority were black and 18 were diabetic. Many, but not all, had had several previous access operations. Most upper-arm graft recipients were sedated with intravenous propofol (Ditropan) and locally anesthetized with 1/2% lidocaine. Thigh graft recipients were given general or spinal anesthesia.

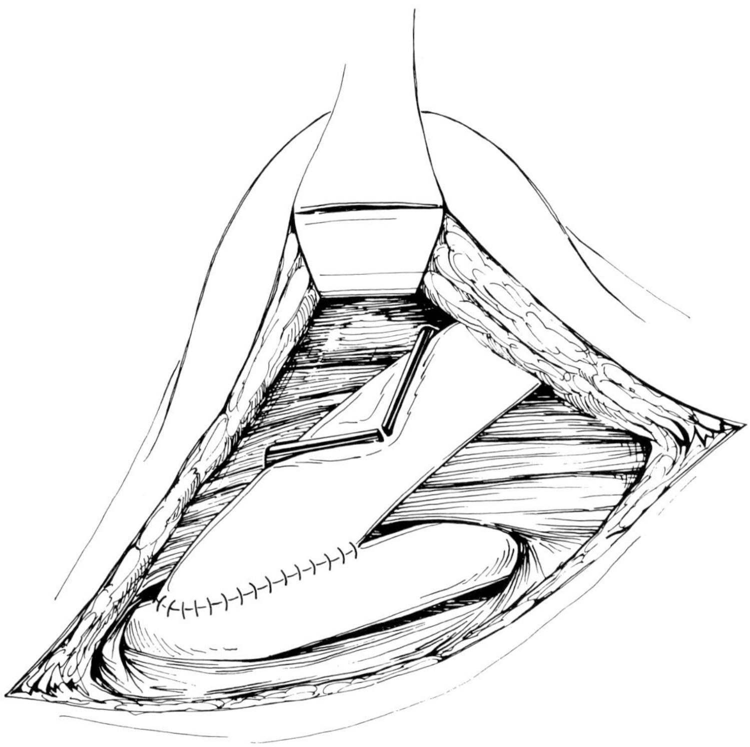

Figure 20-1. If clips are needed, it is recommended that they be placed on the graft as shown. The gentle slopes provided by this delta configuration should minimize possible turbulence.

Operative Technique

The brachial artery just above the elbow was isolated for 4 or 5 cm and bathed in papaverine. To expose the axillary vein, we used a transverse incision high in, and proximal to the deepest part of, the axilla. The pectoralis minor muscle was retracted medially. The axillary vein was usually 8-12 mm in diameter. Vessel loops were used to elevate the axillary vein, and a C-shaped vascular clamp applied. A standard reinforced 8-mm expanded polytetrafluoroethylene (GORE-TEX, W.L. Gore & Associates) graft was used.[1] The graft was sutured with 5-0 or 6-0 polypropylene suture. Intravenous heparin was given. An 8- to 15-mm arteriotomy was made and the obliquely cut graft sewn with a 6-0 suture. After there was flow in the graft, the radial pulse was checked. If indicated, an ultrasonic Doppler flow detector was used to help judge whether flow through the graft was excessive and producing a steal syndrome. If deemed necessary, two 13-mm Weck clips (Hemoclip hemostatic clips, Edward Weck & Co., Research Triangle Park, North Carolina) were placed across 3 or 4 mm of the graft to narrow the lumen until the Doppler signal seemed adequate (figure 20-1). In our one experience, in which a small clip was placed, it was later found to have fallen off. A large, bulky dressing from fingertips to axilla splinted the arm for three days. One baby aspirin was prescribed indefinitely. The graft was not used for at least eight days.

For patients whose subclavian veins were stenotic or whose brachial arteries were very small, we placed the graft from the superficial femoral artery just above the adductor canal out laterally in a V-shape and then back to the femoral vein in the groin. With this distal arterial anastomosis there was less dead space and foreign body in the vulnerable groin area.

Results

Clip Not Applied Initially to 29/36 Grafts

Six patients developed a steal and required a clip to the graft. Clips were applied at day one (radial pulse present subsequently but another clip applied at two weeks because of persistent mild numbness); day two (graft clotted two days later); one week, two weeks, and four weeks (for this patient, another clip was needed because of coolness of the foot at three months).

One patient was a blind, type 1 diabetic who had had two Permacath (Quintom, Seattle, Washington) dialysis catheters that had become infected and an arm graft that had clotted. Two months after placement of a thigh graft, all the toes became purple. Despite ligation of the graft, a below-knee amputation became necessary. She died one month later.

Three patients developed nonthrombotic complications. One cirrhotic patient, with anasarca, developed a lymph leak from both thigh incisions. The graft became infected and was removed. One diabetic patient developed arm swelling and a lymph leak for 10 days. A 68-year-old diabetic patient with poor left ventricular function died from congestive heart failure eight days postoperatively. A total of nine patients have died. It was not thought that excessive flow through the graft was the cause of death in any other patient.

Branham tests have been done in eight patients with no clip on their grafts. Six patients showed no change. One demonstrated a heart rate decrease from 110 to 104 beats/min and the other a decrease from 108 to 100 beats/min. Twenty-four grafts were never clipped and none thrombosed.

Clip Applied at Initial Operation to 7/36 Grafts

One thigh graft clotted at three months. The arterial end was declotted only after the clip was removed. One month later, a steal syndrome required graft ligation, and peritoneal dialysis was started. One arm graft was declotted at three weeks in a patient following a liver transplant. The graft had to be clipped on two subsequent occasions. A fungal infection in the graft required its eventual removal. One thigh graft clotted at three months; it was declotted and has remained open.

Discussion

We have optimized the arterial anastomosis in order to maximize flow through the graft, to minimize chances of clotting, and, as an extra dividend, to assure the ability to perform high-flux hemodialysis. If the hand or foot appeared to be in jeopardy, clips were applied to narrow the graft at the primary operation or at a subsequent operation.

We were surprised that 24/36 grafts have never needed a clip. The fact that none of these clotted would seem to justify the approach. Although the high flow might later induce intimal hyperplasia in the large axillary or femoral vein, this has not been observed. However, other complications have occurred and were potentially due to the high blood flow. This requires careful follow-up so that if the graft needs to be clipped, it can be done expeditiously. One diabetic still complains of mild paresthesias median nerve distribution despite a palpable radial pulse that was made stronger by use of a clip.

To judge whether high flow is deleterious to the heart is difficult to assess. High flow through the graft may have contributed to at least one instance of heart failure and death. But of eight patients with unclipped grafts examined recently with the Branham test, only two had a (mildly) positive test. Parfrey et al. concluded in 1991 that the excess mortality from cardiovascular disease in the dialysis population is not fully explained.[4] Surprisingly, they never once mentioned A-V fistulas. The increased flow through the graft might be balanced by the decreased flow to the kidneys in dialysis patients.

The main advantage of the clip is that it is simple to apply and easy to adjust the degree of narrowing by trial and error until flow is maximized. We have used an ultrasonic Doppler flow detector to determine whether the signal is triphasic or biphasic and to provide an estimate of flow to the hand or foot. We have not yet used portable angiodynography, which would visually reveal reversal of flow in the distal artery, as described recently by Jain et al.[5] These authors described the use of polypropylene sutures to band a graft.

Although a 9- to 15-mm arteriotomy would seem a priori to place the native artery itself at greater risk, the extra risk must be small. The anastomosis is technically easier. There may be an increased chance of a false aneurysm, but we have had none since 1976. Because the critical parts of any arteriotomy are its two ends, the short arteriotomy is almost as risky as a long one. If an infection requires graft removal and a vein patch for the artery, the suture line will be longer. In our one experience, the extra 6- to 9-mm length of vein patch has not been a problem. It is possible that the placement of a single clip early in our experience caused increased turbulence on the distal side of the clip and thus predisposed the graft to thrombosis. It is not clear. Possibly, the clip converts a round graft into a flattened graft. Conversely, the large 8-mm graft may be flattened until the clip is applied, and the faster flow through the narrowed graft may make the lumen become circular. Theoretically, placement of the clip at right angles to the artery across the toe of the graft might avoid excessive turbulence. When we tried this method, however, the clip narrowed the distal artery itself. Thus, we recommend two clips in the shape of a delta as shown in figure 20-1. Even if an encircling band were used, the lumen might be irregular from infolding tucks and wrinkles of the nonelastic PTFE. Ebeld and Saranchak have made the point that a wide encircling band permits the lumen to be narrowed less, thus causing less turbulence.[6] Our delta-shaped clips, although not encircling, do provide a band with gentle slopes.

Another advantage of the clip became evident when grafts clotted. For one graft, the balloon catheter did not extract the thrombus from the arterial end until the clip was removed. For another, the "estuary" created by the large arterial anastomosis was not clotted, so passage of the balloon was not needed. When a declotting operation was done, not only was the clot removed, but the clip was reapplied in a way not to narrow the graft as much. Had the original arteriotomy been small, a new anastomosis would have been required.

It is true that several patients had to return to the operating room once or twice for application of clips. However, a greater number of patients were probably spared a more serious declotting operation, and perhaps some patients were spared the use of anticoagulants. Although Vanderwerf et al.[7] ascribed many graft problems to excessively high flows, we believe our results justify a continuing trial.

Conclusion

Large anastomoses to a large artery and a large vein have made graft clotting unlikely. None of the 24 grafts not clipped in this series has clotted so far. Such an approach is especially indicated for the patient who has had clotted grafts previously. Adjustment of flow with clips on the graft was simpler and more precise than guessing what the original diameter of the anastomosis should have been. We conclude that this method is beneficial. Complications that may be due to excessive flow make us also conclude that we should use the clip more frequently at the initial operation or, based upon frequent postoperative observations, at a subsequent operation.

References

1. Humphries AL, Hamilton WF, Wynn JJ, Nesbit RR, Caruana RJ, Wray CH. Alternative plans for vascular access for hemodialysis. In: Sommer BG, Henry ML, eds. Vascular access for hemodialysis. Chicago:W.L. Gore & Associates, Inc., and Pluribus Press, Inc., 1989;95-113.
2. Taylor RS, Loh A, McFarland RJ, Cox M, Chester JF. Improved technique for polythetrafluoroethylene bypass grafting: Long-term results using anastomosis vein patches. Br J Surg 1992; 79:348-354
3. Braunwald NS, Castanedo AR. Use of the doubly tapered graft for the creation of a systemic-pulmonary arterial shunt. Ann Thorac Surg 1976; 239-244.
4. Parfrey PS, Harnett JD, Barre PE. The natural history of myocardial disease in dialysis patients. J Am Soc Nephrol 1991; 2:2-12.
5. Jain KM, Simoni EJ, Munn JS. A new technique to correct vascular steal secondary to hemodialysis grafts. Surg Gynecol Obstet 1992;175:183-184.
6. Ebert A, Saranchak HJ. Banding of a PTFE hemodialysis fistula in the treatment of steal syndrome. Clin Exp Dial Apheresis 1981; 5: 251-257.
7. Vanderwerf BA, Williams T., Koep LJ. Haemodynamics of arteriovenous fistulas. In: Kootstra G, Jörning PJG, eds. Access surgery. Ridgewood, N.J.: Bogdon, 1983;29-133.
8. Sumner DS, Kumpe DA. Hemodynamics and diagnosis of arterial disease: Basic tenchiques and applications. In: Rutherford RB, ed. Vascular surgery. Philadelphia: Saunders, 1989; 17-41.

DISCUSSION

Moderator:
Ronald M. Ferguson, M.D., Ph.D.
Panelists:
Richard C. Dillihunt, M.D.
Leo Hofstra, M.D.
Arthur L. Humphries Jr., M.D.
José R. Polo, M.D.
Jeffrey J. Sands, M.D.

Discussant: Dr. Sands, the problem I have with my radiologists is they cannot measure flow for me. They tell me they can measure velocity. Can you tell me how you can get such reliable flow measurements?

Dr. Sands: Our experience with ultrasound has been that if you have to use a radiologist, you've got a problem. In my institution, the radiologists generally are not interested in dialysis access, and the time it takes to get the information translated into action is too long. We do it ourselves. Nephrologists read the ultrasound. Procedures are done within or next to the dialysis unit. We calculate a flow volume by using a cross-section of the area of the access and the mean velocity over three cardiac cycles. It gives you an index. I do not believe that the flow volumes correlate exactly with a flowmeter, but what we have shown in other studies is that those Doppler measurements correlate with clotting. I want to be able to predict which accesses are going to clot. Also, if I intervene in those accesses, can I improve outcome? The bottom line, as far as I am concerned, is improving access outcome.

Discussant: In patients who have stenosis, at what flow rate or percentage narrowing do you intervene?

Dr. Sands: In our setting, if you look at grafts with flows of 1,000 cc or less per minute, those all clot within six months. If you look between about 1,000 and 1,200 cc, there is about a 40-50% clotting rate within six months. And then over 1,300 cc it goes way down. We do look at accesses with low flows and look for areas of stenosis. Those patients are then sent to radiology for angioplasty. In our facility, when I or one of my colleagues see an abnormal ultrasound, the first call is to the dialysis unit. That patient is then scheduled for a fistulogram, and if necessary, an angioplasty. One of the problems we have had in the past is that if you wait a week, things happen quickly and you lose a lot. The second problem we have had is a very high re-thrombosis rate in the first week and month and two months. One of the limitations with what we have been doing with screening is we have not been following those patients closely enough. We have been looking six months apart or three months apart, but you really need to look much more frequently after you thrombectomize them or use thrombolysis. Our PTFE grafts that clot all go for thrombolytic therapy, and it is done on an outpatient basis. It is a two-hour turnaround time.

Discussant: Dr. Sands, how do you know you have not selected a different group of patients, like group 2 and group 3, that are thrombosed?

Dr. Sands: That is the problem. What I can tell you is when I have looked at it, the interval in time between placement of the graft and when the intervention was made is not statistically different. The flow characteristics and the sonographic characteristics are not different. The age and the quality of patients are not different.

It is not a perfectly clean study. It is not a prospective study, the way I would like to do. I cannot do that in my institution. However, I can tell you that the incidence of thrombosis has gone way down. The incidence of inhospital dialysis has dropped 25%, and the incidence of surgical revisions and thrombectomies is going way down. All of the data that I have seem to show that it works. I think the bias actually is in favor of the group that clots rather than in the group that is revised, because we missed a lot of things. The number of patients who were electively revised is a much higher percentage of those that are still dialyzing. If you pull out that subset, those grafts have lasted much longer. If you keep going with the data in any length, it is going to make those numbers increase.

Dr. Ferguson: It seems as though you are saving a considerable amount of cost as well as morbidity by having color Doppler. What you are really doing is spending the capital investment for instrument up front, but what are the ongoing costs?

Dr. Sands: I am still in the process of getting those data together. To talk about costs, we need to look at them in a multifactorial way. Doing a surgical thrombectomy at my institution results in about $12,000 in charges, including all of the complications. The cost of doing a thrombectomy using urokinase in radiology is $4,500 to $5,000. If you do screening, and it costs you $150 or $200 or even $300 per screen, you do not have to prevent a whole lot of clotting to make it a lot cheaper. One of the criticisms I have heard is, "You are only picking up five or six or seven episodes of clotting in all of these tests." Even if you pick up only five episodes of thrombosis with the screening, it is still cheaper, not to mention the impact on patients. It is a whole lot different for our patients to have two fewer surgeries a year.

Discussant: Dr. Humphries, what kind of flow rate do you have through an 8-mm graft with 1.5-mm anastomoses?

Dr. Humphries: I do not know. We have not put flowmeters on the artery. You cannot put a flowmeter on the graft.

Discussant: Dr. Dillihunt, I am thankful that I have not had those complications that you have had. Over the past 20 years, I have put in a lot of thigh grafts. The only thing that I saw that I do differently is that I make a loop graft just as you did, but I use the superficial femoral just distal to the profunda takeoff with the idea that perhaps I will not steal as much blood from the distal leg. I come in on the vein side to the saphenous just prior to the junction with the femoral. If the graft clots, you still have a little bit of saphenous left to move up. Eventually, you may have to move up to the femoral vein. I have not seen that complication, and maybe it is the higher flow from the common femoral and the fact that you are going into the femoral vein. I do not know, but that is one thought.

Dr. Dillihunt: I appreciate that as a possibility. Formerly, we plugged the venous end into the end of the saphenous vein, but we found a different set of complications occurring there. And that was stenosis at the venous anastomoses in the region of the saphenous requiring revisions and patch angioplasty. Has that been your experience?

Discussant: Yes, that has been my experience over a period of time, but some of them will last two or three years. I have not seen the femoral or iliac vein stenosis, and we have done a lot of thigh grafts over the years. We use either a 4-7-mm or 6-mm graft. There is no question that any time you go into a vein with an access graft you eventually will get a stenosis at the venous anastomosis.

Discussant: Dr. Sands, on the question of costs, whose equipment are you using?

Dr. Sands: In my case, it is mine.

Discussant: So it is dedicated to your unit?

Dr. Sands: We originally tried to do this with the radiologist in the hospital. The technicians did not really know what they were doing and the radiologists were not quite sure what they were looking at and were not very interested. So I hired a radiology technician, bought an ultrasound machine, and started doing it myself. I can now get ultrasounds very easily. That is not the universal experience.

Discussant: I think capital investment is going to be the limiting factor for most people.

Dr. Ferguson: What is the cost of a machine?

Dr. Sands: A high quality machine costs more than $100,000. The way it can be done in a larger sense is by setting up a method of screening so that you are doing multiple dialysis units and you are doing them at intervals such that you are in the unit often enough that it is useful. You are absolutely right, that is a problem.

Discussant: Dr. Hofstra, back in the early 1970s, a group of investigators looked at compliance mismatch in composite grafts connecting either a Dacron or GORE-TEX to the saphenous vein for extending the grafts down the lower extremity when the vein was inadequate. They found that you could attenuate a compliance mismatch by making a long, tapering anastomosis between the larger Dacron or GORE-TEX graft and the vein. If you did that and tapered the anastomosis so that the length of it was at least twice the diameter of the larger tube, you attenuated that compliance mismatch and the alterations in shear forces, rather than just making an end-to-end anastomosis between the tube. We have tried to do this in some of our synthetic dialysis grafts and made long, tapering venous anastomoses. This seems to extend the life of the graft and prolongs the interval before fibrous hyperplasia produces a stenosis, although it does not totally prevent it. I would offer it to you for your consideration.

Dr. Hofstra: Yes, there is no question about your comment. I do want to stress that the data that I have presented are just a simplification of the complexity of the flow and pressure situation in A-V fistulas. I think modifications of the venous anastomosis such as placement of a Miller cuff or a Child cuff may attenuate compliance mismatch and lead to increased patency rates.

Discussant: Dr. Sands, have you compared Doppler ultrasound with other techniques of screening, such as venous pressures, Kt/V, and recirculation? How can we put this technique in context so we can compare it? What is its margin of utility compared with the techniques we have that are cheaper?

Dr. Sands: I have not compared it adequately. I was not trying to present Doppler as the do-all and the end-all. What I really wanted to show was that if you screen people and electively revise them, it has an impact. Unless you can show that, screening goes out the window. I was also interested in showing that we are not doing it for convenience, but that it has a long-term impact. You do not have to do an emergency procedure at a bad time. I think we are headed toward doing a blend of screening. The problem I have with venous pressures through the machine is that you end up doing far too many dye studies that do not show anything. You see stenoses, but those do not necessarily predict clotting. We and others have shown that just as stenosis is not good enough to predict clotting, flow is a much better predictor. When we have used recirculation, we again were sending far too many patients for dye studies and we were not getting enough positives. Ultimately, we need to do a trial comparing different methods of screening, not only showing that these methods have a predictive power in terms of stenosis, but that they also improve outcome. We then need to compare the costs and see how much invasive therapy you are doing in order to find out which of these techniques actually work and what the intervals between them should be. What are the subsets of patients that have to be studied more often? I believe that PTFE grafts that fail once have to be studied much more often than fistulas. Then we begin to set up protocols in a more uniform fashion that is a blend of all of those therapies. I am currently in the process of trying to do this, because we miss all too many episodes of thrombosis using Doppler alone. I do not want to restrict myself to one technique. All I care about is patient outcome—not what technique is used.

Dr. Polo: Over the past five years, we have checked every three months in our dialysis unit Kt/V, recirculation, and venous dialysis pressure, and it works perfectly for the use of cephalic fistula. In prosthetic grafts, in more than 50% of the cases with thrombotic episodes we found venous graft stenosis. I think we need other parameters, perhaps color flow Doppler, or need to change the level of the parameters.

Dr. Sands: In addition to that, using Kt/V or URR has been very helpful. If we see the urea reduction rate dropping, we believe it and get an ultrasound or some study to look at that access unless we have a very good explanation of what is going on there. We do that very promptly. That has added a lot in terms of picking up things in between.

SECTION VII

21

WALLSTENTS FOR THE FAILING HEMODIALYSIS ACCESS

Richard J. Gray, M.D., Keith M. Horton, M.D.,
Bart L. Dolmatch, M.D., John H. Rundback, M.D.,
David Anaise, M.D., Alejandro O. Aquino, M.D., Charles B. Currier, M.D.,
Jimmy A. Light, M.D., and Truman M. Sasaki, M.D.

FOR YEARS, THE STANDARD TREATMENT FOR FAILING HEMODIALYSIS ACCESS has been surgical revision. Over the past decade, balloon angioplasty has become an accepted alternative treatment for venous stenoses that commonly cause dialysis failure. Recurrence rates at six months following balloon angioplasty for peripheral venous stenoses near the hemodialysis access are 30-40%.[1-3] Relative to peripheral lesions, central vein stenoses respond poorly to balloon dilatation,[3] and angioplasty for complete catheter-related vein occlusions has been reported only sporadically and usually fails.[4] Investigations of other percutaneous techniques, including atherectomy[5-7] and thrombolysis,[8] have been undertaken in an attempt to improve the results. Herein, we report our experience using the Wallstent (Schneider, Minneapolis, Minnesota) wire mesh biliary endoprosthesis for hemodialysis-related venous stenoses and occlusions.

The authors would like to express appreciation to Theresa Kowal, R.N., the project's clinical coordinator; Cory Anger, B.S., for statistical support; Peter Brandt for preparation of the photographs; and Mrs. Nancy Carnes for preparation of multiple manuscript drafts.

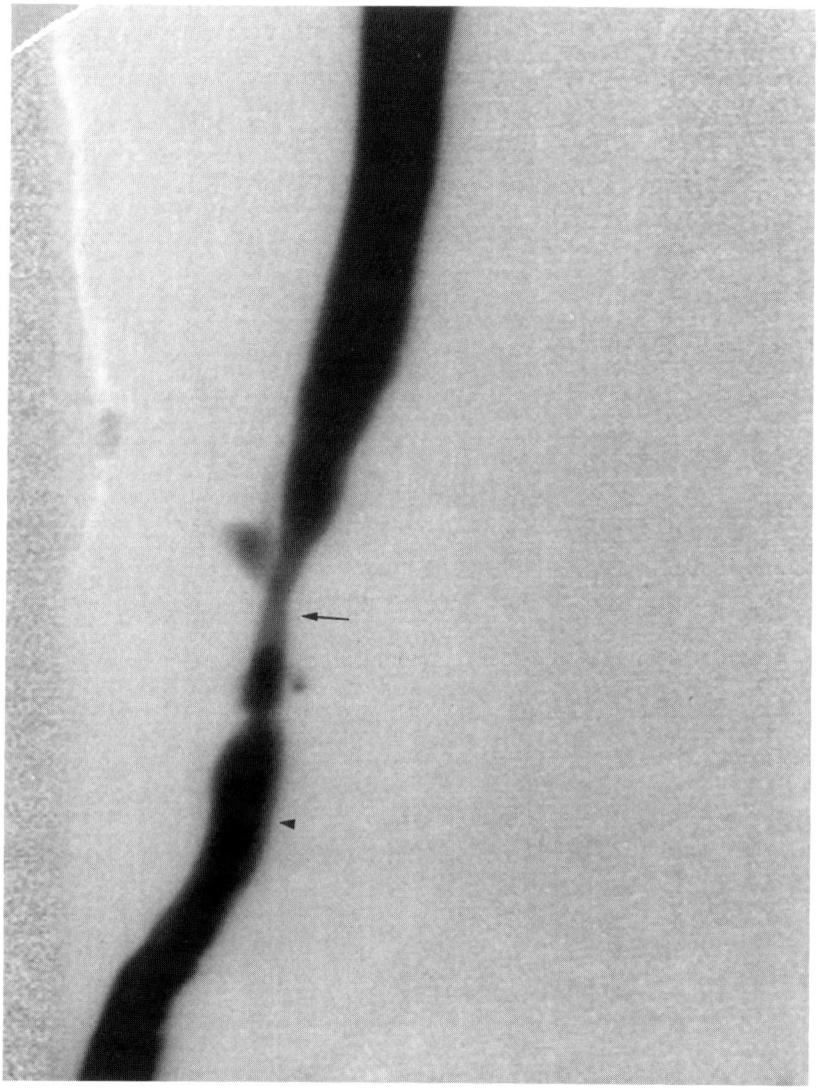

Figure 21-1A. Angiogram following surgical thrombectomy shows a high-grade stenosis (arrow) at the venous anastomosis of a PTFE graft (arrow).

Material and Methods

Patient Selection

From December 1991 through December 1993, the Wallstent biliary endoluminal prosthesis was used to treat 56 lesions in 52 patients. There were 27 females and 25 males with a mean age of 62 years (range: 30-90 years). There were 24 peripheral lesions located at the venous anastomosis (21 stenoses) or in the outflow vein proximal to the anastomosis (3 stenoses). There were 32 central lesions located in the subclavian (11 stenoses, 5 occlusions), innominate (3 stenoses, 7 occlusions), subclavian extending into the innominate (1 stenosis, 2 occlusions), and iliac (3 stenoses) veins. Each central lesion was preceded by placement of a central dialysis catheter months to years prior to treatment. Two central lesions with acute superimposed phlebothrombosis were treated by catheter-directed urokinase (UK) prior to angioplasty and stent placement. The mean length of the peripheral lesions was 43 mm (range: 5-96 mm), and the mean length of the central lesions was 31 mm (range: 10-75 mm). The overall mean length was 36 mm (range: 5-96 mm).

Preliminary digital subtraction angiography was performed for the following clinical indications: recent hemodialysis access thrombosis (n=18), extremity edema (n=22), recent hemodialysis access thrombosis concurrent with extremity edema (n=5), recirculation (n=4), increased venous dialysis pressures (n=4), and routine surveillance following angioplasty (n=3). Stenoses of ≥ 50% on orthogonal views or >70% on a single view were considered significant if the stenosis location correlated with the clinical indication. In each case, the hemodialysis access was a 6-mm polytetrafluoroethylene (PTFE) graft. The only available Wallstents during the course of this study were the 10-mm x 42-mm and 10-mm x 68-mm biliary stents. All procedures were performed following an Institutional Review Board–approved protocol and with the patients' informed consent.

Angioplasty was attempted in 39 lesions immediately prior to stent placement; two of these had also failed directional atherectomy (figures 21-1A—21-1E). These were considered angioplasty failures due to a 30% or greater residual stenosis.[9] In four other lesions, a re-stenosis had occurred less than one month following a technically successful (<30% residual stenosis) angioplasty. Of the 13 other lesions, 8 were considered unsuitable for angioplasty or atherectomy: 7 were complete subclavian (n=4) or innominate (n=3) occlusions (figures 21-2A and 21-2B), and one was a 7-cm iliac stenosis. The remaining five were treated at the operator's discretion with primary Wallstent placement following predilatation; three were subclavian stenoses and two were venous anastomotic stenoses.

Procedure

Percutaneous intervention was performed through a no. 7 Fr vascular sheath placed into the synthetic graft. Grafts were punctured at an obtuse angle to enhance hemostasis after sheath removal. All procedures were performed by one of five interventional radiologists with either fellowship training or more than 15 years of experience. The Wallstent is a flexible wire mesh cylinder composed of fine steel filaments. It is deployed by retracting a plastic membrane that allows the stent to be released from a no. 7 Fr delivery catheter. When deployed, the stent shortens as it expands. Stent size (10 mm x 42 mm or 10 mm x 68 mm) was selected by matching the lesion length as closely as possible to the predicted stent length at the anticipated final stent diameter. For example, the mean length of a 42-mm stent expanded to 6, 8, or 10 mm is 63, 46 and 24.5 mm, respectively.[10] The anticipated final stent diameter was based either on measurements of the normal vein diameter adjacent to the lesion or on observation of balloon size relative to the adjacent normal vein

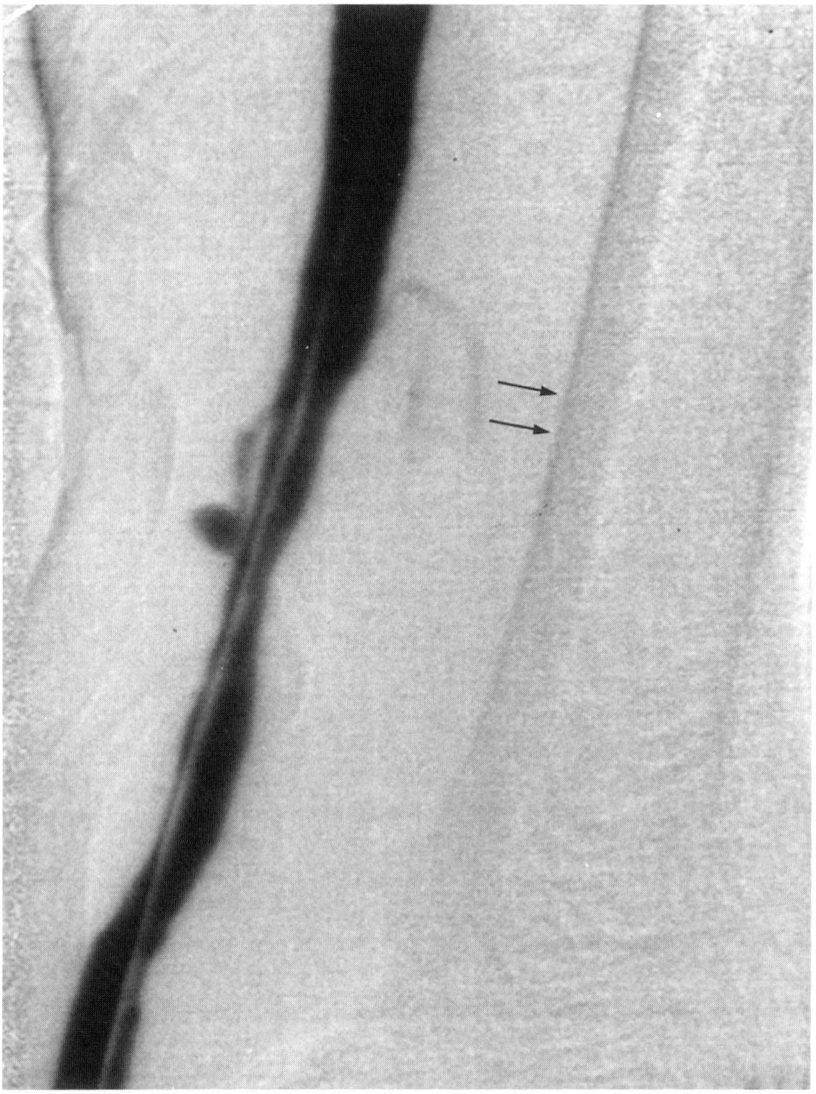

Figure 21-1B. Diagnostic study following complete expansion of a 7-mm angioplasty balloon across the stenosis shows a residual 50% stenosis. The humerus is faintly seen (arrows).

using digital road-mapping. Vein size was extrapolated from the dialysis access graft by assuming a graft diameter of 6 mm (the standard graft size implanted at our institution). Fifty-four of 56 lesions were dilated prior to stent deployment, either during attempted angioplasty (n=39) or as an intended predilatation (n=15). In each case, the guide wire tip was positioned in the inferior vena cava during stent deployment to avoid losing control of the stent should immediate migration occur.[11] Following deployment, 53 of 56 (94%) Wallstents were dilated to the anticipated final stent diameter.

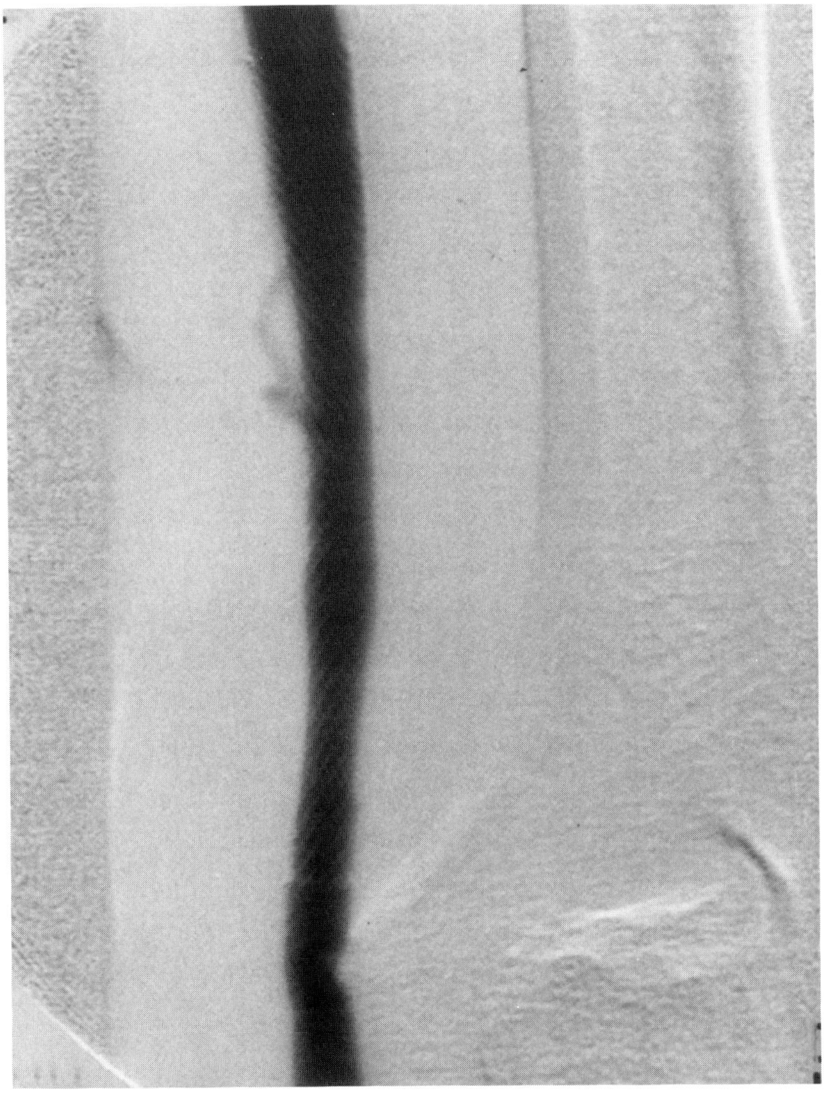

Figure 21-1C. Following deployment of a 10-mm x 42-mm biliary Wallstent and stent dilatation to 7 mm, the venous outflow is widely patent.

Procedural medication was at the discretion of the operator. All graft percutaneous puncture sites were anesthetized with 2% lidocaine. Thirty-four patients received 2,000 U units of heparin. Nitroglycerin was administered to 12 patients in 100-200 µg aliquots as needed to prevent spasm. Patients were given 25-50 µg fentanyl and 1-2 mg Versed (n=13), 50 mg Demerol (n=4), 50 mg Demerol and 2 mg Valium (n=4), or 2 mg morphine sulphate (n=1). The other 26 patients received no sedation or systemic analgesia. No antibiotics were administered to any patient.

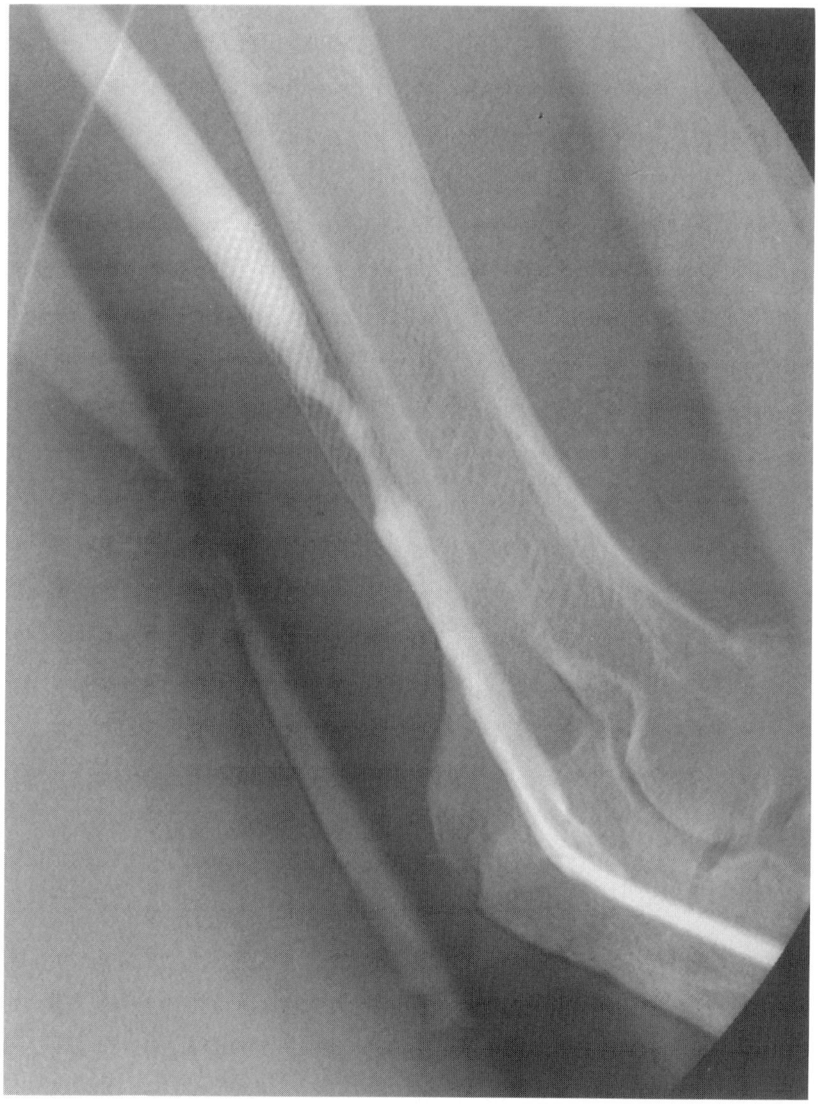

Figure 21-1D. Digital subtraction image nine months later shows significant intrastent stenosis.

Following the procedure, manual compression was maintained at the percutaneous puncture site until hemostasis was achieved. One patient was given protamine. The patients were discharged from the interventional radiology recovery room after a two- to three-hour observation period.

Follow-Up

Thirty-eight treatment sites were followed clinically and with repeat subtraction arteriography at about 1, 3, 6, 9, and 12 months following treatment. Follow-up of

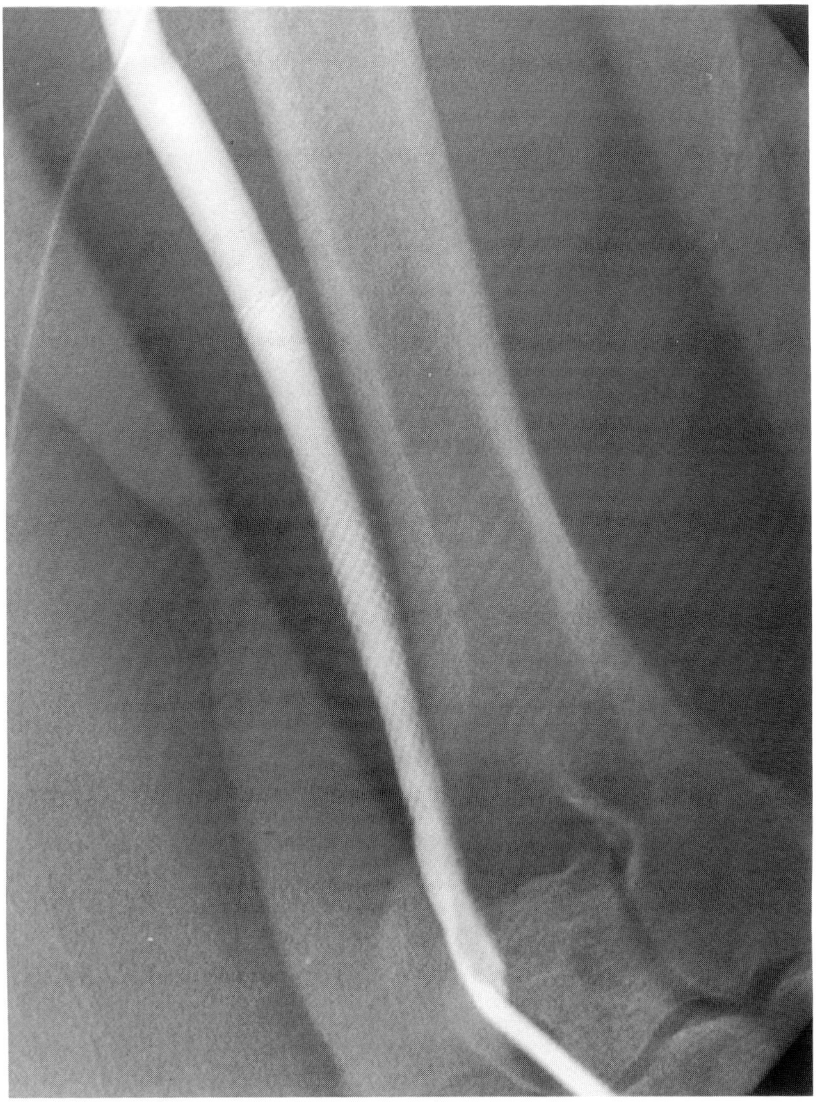

Figure 21-1E. Following treatment with a no. 9 Fr directional atherectomy catheter and dilatation to 7 mm, the stent is now widely patent.

the other 18 was clinical only and was obtained at similar intervals. Initial procedural success was defined as <30% residual stenosis[9] on orthogonal views and by resumption of dialysis with normal venous dialysis pressures and no recirculation or arm swelling. In all cases, an attempt was made to leave no residual stenosis. Significant re-stenosis was determined by recurrent signs or symptoms of dialysis malfunction and/or ≥50% stenosis (orthogonal views) or >70% stenosis (single view) on angiography.

Whenever significant re-stenoses occurred, an additional percutaneous procedure, if possible, was performed to maintain the viability of the hemodialysis access (figure 21-2). These procedures included angioplasty (n=3), directional atherectomy

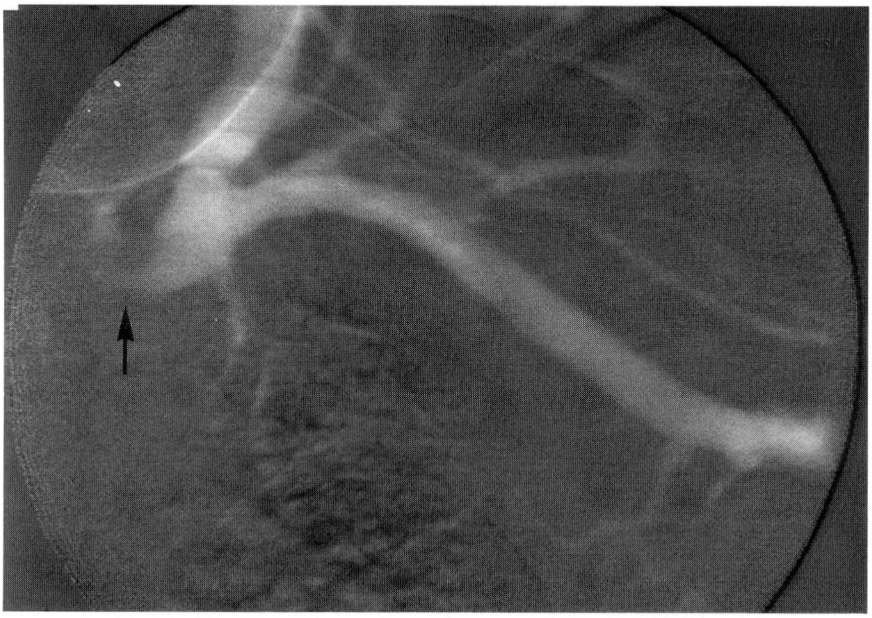

Figure 21-2A. Digital subtraction image in a patient with massive left upper extremity swelling and a left arm dialysis graft shows complete occlusion (arrow) of the innominate vein.

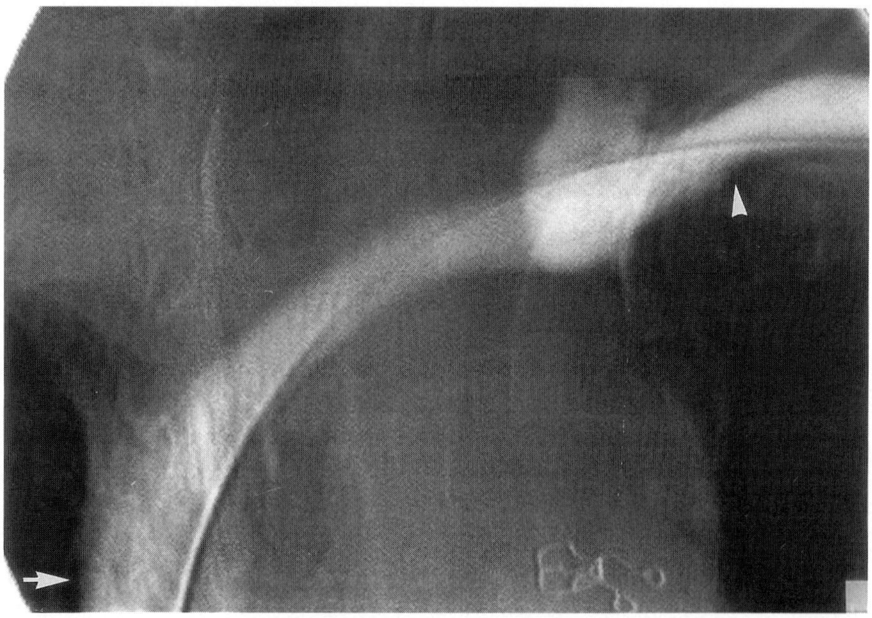

Figure 21-2B. The innominate occlusion was negotiated with a guide wire and predilated with a 10-mm balloon. Following 10-mm dilatation of a 10 mm x 68 mm Wallstent, there is free flow from the subclavian (arrow) to the superior vena cava (arrow). The patient's arm swelling resolved completely.

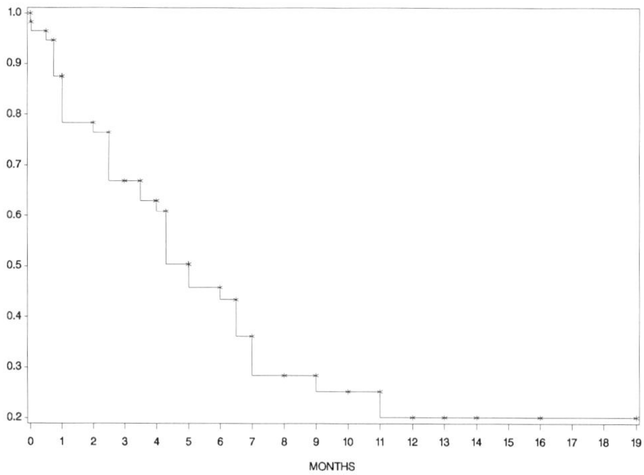

Figure 21-3. Primary patency.

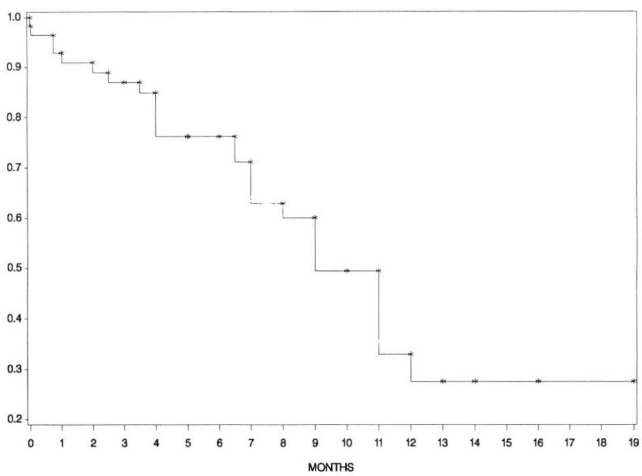

Figure 21-4. Assisted patency.

(n=3), directional atherectomy followed by angioplasty (n=2), and additional Wallstent deployment (n=11).

Life tables of the primary and assisted patencies for all 56 lesions were constructed using the Kaplan-Meier method. Life tables for the primary and assisted patencies were also constructed separately for the central stenoses, peripheral stenoses, and complete occlusions (all central lesions). Separate life tables were also constructed for the lesions subdivided by length (< 2 cm, 2.1-4 cm, > 4 cm). The Wilcoxon test was used to compare the primary and assisted patencies of these subgroups.

Because only two stent lengths were available, some lesions matched the stent length well while other lesions were much shorter than the stent. Life tables were constructed for the primary and assisted patencies of lesions with 1-33% stent involvement by lesion, 34-67% stent involvement by lesion, and 68-100% stent involvement by lesion. The Wilcoxon test was performed to compare the patencies of these subgroups.

Results

Once the decision was made to place a Wallstent, the immediate procedural success was 96% (54/56). Three lesions were treated with two stents to achieve complete lesion coverage by stent. One procedural failure occurred in a patient with arm swelling related to tandem central venous lesions when a subclavian stenosis was successfully stented, but an innominate occlusion could not be negotiated with a guide wire. The other procedure failure involved a patient with upper extremity swelling, a 90% subclavian stenosis, and an adjacent subclavian vein diameter measuring 14 mm; placement of a 10-mm x 42-mm Wallstent dilated to 10 mm failed to resolve the patient's arm swelling, presumably due to the undersized stent.

The six-month primary patency was 46% (n=48); however, with retreatment, the six-month assisted patency was 76% (n=47). The 12-month primary patency was 20% (n=41), and the assisted patency was 33% (n=30).

The Wilcoxon test revealed no significant difference in the primary (p=0.65) and assisted patencies (p=0.59) for central versus peripheral lesions. There was also no significant difference in the primary (p=0.88) and assisted patencies (p=0.61) for central occlusions versus central stenoses versus peripheral stenoses.

The primary (p=0.33) and assisted patencies (p=0.29) for lesions < 2 cm (n=17), 2.1-4 cm (n=20), and > 4 cm (n=17) were not statistically different. There was no difference in the primary (p=0.77) or assisted patency for stents with 1-33% stent involvement by lesion (n=16), 34-67% stent involvement by lesion (n=25), and 68-100% stent involvement by lesion (n=15). Finally, there was no significant difference (p=0.06) in patency following retreatment of recurrent stenoses by directional atherectomy with or without supplemental angioplasty (n=5), angioplasty alone (n=3), or additional stent placement (n=11), although the sample sizes were small.

Documented causes of recurrence included intrastent stenosis (n=11), stenosis immediately adjacent to the stent (n=8), and a new stenosis remote from the stent (n=2). Eleven patients (7 thrombosed grafts, 4 recurrent symptoms/signs) had recurrences that were not angiographically studied. In four other patients, the stent slipped slightly (up to 1 cm) central to the initial deployment site and foreshortened to uncover the lesion (figures 21-5A—21-5C). Two other stents moved slightly central relative to the initial deployment site without uncovering the lesion. Four of these stents were in central veins and two were in peripheral veins. Of the six stents that moved slightly, three appeared to be undersized relative to the adjacent vein and three appeared to be adequately sized.

One complication was directly related to the stent. This was a 2.4-cm pseudoaneurysm that developed 10 months after placement of a 10-mm x 42-mm Wallstent across a stenosis just above the venous anastomosis of a PTFE graft. This graft was ligated and replaced. In one procedure-related complication, a patient went into pulmonary edema due to excessive administration of I.V. fluids before and during the stenting procedure. This patient was treated by dialysis.

Two complications were related to subsequent procedures. These were two subclavian stents that were dislodged and embolized to the pulmonary artery when a

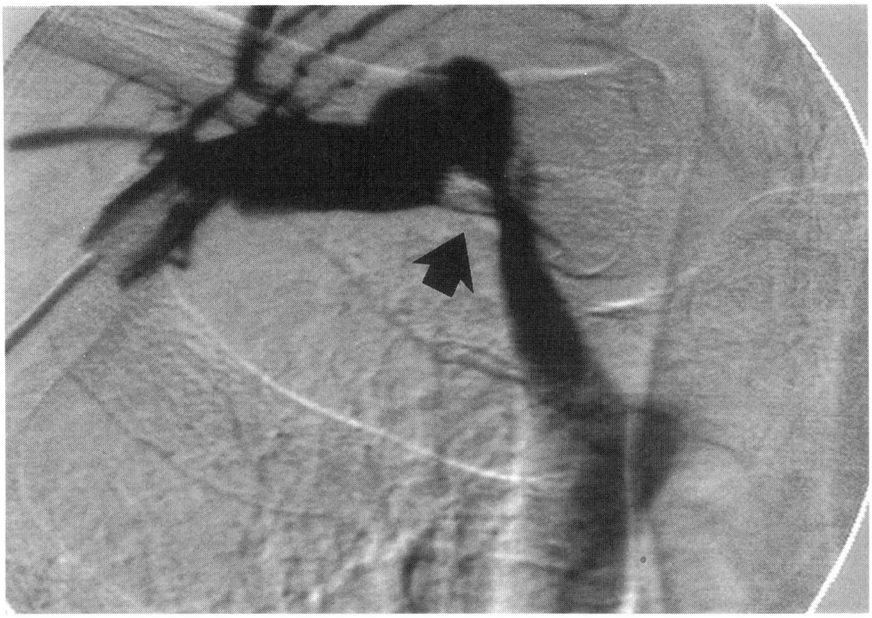

Figure 21-5A. Digital subtraction image shows a high-grade innominate stenosis (arrow) in a patient with arm swelling and an ipsilateral dialysis graft.

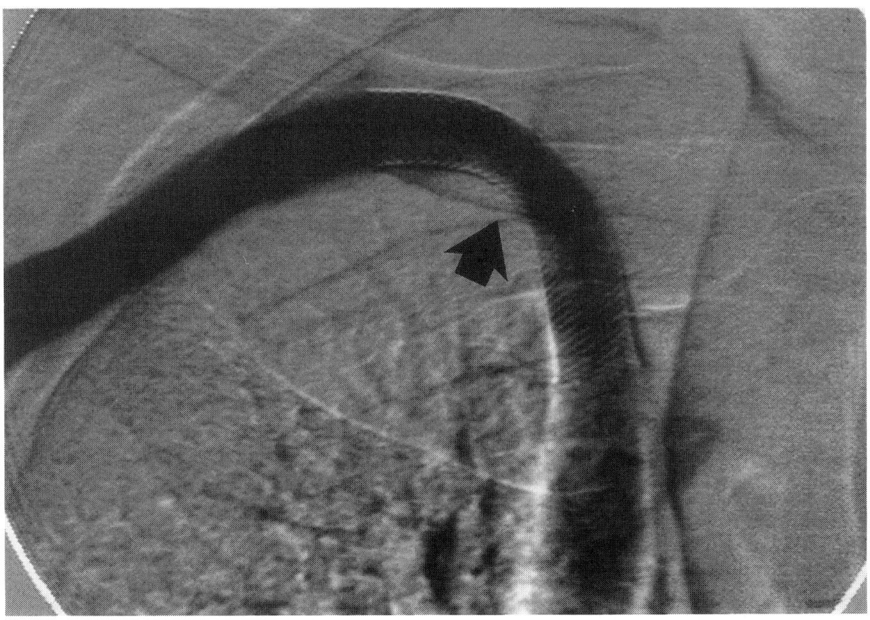

Figure 21-5B. Following deployment of a 10 mm x 42 mm Wallstent dilated to 10 mm, there is minimal residual stenosis (arrow)

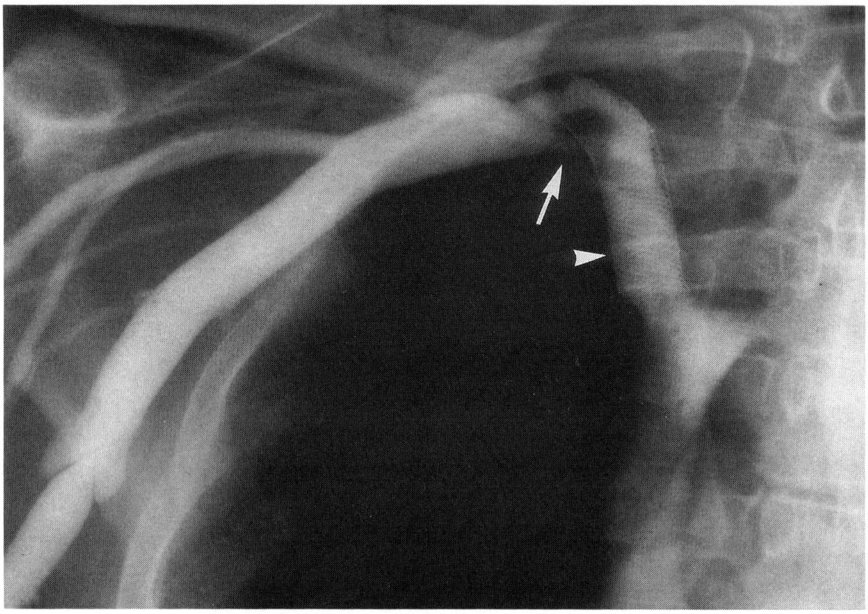

Figure 21-5C. When the patient's arm swelling recurred, a diagnostic study revealed a re-stenosis (arrow). Note foreshortening of the stent with crowding of the stent interstices (arrow). Compare with figure 21-5B. This patient was retreated successfully with a second Wallstent.

dialysis catheter was introduced into the subclavian vein (figures 21-6A—21-6C). Both stents were snared from a femoral approach using a 25-mm Nitinol snare (MicroVena, Vadnais Heights, Minnesota). One stent was withdrawn into a no. 24 Fr sheath and removed. The other stent was mangled by the subclavian dialysis catheter and by the snaring procedure; this stent lodged in the right common iliac vein and required surgical removal via a retroperitoneal approach.

Discussion

Surveillance of hemodialysis fistulas for signs of venous stenosis is done in a variety of ways, including hemodialysis venous pressure monitoring,[12] recirculation testing,[13] color flow Doppler,[14] and physical examination.[15,16] Regardless of the screening technique, aggressive treatment of venous stenoses has been shown to improve the life expectancy of hemodialysis access.[12] Repetitive percutaneous angioplasty has resulted in patencies up to 70% at three years.[17] Despite this record of success, technical failures of balloon angioplasty may occur despite full expansion (i.e., no waist) of the angioplasty balloon. Such failures are usually due to elastic recoil that is minimized by using intentionally oversized balloons,[18] thereby disrupting the elasticity of the treated vein wall segment. For these angioplasty failures, deployment of an endoluminal stent is a logical therapeutic maneuver because

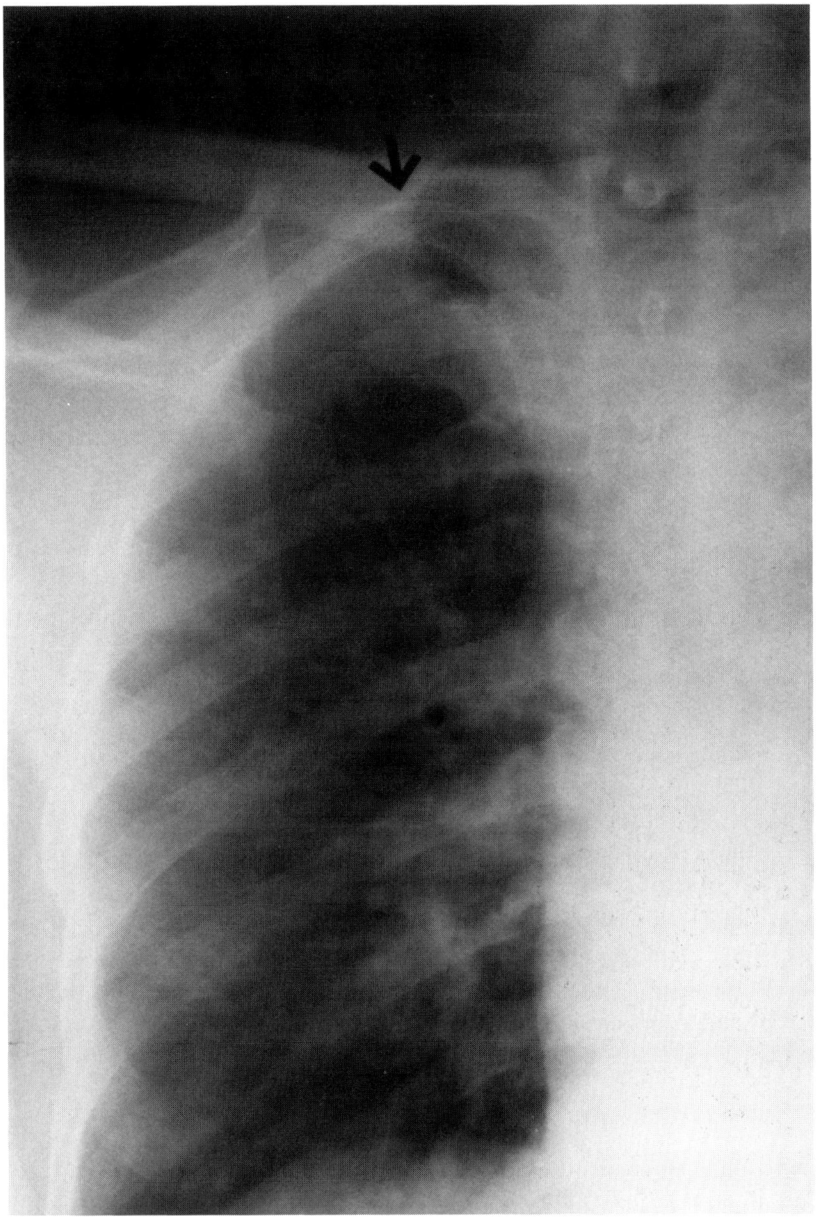

Figure 21-6A. Chest x-ray shows Wallstent (arrow) one month after deployment.

elastic recoil is prevented. We did not deploy stents for lesions resistant to high-pressure balloons; however, in our experience, these lesions are not common.

A number of reports describe endoluminal stenting in the dialysis population, including Palmaz,[19] Wallstents,[20,21] and Gianturco[22,23] stents. However, several of these series are very small,[19,20] and/or have not undergone peer review.[19-21] In the largest peer-reviewed series, Beathard[22] prospectively compared angioplasty with

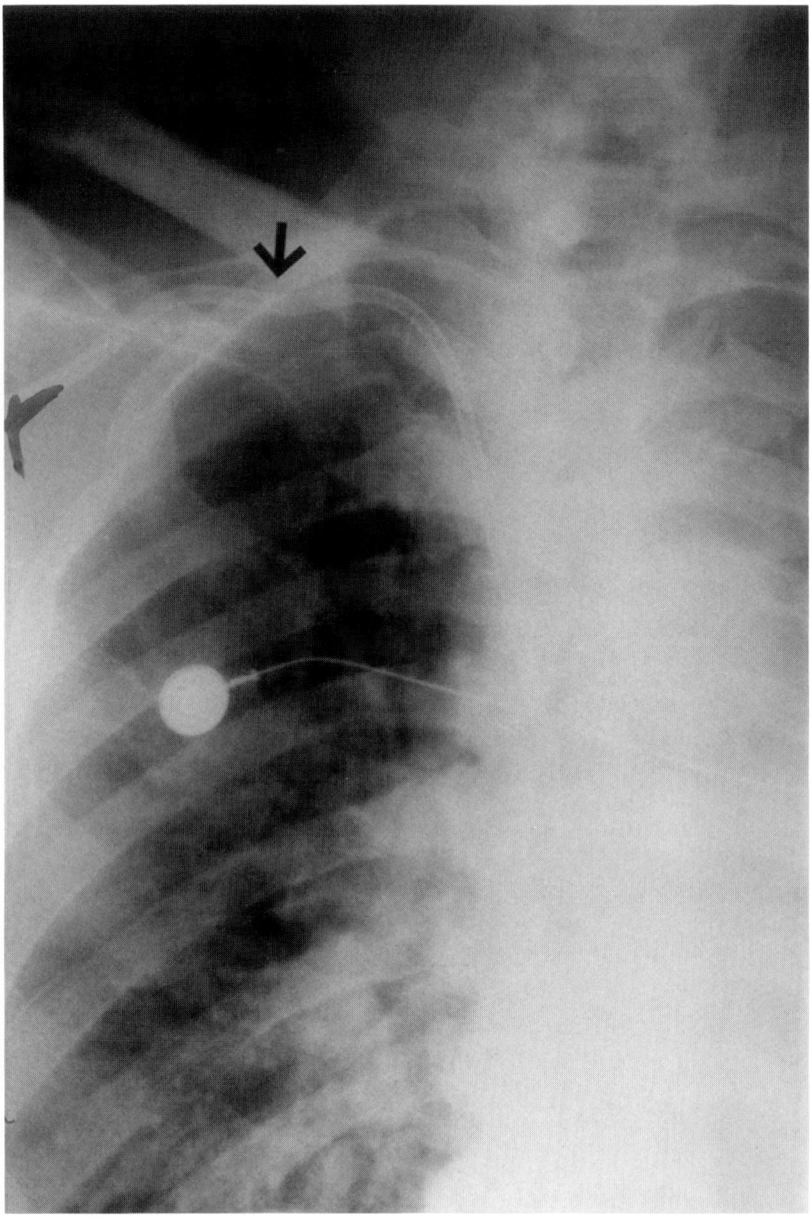

Figure 21-6B. Repeat chest x-ray two hours later shows central line (arrow). The stent had migrated into the pulmonary artery.

Gianturco stents (Cook, Bloomington, Indiana) for PTFE venous anastomotic stenoses in 58 patients and found no significant difference. In another series, Quinn et al.[23] treated 25 venous lesions in 19 patients with the Gianturco stent and reported a 25% primary patency at two years; however, fewer than 10 patients were followed after the first year, casting doubt on the validity of these two-year patency figures. The results of both of these studies must be questioned, since the Gianturco stents in

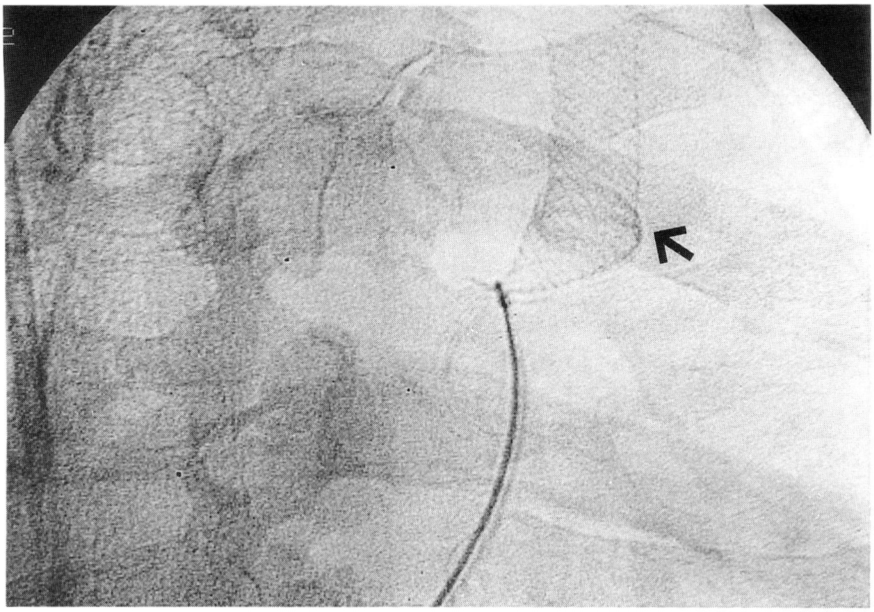

Figure 21-6C. The stent has been captured with a Nitinol snare. Note deformation (arrow) of the stent, probably related to the subclavian puncture needle.

both were made in the investigator's institutions with no description of quality control given.

In the only other peer-reviewed publication identified, Schoenfeld et al.[24] treated 19 central venous lesions with commercially available Wallstents (Schneider, Minneapolis, Minnesota) and/or Palmaz stents (Johnson & Johnson Interventional Systems, Warren, New Jersey). They reported a 68% primary and a 93% secondary patency at 17 months; however, only five patients were followed beyond six months.

To our knowledge, our study is the first published report with long-term follow-up of a commercially available stent in a sizable hemodialysis series. Our results indicate that biliary Wallstents are useful for salvaging and maintaining patency of hemodialysis access when angioplasty is unsuccessful or is unlikely to succeed. Given an expected 21-month mean PTFE graft life,[25] an additional 6 to 12 months patency is important. When larger diameter Wallstents become available, the patency for central stenoses may improve because slippage of the stent may be prevented. Another way to improve the patency may be overdilation of the Wallstent, as recently reported for transjugular intrahepatic portosystemic shunt placement.[26] Since only a small number of our patients were treated by de novo stent placement, we did not address the issue of Wallstent versus balloon angioplasty patency. This comparison will require a prospective, randomized series. The results of Wallstent placement may be better if used for the initial stenosis rather than angioplasty failures and re-stenoses. Due to small numbers, we could not determine the best treatment for recurrent stenoses following Wallstent placement.

Significantly, we had no spontaneous migrations from the stent deployment site; this was in contrast with our experience using the Palmaz stent.[11] This is probably due to the sharp flared ends of the Wallstent. The ability of the Wallstent to reexpand if compressed may also contribute to positional stability. Furthermore, unlike previous reports on the Palmaz stent,[27] we had no occlusion from stent compression in our series. We did have six slippages of the stent, with resultant foreshortening, which may have resulted from external compression. This small movement (relative to migration) is similar to movement of an angioplasty balloon dilated with a resistant stenosis toward one end of the balloon. Significantly, we did not have any such slippages if the stent was well centered or if the stenosis was toward the leading edge of the stent (relative to upper extremity graft percutaneous access) so that the portion of the stent uninvolved by the lesion was in a vein of smaller diameter. Larger stents may decrease the incidence of stent slippage through better contact with the vein wall by the flared filamentous ends.

Our most significant complications were the two migrations to the pulmonary artery related to subsequent central line placement into the stented subclavian vein. Percutaneous retrieval of Palmaz and Wallstents from the pulmonary artery or right heart has been previously described.[11,28-31] Our migrations occurred despite having advised patients and referring physicians against placing ipsilateral central lines in patients with central vein stents. Because we are a large tertiary care referral center, resident physicians frequently care for patients and may be unaware of the stent, as in our two cases. We now advise all patients to purchase a Medic Alert bracelet that describes the stent location and contraindicates ipsilateral central line placement. Nothing is lost regarding access, since a central line placement would not be attempted if the subclavian is known to be stenosed or occluded. Although we have not routinely placed central lines through innominate stents, this could be done if necessary, but only under fluoroscopic control.

Because central stenoses or occlusions usually contraindicate any future permanent upper extremity dialysis access, our ability to salvage angioplasty failures and treat occlusions in these veins with Wallstents contributes significantly to the care of these patients. These lesions are not rare; up to 50% of dialysis patients with prior subclavian dialysis catheters have a significant subclavian vein stenosis.[32,33] When placing a stent in a subclavian vein, the internal jugular origin should be crossed only if necessary. Leaving the internal jugular-subclavian vein junction patent allows two potential future options: (1) an axillojugular veno-veno bypass[34] or a brachiojugular PTFE dialysis graft[35] may be performed if the stent occludes and cannot be retreated, or (2) an internal jugular temporary dialysis catheter can be placed if no permanent access is available.

Wallstents are useful for salvaging balloon angioplasty failures and for treating catheter-related central vein occlusions. Wallstents appear to be safe unless surgically manipulated after placement. In contrast to Gianturco stents,[36] we have seen no breakdown of the Wallstents, although the fate of the stent at 5, 10, or 15 years is unknown. Surveillance and repetitive treatments are necessary for continued Wallstent patency; however, their patency beyond 12 months is attainable only in a minority.

References

1. Saeed M, Newman GE, McCann RL, et al. Stenoses in dialysis fistulas: treatment with percutaneous angioplasty. Radiology 1987; 164:693-697.
2. Glanz S, Gordon DH, Butt KMH, Hong J, Lipkowitz GS. The role of percutaneous angioplasty in the management of chronic hemodialysis fistulas. Ann Surg 1987; 206:777-781.
3. Beathard GA. Percutaneous transvenous angioplasty in the treatment of vascular access stenosis. Kidney Int 1992; 42:1390-1397.
4. Glanz S, Gordon D, Butt KMH, Hong J, Adamson R, Sclafani SJA. Dialysis access fistulas: treatment of stenoses by translumenal angioplasty. Radiology 1984; 152:637-642.
5. Zemel G, Katzen BT, Dake MD, Benenati JF, Lempert TE, Moskowitz L. Directional atherectomy in the treatment of stenotic dialysis access fistulas. JVIR 1990; 1:35-38.
6. Gray RJ, Dolmatch BL, Buick MK. Directional atherectomy treatment for hemodialysis access: early results. JVIR 1992; 3:497-503.
7. Gaylord GM, Taber TE, Ehrman KO, Brown PO. Angioplasty versus directional atherectomy of dialysis graft venous anastomotic strictures (abstr). JVIR 1994; 5:49.
8. Roberts AC, Valji K, Bookstein JJ, Hyde RJ. Pulse-spray pharmacomechanical thrombolysis for treatment of thrombosed dialysis access grafts. Am J Surg 1993; 166:221-226.
9. Ahn SS, Rutherford RB, Becker GJ. Reporting standards for lower extremity arterial endovascular procedures. J Vasc Surg 1993; 17:1103-1107.
10. Haskal ZJ, LaBerge JM, Gordon RL, Gonzales J. Response of Wallstents to dilation: therapeutic implications. JVIR 1993; 4:635-637.
11. Gray RJ, Dolmatch BL, Horton KM, Romolo JL, Zarate AR. Migration of Palmaz stents following deployment for venous stenoses related to hemodialysis access. JVIR 1994; 5: 117-120.
12. Schwab SJ, Raymond JR, Saeed M, Newman GE, Dennis PA, Bollinger RR. Prevention of hemodialysis fistula thrombosis. Early detection of venous stenoses. Kidney Int 1989; 36:707-711.
13. Windus DW, Audrain J, Vanderson R, Jendrisak MD, Picus D, Delmez JA. Optimization of high-efficiency hemodialysis by detection and correction of fistula dysfunction. Kidney Int 1990; 38:337-341.
14. Dousset V, Grenier N, Douws C, et al. Hemodialysis grafts: color Doppler flow imaging correlated with digital subtraction angiography and functional status. Radiology 1991; 181:89-94.
15. Trerotola SO, Scheel PJ, Powe N. Physical examination vs. color flow Doppler US for detecting impending vascular graft failure (abstr). JVIR 1994; 5:39.
16. Beathard GA. Physical examination of AV grafts. Dialysis Clinic Feb 14, 1992; 74.
17. Turmel-Rodrigues L, Pengloan J, Blanchier D, et al. Insufficient dialysis shunts: improved long-term patency rates with close hemodynamic monitoring, repeated percutaneous balloon angioplasty, and stent placement. Radiology 1993; 187:273-278.
18. Hunter DW, Castaneda-Zuniga WR, Coleman CC, et al. Failing arteriovenous dialysis fistulas: evaluation and treatment. Radiology 1984; 152:631-635.
19. Ehrman KO, Reed JD, Gaylord GM, Harris VM. Use of the Palmaz balloon-expandable stent in subclavian/brachiocephalic vein stenosis. JVIR 1992; 3:13 (abstr).
20. McNamara TO, Goodwin SC. Initial and long-term results of thrombolysis, percutaneous translumenal angioplasty, and stents for central vein obstruction in patients with ipsilateral dialysis access graft (abstr). Radiology 1993; 189:200.

21. Vorwerk D, Guenther RW, Bohndorf K, Gladziwa U, Kistler D. Self-expanding stents in peripheral and central veins used for arteriovenous shunts: five years of experience (abstr). Radiology 1993; 189:174.
22. Beathard GA. Gianturco self-expanding stent in the treatment of stenosis in dialysis access grafts. Kidney Int 1993; 43:872-877.
23. Quinn SF, Schuman ES, Hall L, et al. Venous stenoses in patients who undergo hemodialysis: treatment with self-expandable endovascular stents. Radiology 1992; 183:499-504.
24. Shoenfeld R, Hermans H, Novick A, et al. Stenting of proximal venous obstructions to maintain hemodialysis access. J Vasc Surg 1994; 19:532-539.
25. Zibari GB, Rohr MS, Landreneau MD, et al. Complications from permanent hemodialysis vascular access. Surgery 1988; 104:681-686.
26. Valji K, Bookstein JJ, Roberts AC, Oglevie SB, Royster AP, Varney RR. Overdilation of the Wallstent to optimize portal decompression during transjugular intrahepatic portosystemic shunt placement. Radiology 1994; 191:173-176.
27. Bjarnason H, Hunter DW, Crain MR, et al. Collapse of a Palmaz stent in the subclavian vein. AJR 1993; 160:1123-1124.
28. Saeed M, Knowles HJ Jr., Brems JJ, Takiff H. Percutaneous retrieval of a large Palmaz stent from the pulmonary artery. JVIR 1993; 4:811-814.
29. Zemel G, Brown JA, Becker GJ, et al. Transjugular intrahepatic portosystemic shunts: long-term follow-up (abstr). Radiology 1992; 185(p):166.
30. Sanchez RB, Roberts AC, Valji K, Lengle S, Bookstein JJ. Wallstent misplaced during transjugular placement of an intrahepatic portosystemic shunt: retrieval with a loop snare. AJR 1992; 159:129-130.
31. Cohen GS, Ball DS. Delayed Wallstent migration after a transjugular intrahepatic portosystemic shunt procedure: relocation with a loop snare. JVIR 1993; 4:559-560.
32. Surratt RF, Picus D, Hicks ME, Darcy MD, Kleinhoffer M, Jendrisak M. The importance of preoperative evaluation of the subclavian vein in dialysis access planning. AJR 1991; 156:623-625.
33. Cimochowski GE, Worley E, Rutherford WE, Sartain J, Blondin J, Harter H. Superiority of the internal jugular over the subclavian access for temporary dialysis. Nephron 1990; 54:154-161.
34. Currier CB, Widder S, Ali A, Kuusisto E, Sidawy A. Surgical management of subclavian and axillary vein thrombosis in patients with a functioning arteriovenous fistula. Surgery 1986; 100:25-28.
35. Polo JR, Sanabia J, Calleja J. Brachiojugular PTFE grafts for dialysis (abstr). Dialysis Access IV 1994;38.
36. Carrasco CH, Charnsangavej C, Wright KC, Wallace S, Gianturco C. Use of the Gianturco self-expanding stent in stenoses of the superior and inferior venae cavae. JVIR 1992; 3:409-419.

22

THROMBOSED DIALYSIS GRAFTS: PERCUTANEOUS BALLOON THROMBECTOMY VERSUS THROMBOLYSIS

Michael R. Middlebrook, M.D., Michael C. Soulen, M.D., Ziv J. Haskal, M.D., Richard D. Shlansky-Goldberg, M.D., Constantin Cope, M.D., and Michael J. Pentecost, M.D.

MORE THAN 120,000 PATIENTS RECEIVE HEMODIALYSIS in the United States each year. The number of patients beginning hemodialysis is increasing yearly, as is the long-term survival of these patients.[1,2] Prolonged patient survival has added new importance to the extension of arteriovenous (A-V) graft life,[3] a process that has evolved over the past decade from a surgical problem to one that involves interventional radiologists, nephrologists, and surgeons in a team approach incorporating graft surveillance, angioplasty, and thrombolysis of occluded grafts.[2]

Fibrinolytic therapy has changed from a procedure of questionable utility or cost-effectiveness[4-6] to a well-accepted procedure used routinely in the care of occluded grafts.[7-13] The cost of urokinase (UK) is high, and complications, although few, still occur during thrombolysis.[5,7,8,10-13] These two reasons have prompted some to advocate mechanical thrombectomy and angioplasty over thrombolysis.[4] Experimental work has been done regarding devices that would allow percutaneous mechanical aspiration thrombectomy,[14] but no devices are commercially available in the United States. A technique of percutaneous mechanical graft declotting using readily available balloon catheters has been described, and preliminary results show it to be effective and safe.[15] We describe our results using this technique and compare it to thrombolysis.

Patients and Methods

Forty-five patients treated for occlusion of polytetrafluoroethylene (PTFE) arm grafts between January 1, 1991, and August 1, 1993, underwent 65 procedures during the 19-month period. These procedures were performed under the direction of one of four staff members who rotated through the clinical laboratories weekly. Two of these staff members used the pulsed-spray thrombolysis technique, and two used the mechanical declotting method. Patients were treated randomly by the technique used by the staff member on duty when they presented for treatment. Patients who were treated more than one time did not necessarily receive the same method of declotting each visit. Thrombolysis was performed in 31 patients, and 34 patients received mechanical declotting of their occluded graft. Average age in both groups was 55 years. Almost all patients received heparin 2,000-7,000 U I.V. as a bolus, and I.V. sedation and supplemental oxygen were used as needed.

Hemodynamic monitoring included continuous pulse-saturation oximetry, EKG, noninvasive blood pressure, and nurse observation during the procedure. Data collected included heparin dose, UK use and dose, procedure duration, complications, graft function postprocedure, and interval until next graft intervention (surgical or radiological) or abandonment for any reason. Initial technical success was defined as the percentage of patients with patent grafts at the end of their procedure. Clinical success was defined as the graft being used successfully for hemodialysis three times or remaining patent for one week.[15] Primary patency was measured as the number of days from the date of the procedure until the patient required another graft-related intervention (surgical or radiological) for thrombosis or decreased flow rates, or until the graft was abandoned and dialysis was performed using a different access. None of the patients in this study underwent renal transplantation or died. Procedure time was defined as the period of time the patient occupied the procedure room. This figure was chosen because it is used when calculating average room time charges per procedure.

Procedure

All grafts were initially punctured near the arterial anastomosis with the needle directed centrally. A guide wire was passed centrally in all cases, followed by a multihole catheter. Venography was performed to evaluate the venous anastomosis and central vessels.

Thrombolysis

A second puncture was then made in the graft near the venous anastomosis directed peripherally and a guide wire and catheter were advanced, with the tip ending near the arterial anastomosis. Gentle contrast injection was used to evaluate the arterial anastomosis. Care was taken to avoid reflux of thrombus into the native artery.

Thrombolysis was performed through the crossing catheters.[11] The Mewisson catheter (Meditech, Watertown, Massachusetts) and the Cook multiside hole infusion catheter (Cook Inc., Bloomington, Indiana) were commonly used. These catheters have multiple side holes that span a preselected length, usually 5 or 10 cm. The side holes are buried within the clot and UK pulsed through the side holes after a guide wire is placed to occlude the end hole. UK (Abbokinase, Abbott

Pharmaceuticals, North Chicago, Illinois) was typically mixed 250,000 U/50 cc normal saline and forcefully pulsed equally through both catheters over 20-30 minutes at a rate of 0.5 cc per catheter every 30 seconds. Clot maceration was performed during the procedure by manually massaging the graft. Additional UK was used in a similar fashion if residual clot was present. Residual clot was often found near the arterial anastomosis and sometimes in the midgraft near areas of frequent needle puncture. If these persisted following additional UK, an angioplasty balloon was used to dilate the area and dislodge the thrombus in order to reestablish flow. Angioplasty of venous or graft stenoses was performed as needed, and final angiography was performed to confirm a good result.

Mechanical Declotting

After the initial venogram, all significant venous stenoses were dilated. This included the venous anastomosis most commonly and any more central native venous narrowings that would limit flow. An 8.5- or 11-mm occlusion balloon (Meditech) was placed in the graft over the indwelling guide wire and inflated. The balloon was then pushed centrally from the graft, through the arm vein and into the central subclavian vein. The partially inflated angioplasty balloon was sometimes used, thus saving the step of exchanging for the occlusion balloon.

A second puncture was then made in the graft near the venous anastomosis directed peripherally and a guide wire and catheter advanced with tip ending near the arterial anastomosis. Gentle contrast injection was used to evaluate the arterial anastomosis avoiding reflux of thrombus into the native artery. Because arterial anastomotic lesions are uncommon, and since many arterial anastomoses contain a plug of thrombus that can be readily removed,[13] angioplasty was rarely performed prior to mechanical declotting.

An occlusion or angioplasty balloon was then passed into the native artery over the guide wire. The balloon was inflated and pulled back, bringing the clot back into the graft . Frequently, removal of the focal plug of clot from the arterial end allowed prompt restoration of flow. External massage of the graft with a contrast-lubricated finger, in a stripping motion from the arterial end centrally, or brisk injection of a burst of saline into the graft, would also aid the resumption of flow. If no thrill was present or slow flow with residual thrombus was present angiographically, the maneuvers were repeated.

Once flow was restored, all catheters were removed and gentle pressure held over the two puncture sites until hemostasis was obtained. Patients either went immediately to dialysis or were observed one to two hours and discharged home.

Results

Twenty-eight of 30 patients (93%) in the thrombolysis group and 31/33 patients in the mechanical group (94%) left the department with a patent graft. Three of the four failures were secondary to persistent outflow lesions. A specific reason for failure was not found in one thrombolysis patient. Clinical success was achieved in 88% of the grafts treated mechanically and 90% of those treated with thrombolysis.

The mean primary patency in both groups was 76 days (0-512 days). Probability of primary patency (mechanical versus thrombolysis) was 36% versus 36% at three months, 32% versus 26% at 6 months and 16% versus 6% at 12 months (p=N.S.). The mean total procedure time for patients undergoing thrombolysis was 3.5 hours and 2.2 hours for mechanical declotting ($p < .05$). Average total dose of UK was 340,000 U.

No difficulties were encountered related to the procedures. No patient complained of chest pain, shortness of breath, or pleurisy during the procedure. Peripheral O_2 saturation remained stable. Two patients who had not undergone dialysis in several days presented with dyspnea and were treated, with the table in reverse-Trendelenburg position. These two patients had no acute changes during the procedure and returned to their usual baseline respiratory status after dialysis. No patient developed any clinical signs suggesting pulmonary embolism following the procedure nor any time during the follow-up period.

No major complications occurred in either group. One patient developed distal embolization to the hand during thrombolysis, with associated pain and loss of the ulnar pulse. With continued UK infusion, the patient's symptoms resolved, but the pulse never returned to normal. Another patient undergoing thrombolysis was noted to have a small amount of contrast extravasation into the soft tissues adjacent to the graft with no palpable hematoma. The procedure was continued uneventfully. Four patients required prolonged manual compression of puncture sites following completion of the procedure (≥30 minutes), three in the thrombolysis group and one in the mechanical group. None of these had any further bleeding once hemostasis was achieved.

Comments

Mechanical declotting of thrombosed hemodialysis grafts combined with percutaneous angioplasty provides a reliable and potentially safe way to restore flow to failed access that does not differ significantly in immediate or long-term success from results achieved with thrombolysis in individuals selected randomly from the same population of hemodialysis patients. The technique offers time and cost benefits compared to thrombolysis. With a probability of access thrombosis over a 12-month period of > 30% in patients with PTFE grafts, hospital admissions just for access-related problems become a significant source of lost time and medical cost.[1,2] Although UK thrombolysis is a timely, safe and, cost-effective alternative to surgical thrombectomy,[2,5,9,13] mechanical declotting offers further reductions in cost and procedure time.

Mechanical declotting of grafts produces small pulmonary emboli. Our data and those reported by Trerotola support the preliminary conclusion that mechanical declotting is safe in the acute setting. There is also support for this in the literature. In his now classic paper, Gorham reported that the majority of patients (85%) with sudden death secondary to pulmonary embolism had massive bilateral emboli.[16]

Many of the remaining 15% had coronary artery sclerosis, myocardial changes, and severe fatal underlying disease, especially of the heart or lungs. Those who died with small emboli and less severe underlying pathology generally had advanced cardiac disease with pulmonary hypertension and right heart failure or other primary lung disease that reduced pulmonary capillary reserve.

Even with theoretical maximum clot sizes of 8.4 cc, mechanical declotting should not be expected to cause massive embolism and sudden death.[15] Mechanical declotting would, however, be contraindicated in patients with underlying pulmonary disease or advanced heart disease (particularly right heart disease), and it probably should not be performed without the administration of heparin. Paradoxical embolism (arterial embolism arising from venous source), most commonly through a patent foramen ovale, is a rare entity; with only 128 cases in the literature since the late 1800s, it is most likely not a significant concern.[17,18]

Overall, given the large numbers of patients who will be on chronic hemodialysis, the success of which depends upon maintaining reliable vascular access, the potential benefit of our technique is measured not only in dollars saved, but in convenience for the patient. This justifies further investigation to prove its safety and efficacy. A prospective series quantitating pulmonary embolism and other clinical parameters over time should be possible in this group of patients receiving chronic hemodialysis.

References

1. Churchill DN, Taylor DW, Cook RJ, et al. Canadian hemodialysis morbidity study. Am J Kidney Dis 1992; 19(3):214-234.
2. Gaylord GM, Taber TE. Long-term hemodialysis access salvage: problems and challenges for nephrologists and interventional radiologists (edit). J Vasc Interv Radiol 1993; 4(1):103-107.
3. Bell DD, Rosental JJ. Arteriovenous graft life in chronic hemodialysis. A need for prolongation. Arch Surg 1988; 123(9):1169-1172.
4. Smith TP, Cragg AH, Castaneda F, Hunter DW. Thrombosed polytetrafluoroethylene hemodialysis fistulas: salvage with combined thrombectomy and angioplasty. Radiology 1989; 171(2):507-508.
5. Summers S, Drazan K, Gomes A, Freischlag J. Urokinase therapy for thrombosed hemodialysis access grafts. Surg Gynecol Obstet 1993; 176(6):534-538.
6. Young AT, Hunter DW, Castaneda-Zuniga WR, et al. Thrombosed synthetic hemodialysis access fistulas: failure of fibrinolytic therapy. Radiology 1985; 154(3):639-642.
7. Schilling JJ, Eiser AR, Slifkin RF, Whitney JT, Neff MS. The role of thrombolysis in hemodialysis access occlusion. Am J Kidney Dis 1987; 10(2):92-97.
8. Davis GB, Dowd CF, Bookstein JJ, Maroney TP, Lang EV, Halasz N. Thrombosed dialysis grafts: efficacy of intrathrombic deposition of concentrated urokinase, clot maceration, and angioplasty. Am J Roentgenol 1987; 149(1):177-181.
9. Ehrman KO, Gaylord GM. Thrombolytic therapy for occluded dialysis access grafts. Semin Interv Radiol 1992; 9(3):190-194.
10. Bookstein JJ, Fellmeth B, Roberts A, Valji K, Davis G, Machado T. Pulsed-spray pharmacomechanical thrombolysis: preliminary clinical results. Am J Roentgenol 1989; 152(5): 1097-1100.

11. Valji K, Bookstein JJ, Roberts AC, Davis GB. Pharmacomechanical thrombolysis and angioplasty in the management of clotted hemodialysis grafts: early and late clinical results. Radiology 1991; 178(1):243-247.
12. Brunner MC, Matalon TA, Patel SK, McDonald V, Jensik SC. Ultrarapid urokinase in hemodialysis access occlusion. J Vasc Interv Radiol 1991; 2(4):503-506.
13. Roberts AC, Valji K, Bookstein JJ, Hye RJ. Pulse-spray pharmacomechanical thrombolysis for treatment of thrombosed dialysis access grafts. Am J Surg 1993; 166(2):221-225.
14. Schmitz-Rode T, Pfeffer J G, Bohndorf K, Gunther R W. Percutaneous thrombectomy of the acutely thrombosed dialysis graft: in vitro evaluation of four devices. Cardiovasc Intervent Radiol 1993; 16(2):72-75.
15. Trerotola SO, Lund GB, Scheel PJ, Venbrux AC, Osterman FA. Thrombosed dialysis access grafts: Percutaneous mechanical declotting without urokinase. Radiology 1994; 191:721-726.
16. Gorham L. A study of pulmonary embolism. Arch Intern Med 1961; 108:76-90.
17. Gleysteen JJ, Silver D. Paradoxical arterial embolism. Collective review. Am Surg 1970; 36: 47-54.
18. Laughlin RA, Mandel SR. Paradoxical embolization. Case report and review of the literature. Arch Surg 1977; 112(May):648-650.

23

VENOUS ANATOMY OF THE UPPER ARM OUTLINED BY VENOGRAPHY: SURGICAL IMPLICATIONS

Lucio Flores, M.D., Warren Shapiro, M.D., Paul B. Haser, M.D., Kathleen Bradbury, S.A., and Gerald Shaftan, M.D.

THE IMPORTANCE OF A FUNCTIONING ARTERIOVENOUS (A-V) access for the end-stage renal disease (ESRD) patient on maintenance hemodialysis cannot be overemphasized. Recently, with the increase in older patients, diabetics, and intravenous drug abusers, the creation of an A-V access has become difficult due to the lack of adequate native blood vessels, and it is frequently necessary to use synthetic graft materials. In this prospective study, we evaluated the venous anatomy of the upper arm outlined by preoperative venography in 225 consecutive ESRD patients who were candidates for upper-arm angio-access (A-V graft), with the venous anastomosis performed 3 cm below the axillary hairline.

Patients and Methods

Between January 1980 and December 1989, preoperative venograms were performed in 225 consecutive ESRD patients who were candidates for upper-arm A-V graft angio-access at the Brookdale Hospital Medical Center, New Rochelle, New York. Patients with prior upper-arm graft angio-access of the same extremity or a history of allergy to radiographic contrast material were excluded from this study.

All venograms were performed in the operating room prior to graft placement. A 25-gauge needle was inserted in the skin as a marker on the medial aspect of the upper arm at the potential site for the venous anastomosis of the A-V graft. Then 20 ml of 60% diatrizoate meglumine (Renografin 60) was injected and a single anterior-posterior radiograph was taken, developed with a soft tissue technique, and

Table 23-1. Results of Venography of the Upper Extremity in 225 Patients

No. veins	No. patients (%)
1	83 (37)
2	105 (47)
3	32 (14)
4	5 (2)
Total	225 (100)

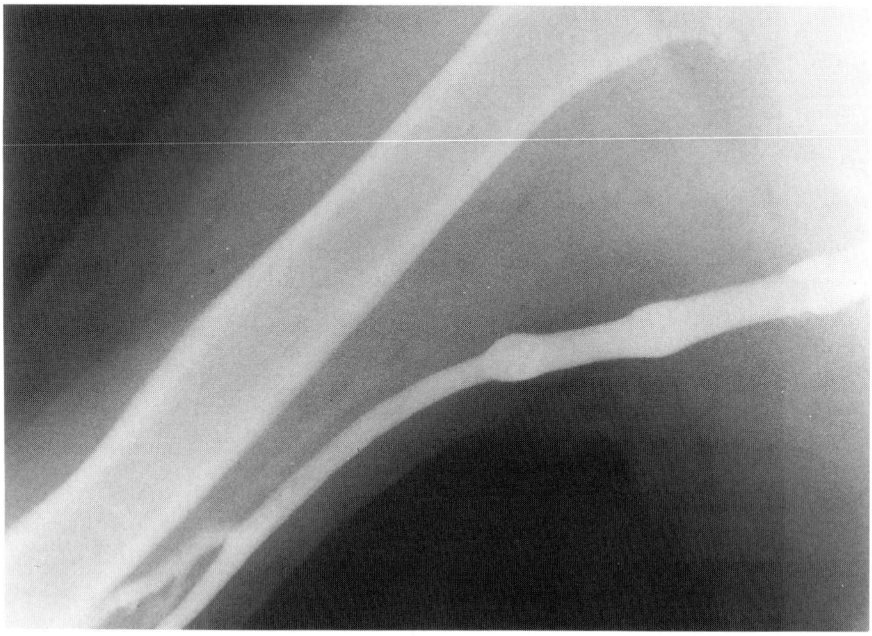

Figure 23-1. Preoperative upper-arm venography showing a single brachial vein.

read by a radiologist. The number and size of the veins visualized in the upper arm at the level of the marker were analyzed.

Surgery

With the patient in a supine position and under local anesthesia, an oblique incision was made over the inner aspect of the arm about 3 cm below the axillary hairline. The subcutaneous tissue and brachial fascia were incised and the neurovascular bundle exposed. When the venogram indicated the presence of a single vein, it was usually situated under the brachial fascia, easily isolated with minimal manipulation of the neurovascular bundle, and the search for other veins was eliminated.

In patients with multiple veins, only the largest was isolated, and its position relative to the neurovascular structures was noted as either medial or lateral (superficial

Table 23-2. **Patients with a Double Venous System and its Relationship to the Neurovascular Bundle**

No. venograms	Dominant veins (%)		Equal veins (%)
	Medial	Lateral	
105	46 (44)	19 (18)	40 (38)

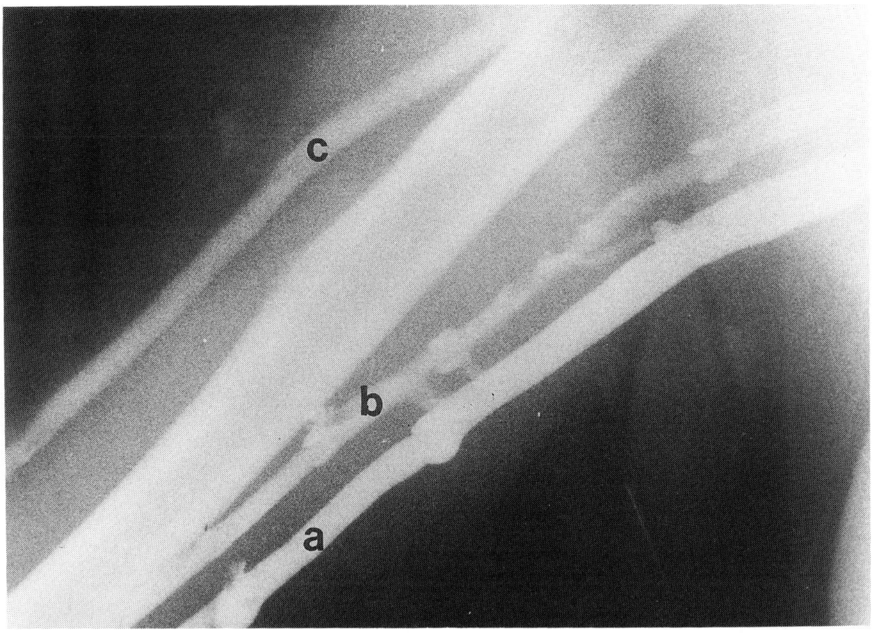

Figure 23-2. Preoperative upper-arm venography showing a double venous system with a dominant medial brachial vein (a = medial brachial vein; b = lateral brachial vein; c = cephalic vein).

or deep). When the venogram indicated that the largest vein was lateral to the neurovascular bundle, the surgical exposure was simplified by incising the brachial fascia near the biceps muscle, followed by lateral retraction of the muscle. This maneuver exposed the vein, which was deeply situated between the muscle and the cords of the brachial plexus. In patients with multiple and nondominant veins, the two most contiguous veins were isolated and employed for double venous outflow using a technique previously described.[1]

Results

The venographic findings are summarized in table 23-1. A total of 225 venograms were performed; in 137 (61%), they conformed to classical textbook description of either two (47%) or three (14%) veins.[2,3] The most common variations

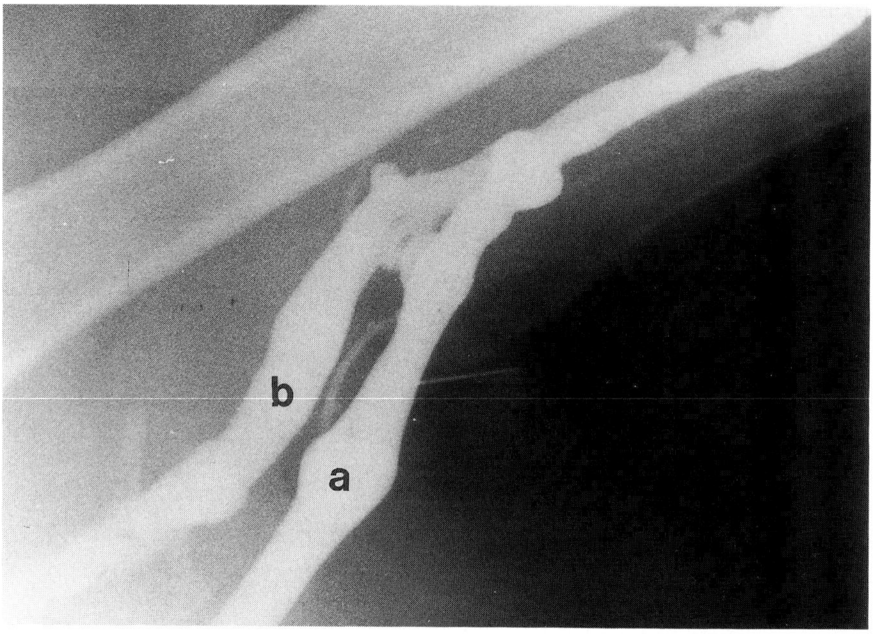

Figure 23-3. Preoperative upper-arm venography showing a double brachial venous system of equal size (a = medial brachial vein; b = lateral brachial vein).

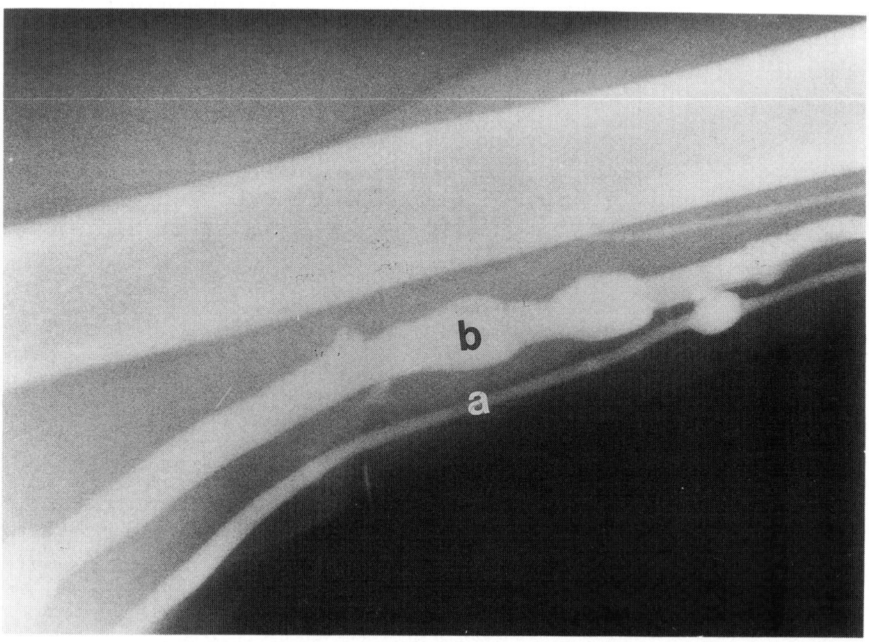

Figure 23-4. Preoperative venography showing double venous system with a dominant lateral brachial vein (a = medial brachial vein; b = lateral brachial vein).

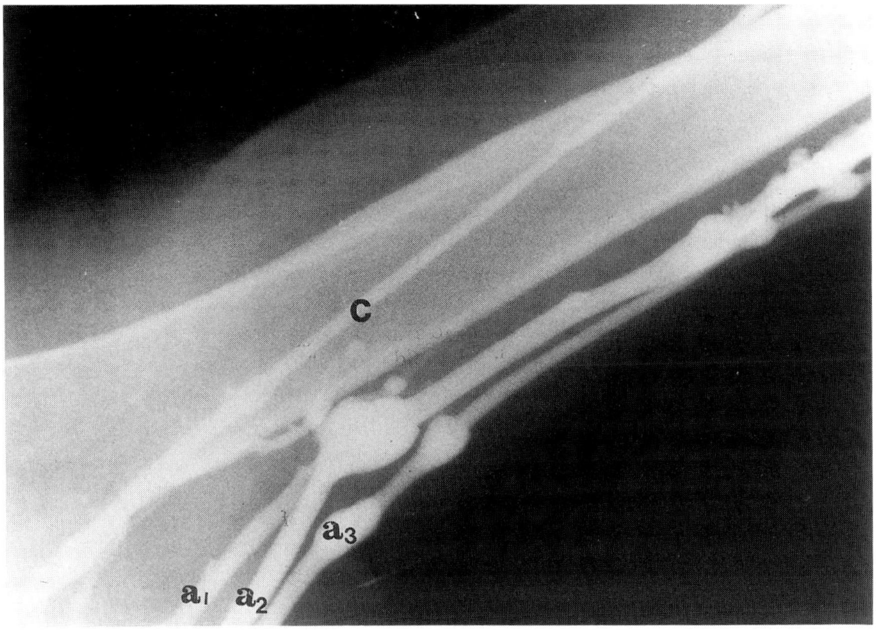

Figure 23-5. Preoperative upper-arm venography showing a triple brachial venous system (a1, a2, a3 = brachial veins; c = cephalic vein).

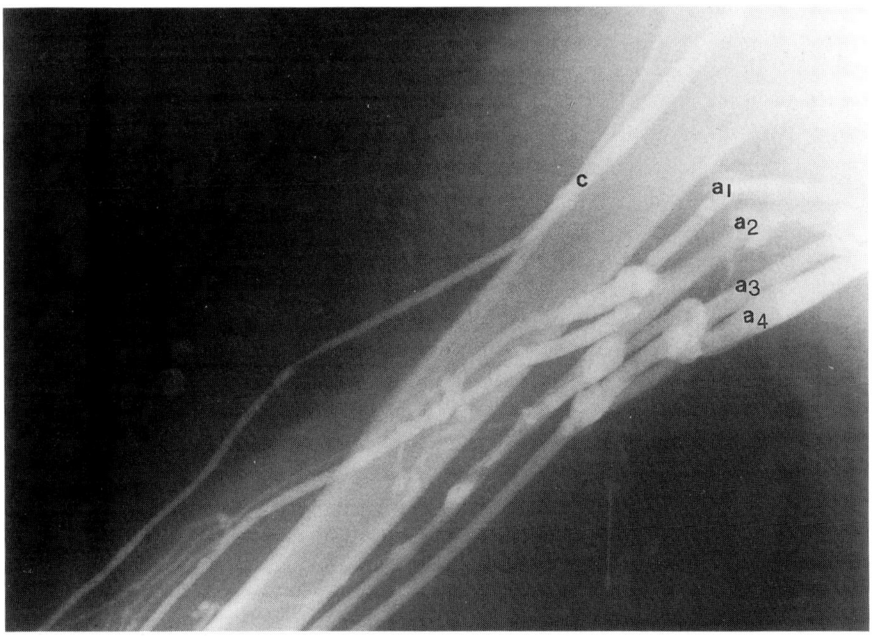

Figure 23-6. Preoperative upper-arm venography showing a quadruple brachial venous system (a1, a2, a3, a4 = brachial veins).

Table 23-3. Patients with Multiple Veins

No. veins	No. patients	Dominant veins (%)		Equal veins (%)
		Medial	Lateral	
3	32	20 (68.75)	4 (12.5)	6 (81.75)
4	5	3 (60)	1 (20)	1 (20)

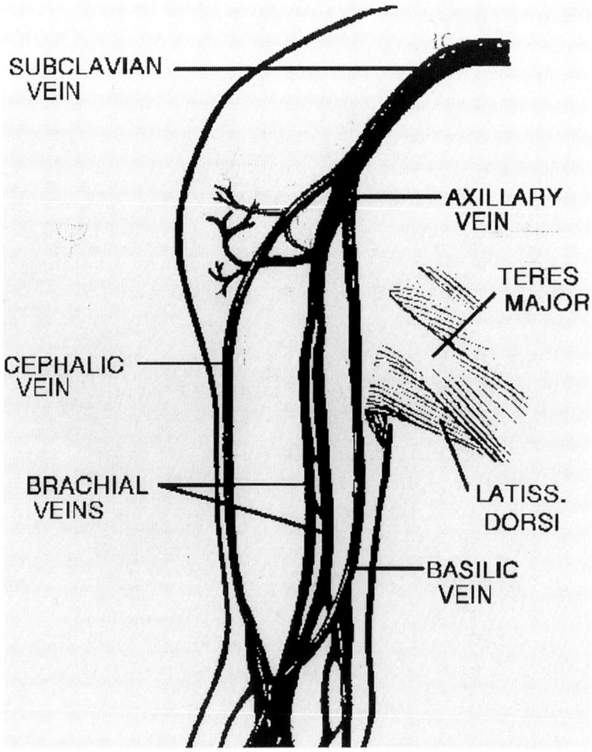

Figure 23-7. Sketch of the description found most frequently in anatomy textbooks.

were a single vein in 37% of the patients (figure 23-1) and four veins noted in five patients (2%).

A more detailed analysis of the venographic findings of those patients with two veins is shown in table 23-2, which outlines the location of the dominant or largest vein relative to the neurovascular bundle. In this group, the most frequent variations were a dominant medial or superficial vein in 44% (figure 23-2) and equal sized veins in 38% (figure 23-3). In the other 18% of the cases, the largest vein was lateral to the brachial plexus, deeply situated between the neurovascular bundle and the biceps muscles and thus not easily accessible to routine exploration of the area (figure 23-4).

In the patients with three veins (figure 23-5) or four veins (figure 23-6), venography was helpful in identifying the presence of a dominant vein; this was situated lateral to the brachial plexus in 12.5% and 20%, respectively (table 23-3). Thus, in 10.66%, (24/225) of the entire series or in 16.9% (24/142) of the patients with two or more veins, the lateral vein is the largest. Allergic reactions were noted in three patients, manifested by itching and maculopapular rash, which resolved with conservative treatment.

Discussion

Venography of the upper extremity has been used extensively in the management of complications of shunts,[4,5] fistulas,[6-8] and A-V graft angio-access.[9-13] This modality has also been useful in patients with previous angio-access procedures or a history of drug addiction.[14] To our knowledge, this is the first study in which the venous anatomy of the upper extremity was routinely delineated by venography prior to graft insertion in upper-arm angio-access surgery.

According to the anatomical descriptions of the upper extremity, the veins can be divided into two systems: superficial and deep, with frequent anastomoses found between the two systems at variable sites. The superficial veins are distributed immediately under the skin, and the deep veins accompany the arteries bearing the same name. In the upper arm, the cephalic vein ascends along the lateral border of the biceps brachii, passing between the pectoralis major and the deltoid muscle, where it pierces the clavipectoral fascia and enters the axillary vein.

The basilic vein continues its upward course superficially along the medial border of the biceps brachii, perforating the deep fascia at variable levels where it becomes a deep vein, ascending on the medial side of the brachial artery and joining the brachial veins to form the axillary vein. If this junction takes place below the lower border of the teres muscle, two major veins will be present, but if the junction occurs above the teres major, three major veins will be present in the brachial axillary area; thus, two or three veins are the most frequent description found in most anatomy textbooks (figure 23-7).

Creation of an A-V fistula provides the access of choice; however, due to the lack of native vessels, graft angio-access is a good alternative. The graft is most frequently placed in the forearm or upper arm in a straight or loop configuration. This study analyzes the venous anatomy for a graft to be placed in the upper arm, with the venous anastomosis near the axillary fossa.

Analysis of our results shows that in 39% of cases, the venous anatomy of the upper arm deviated from the usual textbook description of two or three deep veins. A single brachial vein was the most frequent anatomical variation; it was found in 37% of patients. Four veins were detected in 2% of the cases. Sixty-one percent of our patients had two or three veins (47% and 14%, respectively), which conforms to the textbook description of the normal anatomy of the upper extremity.[2,3]

In the 105 cases in which two veins were visualized, they were of equal size in 38% of the patients, the superficial or medial brachial vein was larger in 44%, and the lateral vein was dominant in 18%.

In patients with three and four veins, venography was helpful in identifying the presence of a dominant vein, and in 12.5% and 20%, respectively, the largest was lateral to the brachial plexus. Thus, in 10.66% of the entire series, (24/225), or in 16.9% of patients with two or more veins (24/142), the lateral vein is the largest; it is not easily accessible to routine exploration and requires dissection between the neurovascular bundle and the biceps muscle.

Our study was not designed to compare graft longevity in patients who had or did not have preoperative venography. However, the findings yield valuable information for surgeons involved in angio-access procedures, demonstrating that the classical textbook description of the venous anatomy is present in only 61% of the cases.

References

1. Flores L, Haser PB, Bradbury K, Carryl S, Shaftan GW. Improved venous outflow by double vein anastomosis in graft angioaccess. Surg Gynecol Obstet 1992; 174:333-334.
2. Gray H. Anatomy of the human body, 30th ed. Philadelphia:Lea & Febiger, 1985;820-825.
3. Hollinshead WH. Pectoral region, axilla and shoulder. In: Hollinshead WEI, ed. Anatomy for surgeons, vol 3: the back and limbs, 2nd ed. New York:Harper & Row, 1958; 264-348.
4. Cohen BJ, Chinitz OL, Sol KH, Ramirez O, et al. Radiological contrast study of arteriovenous dialysis cannulae. Radiology 1970; 94:603-606.
5. Royle JP, Dawborn JK, Thomas DP. The use of radiology in the management of patients with arteriovenous shunts. Med J Aust 1972; 1:529-531.
6. Gilula LA, Staple TW, Anderson CB, Anderson LS. Venous angiography of hemodialysis fistulas. Radiology 1975; 115:555-562.
7. Anderson CB, Gilula LA, Sicard GA, Etheredge E. Venous angiography of subcutaneous hemodialysis fistulas. Arch Surg 1979; 114:1320-1325.
8. Gothlin J, Lindstedt E. Angiographic features of Cimino-Brescia fistulas. Am J Roentgenol Radium Ther Nucl Med 1975; 125:582-590.
9. Thomsen MB, Stenport G. Evaluation of clinical examination preceding surgical treatment of AV-fistula problems. Is angiography necessary? Acta Chir Scand 1985; 151:133-137.
10. Glanz S, Bashist B, Gordon DH, Butt K, Adamson R. Angiography of upper extremity access fistulas for dialysis. Radiology 1982; 143:45-52.
11. Lemaitre P, O'Regan S, Herba M, Kaye M. Complications in expanded polytetrafluoroethylene arteriovenous grafts: an angiographic study. Am J Roentgenology 1978; 131:817-820.
12. O'Reilly RJ, Hanson CC, Rosenthal JJ. Angiography of chronic hemodialysis arteriovenous graft. Am J Roentgenol 1978; 130:1105-1113.
13. Hughes C, Adams FG, Hamilton DN. The radiology of local complications of hemodialysis access devices. Clin Radiol 1980; 31:489-496.
14. Weinbaum FL, Riles TS. Thrombosis of vascular access grafts and its management. In: Waltzer WC, Rapaport FT, eds. Angioaccess: principles and practice. Orlando:Grune & Stratton, 1984:118-123.

24

PNEUMATIC COMPRESSION EXSANGUINATION FOR CREATION OF UPPER EXTREMITY A-V FISTULAS

Carl R. Doerhoff, M.D., F.A.C.S.

PRECISE SURGICAL TECHNIQUE IS REQUIRED to prevent endothelial injury to the native vasculature when placing or revising grafts for arteriovenous (A-V) access. Such an injury can precipitate intimal hyperplasia, embolization, and/or thrombosis. Studies have indicated that all forms of vascular clamps can cause morphological changes to the endothelium.[1-4] Vessel loops also have been shown to cause injury, but to a lesser extent.[5,6] Properly applied tourniquet control is associated with the lowest incidence of ischemic or mechanical injury to native vessels or prosthetic grafts.[4] In addition, the bloodless surgical field provided by pneumatic compression exsanguination (PCE) allows better visualization of the vasculature and requires less dissection of the artery and vein, thus causing less disruption of the vaso vasorum (figures 24-1 and 24-2). Theoretically, PCE should result in a lower incidence of vessel injury and subsequent intimal hyperplasia than either vascular clamps or vessel loops, therefore prolonging graft patency.

Materials and Methods

Since January 1993, PCE has been used in our center in place of traditional vessel loops in 43 procedures on 36 patients, 46% of whom were males and 53% were diabetic. Table 24-1 lists the procedures and their frequencies. Following infiltration of the skin with local anesthesia, minimal exposure of the artery and

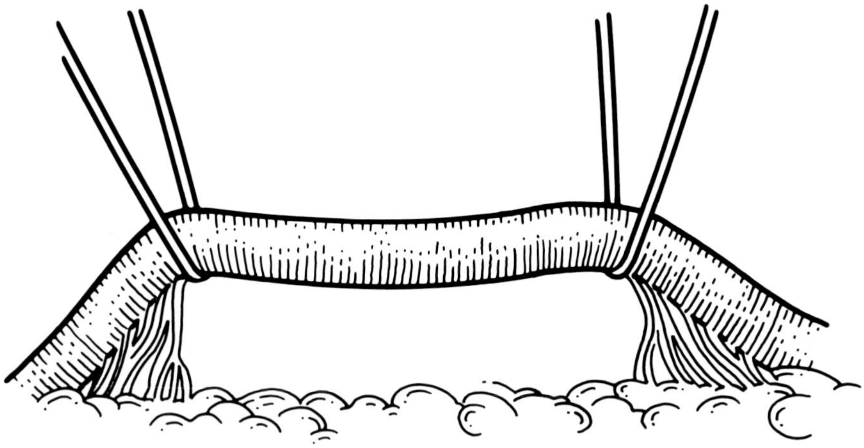

Figure 24-1. Loop exposure with complete vessel dissection from the vaso vasorum.

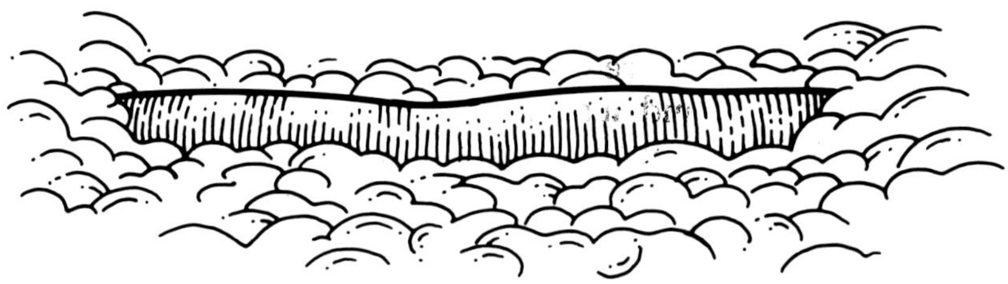

Figure 24-2. Minimal dissection of vessel from vaso vasorum.

Table 24-1. Pneumatic Compression Exsanguination Procedures and Their Frequencies, January 1993—May 1994.

Procedure	No. performed
Straight, forearm graft	17
Forearm loop graft	10
Straight graft, across elbow	1
Straight, upper-arm graft	1
Cimino-Brescia	2
Graft revision	9
Thrombectomy	3

vein is accomplished. The graft is tunneled and 3,500 IU of heparin (unless contraindicated) is administered. The arm is elevated and exsanguinated using an elastic bandage. The tourniquet is then insufflated to 250 mm Hg and the surgical anastomoses are performed (see figure 24-3). After the tourniquet is deflated, flow through the graft or fistula is assessed by palpation, auscultation with a sterile stethoscope, or color flow Doppler (for venous outflow). Target time for initial graft placement is 22 minutes; other procedures, such as graft revision, can take longer.

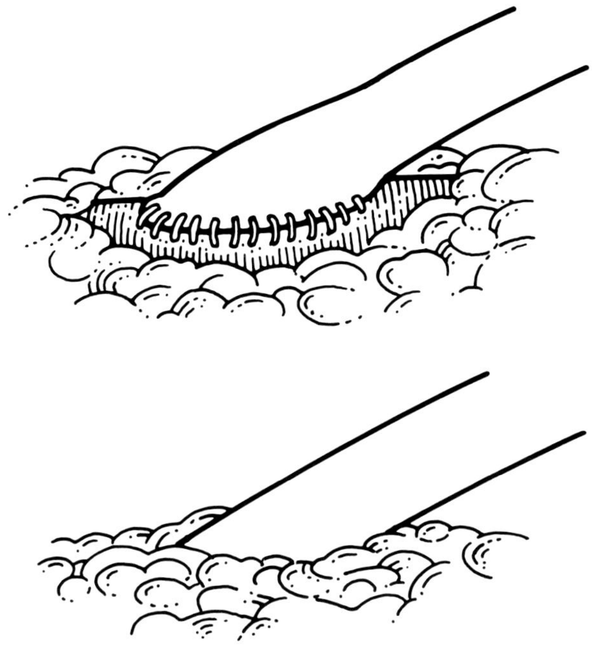

Figure 24-3. After anastomosis is completed (top), the surrounding tissue immediately covers the suture line (bottom).

Results and Discussion

In this series, average tourniquet time was 26.5 minutes (range: 2-65 minutes). All patients tolerated the procedure well, and there have been no complications related to the use of the tourniquet.

PCE was initially used to construct or revise A-V fistulas on patients who could not be given heparin because heparin antibodies were present. Because PCE proved relatively easy to perform with no apparent complications, it has since been used on all patients undergoing A-V access surgery.

PCE offers several advantages over the use of traditional vessel loops. Surgery is performed in a completely bloodless field, allowing better visualization of the anatomy and reducing the time required for the procedure. The incision is much smaller, and minimal dissection of the vein and artery is required. Because the native vessels are not lifted from their underlying bed, they are not compressed or elongated (figure 24-4). This avoids any sort of mechanical or ischemic injury. This technique also limits disruption of the vaso vasorum, ensuring good perfusion of the vessel itself. In addition, PCE allows use of the radial artery as small as 2 mm in diameter (figure 24-5).

Tourniquet control in surgery has been used since Roman times and has been used extensively in orthopedic surgery for many decades. Studies and experience indicate that a tourniquet properly applied at the correct pressure can be used safely for as long as two hours without causing problems or complications.[4,7,8] The target tourniquet time for procedures discussed here is 22 minutes at a

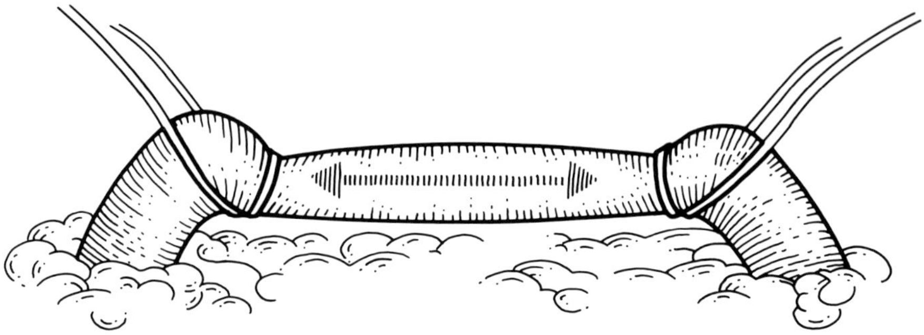

Figure 24-4. The use of loops elongates the vessel, reducing its diameter and potentially causing the mechanical or ischemic damage.

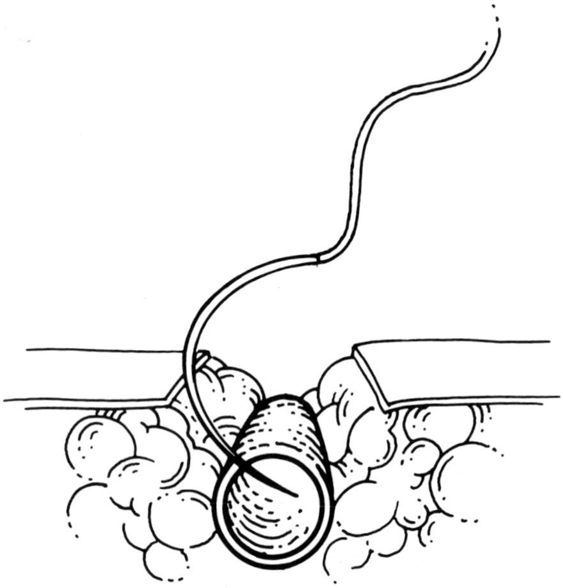

Figure 24-5. Suturing vessels as small as 2 mm in diameter becomes possible when the vessel is left in its tissue bed and the diameter is not reduced by the use of loops.

routine pressure of 250 mm Hg, with an average of 26.5 minutes (range: 2-65 minutes). These times are well within the allowable limits for safety, and none of the patients has experienced complications related to the use of the tourniquet.

Conclusion

The use of PCE for creation of upper extremity A-V fistulas prevents mechanical injury and limits ischemic injury to the vessel. This may decrease subsequent intimal hyperplasia and potentially improve overall graft patency. The minimal exposure of the vessels saves operating time, limiting charges for the operating room and anesthesia, and may reduce the frequency of revisions. Longer follow-up of additional patients is needed to determine the efficacy of PCE.

References

1. Moore WM, Bunt TJ, Hermann GD, Fogarty TJ. Assessment of transmural force during application of vascular occlusive devices. J Vasc Surg 1988; 8:422-427.
2. Moore WM, Manship LL, Bunt TJ. Differential endothelial injury caused by vascular clamps and vessel loops. I. Normal vessels. Am Surg 1985; 51:392-400.
3. Henson GF, Rob CG. A comparative study of the effects of different arterial clamps on the vessel wall. Br J Surg 1956; XLIII:561-564.
4. Collier PE. A traumatic vascular anastomoses using a tourniquet. Ann Vasc Surg 1992; 6:34-37.
5. Dobrin PB, McGurrin JF, McNulty JA. Chronic histological changes after vascular clamping are not associated with altered vascular mechanics. Ann Vasc Surg 1992; 6:153-159.
6. Pabst TS, Flanigan DP, Buchbinder D. Reduced intimal injury to canine arteries with controlled application of vessel loops. J Surg Res 1989; 47:235-241.
7. Sapega AA, Heppenstall RB, Chance B, Park YS, Sokolow D. Optimizing tourniquet application and release times in extremity surgery. J Bone Joint Surg 1985; 67A:303-314.
8. Fletcher IR, Healy TEJ. The arterial tourniquet. Ann Roy Coll Surg Engl 1983; 65:409-417.

DISCUSSION

Moderator:
Mitchell L. Henry, M.D.

Panelists:
Carl R. Doerhoff, M.D., F.A.C.S.
Lucio Flores, M.D.
Richard J. Gray, M.D.
Michael R. Middlebrook, M.D.

Dr. Ferguson: The theoretical basis for using a tourniquet is that you do not want to injure the vessel or predispose that vessel to pseudointimal or myointimal hyperplastic lesions. Dr. Doerhoff, do you have any evidence for that?

Dr. Doerhoff: Several years ago a series was published where tagged studies of the intima were performed. Wherever the saphenous vein was skeletonized *in situ* bypass, complete loss of endothelium occurred. When the vein was covered with subcutaneous fat and an intact vaso vasorum, there was no loss of endothelium.

Discussant: A comment for Dr. Middlebrook. We have presented our experience with a similar protocol, except we used pulsed spray thrombolysis in combination with mechanical thrombectomy percutaneously. We were not as fortunate as you and did not get away with it. Included in that series, we did postprocedural V/Q scans, as well as clinical evaluation on the patients. In the 50 procedures, 80% of the patients had high probability V/Q scans postprocedure and two patients died from pulmonary embolism. One patient had a baseline V/Q scan. The postprocedure V/Q scan in this patient with symptoms was grossly positive, and she expired following treatment. The second patient expired about 24 hours postprocedure. We concluded that you had to be selective and avoid elderly patients and those with poor cardiopulmonary reserve. We felt that those patients were not really candidates for percutaneous thrombectomy because they just didn't have the cardiopulmonary reserve to tolerate a pulmonary embolism. We also concluded that it is not satisfactory to rely on the clinical findings. You must look for pulmonary embolism beyond the clinical findings of pulse oximetry and symptoms.

Dr. Middlebrook: First, we never have intimated at all that patients don't have pulmonary embolism. As a matter of fact, 100% do, we absolutely know that. Second, the cause of death was pulmonary embolism in a patient with severe pulmonary fibrosis, who should not have been done to begin with. The second patient died later of an MI; even though there was a high probability V/Q, there was no documentation that this really was the cause of death. There was no postmortem on either one of those patients that I am aware of. If you screen for patients who have obvious pulmonary disease, such as pulmonary fibrosis or obvious cardiac disease, then no one would do those patients to begin with, and those patients would be spared those kinds of complications and outcomes.

Discussant: Dr. Middlebrook, I have some questions on long-term aspects of this type of procedure. Would there be a higher incidence of pulmonary hypertension on a long-term basis? Our patients require repeated declottings and lysis procedures, and I would be concerned that those micropulmonary emboli might aggregate to be very problematic over a period of time.

Dr. Middlebrook: That is a very good question, but we don't know the answer directly. If you calculate the largest clot load that we could possibly give these patients, say the volume of the graft is 8.5 cc, and we split those up so they are particles that go in fragments. In reality, most of the time when we enter these grafts there is serous fluid, and most commonly, the only really organized thrombus we find is a tiny one at the arterial anastomosis. So in terms of microemboli, we may actually be giving these people much less than we are presuming. The second thing is that there is increasing evidence in the literature that subclinical pulmonary embolism is quite common. There is literature out there where 30% of patients will have emboli and no symptoms. The incidence of chronic pulmonary hypertension is, in fact, decreasing if you look in the literature over the past 50 years. While I have no direct evidence of that, there is at least an anecdotal feeling that it may be not be a problem.

Discussant: In a dialysis unit where the median age is about 69, I have people go through five, six, and seven thrombolytic therapies. Nobody has normal lungs and everybody smokes, so that I have some real concerns about using this on a long-term basis. I think it is an excellent idea if it works, but I am a little scared.

Dr. Middlebrook: Exactly. The idea here is to save time and money for the patients and for the system in general. Obviously, our results are very preliminary and require further work. In our institution we are planning to instigate long-term follow-up with V/Q scanning and other measures of pulmonary function. At this point, we would never advocate this as front line therapy.

Discussant: Dr. Doerhoff, when you are revising a GORE-TEX graft, does your tourniquet get in the way if you need to go high in the axilla?

Dr. Doerhoff: I do not go any higher than the antecubital fossa when I am using the tourniquet. I use conventional means when I am above the antecubital fossa.

Discussant: When you are doing a thrombectomy, you do not always know how high you will need to go. Do you put the tourniquet on to start with and then take it off if you need to?

Dr. Doerhoff: No, I just do not expose the arm higher than that. If I need to run a thrombectomy catheter up above that point, then I will do so. If I believe that I have a proximal stenosis or a central vein occlusion, I will either assess that graft by angioscopy, which I prefer, or by fistulogram. For a single arterial anastomosis in the forearm, you can still use a sterile tourniquet and put it on. If you eliminate that 6% of arterial intimal hyperplasia and graft loss, you have saved hundreds of thousands of dollars per year.

Discussant: Dr. Middlebrook, would it not be easier to take patients with thrombosed grafts to the operating room and spend about one-half hour getting their clot out in a conventional way?

Dr. Middlebrook: If your institution is equipped to do that, yes. At our institution, our surgeons do not have the time to do it, and many times they cannot get to the patients for days, and we end up being the ones who see them most frequently and soonest.

Discussant: Dr. Flores, when I find more than two veins in the axilla, I also find a double arterial system. Is that your experience? Double arterial systems in my experience are 13% of all cases.

Dr. Flores: I have not looked into that, but it is not infrequent to find a double arterial system. I did not pay any attention to correlating the arterial system with the veins, but it is an infrequent observation.

SECTION VIII

25

SUCCESSFUL EARLY USE OF THE STRETCH PTFE GRAFT

John O. Colonna II, M.D., S. John Swanson, M.D., and Timothy R. Shaver, M.D.

PATIENTS WITH CHRONIC RENAL FAILURE not infrequently present in urgent need of an initial or secondary access for hemodialysis. Placement of temporary, percutaneous venous catheters has been used as a bridge until placement and maturation of a permanent access is accomplished. Use of these catheters has been associated with the development of venous strictures that may compromise subsequent access procedures.[1]

Preliminary results with early use of the stretch polytetrafluoroethylene (PTFE) grafts have been favorable.[2-3] Encouraged by these reports, we began to use the stretch-PTFE graft as our primary conduit for all patients in need of hemodialysis access who were not candidates for an autogenous arteriovenous (A-V) fistula. Herein, we report the experience at Walter Reed Army Medical Center, Washington, D.C., with the initial 60 patients.

Materials and Methods

Between September 10, 1992, and February 28, 1994, 60 patients underwent placement of a 4-mm to 7-mm tapered stretch-PTFE graft (Stretch GORE-TEX, W.L. Gore & Associates, Inc., Flagstaff, Arizona) for chronic hemodialysis access. The location and configuration of the grafts were as follows: forearm loop (n=39),

Table 25-1. Early Complications Following Early Use of Graft

	Forearm loop	Upper-arm straight	Thigh loop
Bleeding	0/17	0/14	0/3
Hematoma	0/17	0/14	0/3
Thrombosis	0/17	1/14	0/3
Infection	0/17	0/14	0/3

Table 25-2. Late Complications Following Early Use of Graft

	Forearm loop	Upper-arm straight	Thigh loop
Thrombosis	8/17	1/14	0/3
Steal	1/17	0/14	0/3
Pseudoaneurysm	0/17	2/14	0/3
Infection	1/17	1/14	1/3

upper-arm straight (n=18), and thigh loop (n=3). Forty (66%) of the grafts placed were initial access procedures. The remainder were placed in patients who had undergone one or more previous access procedures.

In 34 patients (57%), the graft was used for dialysis within the first week after implantation. In each case, 16-gauge needles were used, and the initial punctures were performed by an experienced dialysis nurse. Patients were followed from the time of implantation through April 30, 1994, or until the graft was no longer functional (mean: 11 months). Both the patients and their dialysis units were contacted for long-term follow-up of patients whose care was transferred outside our facility. Data were collected on the day of initial use of the access following implantation and on the development of early (<30 days) and late (> 30 days) complications. Results are reported for the 34 patients whose initial access use was within seven days following implantation.

Results

Of the 34 grafts used in the first week after implantation, three were used immediately upon return from the operating room. Nine additional grafts were used within 24 hours after implantation and another 11 within 48 hours. The remaining 11 grafts were used three to seven days after implantation.

Early Complications. Early complications are summarized in table 25-1. None of the patients developed significant bleeding or perigraft hematomas despite early use of the graft, nor were there early graft infections. One patient experienced graft thrombosis 18 days after implantation of an upper-arm straight graft, the fourth access for this patient. Venography revealed subclavian vein occlusion. This patient was converted to peritoneal dialysis.

Late Complications. Late complications are summarized in table 25-2. Nine grafts thrombosed between 90 and 395 days after implantation. Thrombectomy/revision was successful in restoring long-term patency in eight patients. No attempt was made at salvage in the remaining patient, as graft thrombosis followed successful renal transplantation. One patient with severe peripheral vascular disease developed symptomatic steal requiring tapering of the arterial limb of a forearm loop graft. Two patients developed large pseudoaneurysms of upper-arm grafts 8 and 10 months following implantation. Successful "bucket handle" bypasses were performed in both. A high-grade subclavian stenosis identified in one patient may have contributed to the development of pseudoaneurysms. Three grafts were removed for infection at 3, 8, and 10 months after implantation. Three patients died of causes unrelated to their access procedures 6, 12, and 18 months postoperatively.

Discussion

As the U.S. Army's tertiary referral center for the East Coast and Europe, The Walter Reed center is frequently confronted with end-stage renal disease patients who are in need of urgent hemodialysis when first seen. Similarly, patients with thrombosis of an existing graft that fails thrombectomy or revision and patients who have an existing graft removed for infection are in need of a new permanent access. Acute venous hemodialysis catheters can be placed percutaneously in the subclavian, jugular, or femoral locations to temporize. Increased experience with these catheters has shown that this convenience does come at a price.[1] Strictures in the subclavian, innominate, and femoral veins can eliminate the corresponding extremity as a future access site.

Expanded PTFE grafts have become the predominant access for hemodialysis patients who are not candidates for an autogenous A-V fistula.[4] First use of these grafts commonly is postponed for 1-2 weeks to allow the graft to adhere to surrounding tissues. The possibility of prolonged needle-stick bleeding or the development of perigraft hematomas leading to graft thrombosis has led to a hesitancy to use these grafts earlier. In 1985, Taucher reported favorable results with early use of grafts placed with the aid of a tunneling device that had a smaller diameter than the graft, resulting in a tighter tunnel.[5] Eighty-four PTFE grafts were placed and used within 72 hours of implantation. There were only three bleeding complications, nine early thromboses, and two early infections. Despite the availability of several similar tunneling devices, early use of PTFE grafts has not gained wide acceptance. In a panel discussion at the Third Symposium on Vascular Access for Hemodialysis, about 60% of surgeons present had some experience with early use of PTFE, but only a very small minority were advocates.[6]

At the same meeting, two papers were presented on the use of the new stretch-PTFE grafts. Dawidson reported on 12 patients whose grafts were used within seven days.[2] Only one patient had a significant bleeding complication, and no early thromboses were seen. Simoni reported on 15 patients whose grafts were used within 24 hours.[3] All grafts were examined by color flow Doppler imaging at 1-2 weeks and 4-6 weeks after implantation. No perigraft hematomas or pseudoaneurysms were detected. There were, however, seven episodes of early graft thrombosis in five patients.

Our own experience with early use of the stretch-PTFE has been similarly favorable. We observed no episodes of bleeding or perigraft hematoma. The only early thrombosis occurred in a patient with a previously unidentified subclavian occlusion. The unique characteristic of the stretch graft that makes early use possible seems to be the elastic recoil of the additional longitudinal layer.[3] This appears to result in less bleeding upon removal of the dialysis needles. We would also include the use of a 6-mm tunneling device and cannulation done by the "best sticker" in the unit as important factors in successful early use of these grafts.

Conclusion

Our results, along with those previously reported by others, demonstrate that the stretch-PTFE graft can be used safely in the first 48 hours following implantation. This practice can avoid the use of percutaneous, temporary catheters and their attendant morbidity.

References

1. Schwab S, Quarles D, Middleton J, et al. Hemodialysis-associated subclavian vein stenosis. Kidney Int 1988; 33:1156.
2. Dawidson I, Melone D. Preliminary experience with a new PTFE graft for vascular access. In: Henry ML, Ferguson RM, eds. Vascular access for hemodialysis—III. Chicago: W.L. Gore & Associates, Inc., and Precept Press, 1993; 133-136.
3. Simoni EJ, Jain KM, Munn JS. Use of 6 mm stretch PTFE grafts for early use in hemodialysis. In: Henry ML, Ferguson RM, eds. Vascular access for hemodialysis—III. Chicago: W.L. Gore & Associates, Inc., and Precept Press, 1993; 142-145.
4. Ridge, BA. PTFE grafts for hemodialysis. Vasc Forum 1993; 1:55-56.
5. Taucher LA. Immediate, safe hemodialysis into arteriovenous fistulas created with a new tunneler. Am J Surg 1985; 150:212-215.
6. Panel Discussion. In: Henry ML, Ferguson RM, eds. Vascular access for hemodialysis—III. Chicago: W.L. Gore & Associates, Inc., and Precept Press, 1993; 141.

26

STRETCH VERSUS STANDARD EXPANDED PTFE GRAFTS FOR HEMODIALYSIS ACCESS

*Jan H.M. Tordoir, M.D., Leo Hofstra, M.D.,
Denis C.J.J. Bergmans, M.D., Arnold P.G. Hoeks, M.D.,
Karel M.L. Leunissen, M.D., and Peter J.E.H.M. Kitslaar, M.D.*

IN PATIENTS WITH RENAL FAILURE, the autogenous Brescia-Cimino fistula at the wrist is the first option for creation of hemodialysis access. Expanded polytetrafluoroethylene (ePTFE) grafts, implanted as an arteriovenous (A-V) conduit, are widely regarded as an acceptable alternative in case of fistula failure or inability to perform a direct A-V anastomosis in patients with inadequate superficial arm veins. Despite a secondary patency rate of 80% after one year of follow-up, ePTFE A-V grafts have a high rate of thrombotic occlusion, infection, and puncture complications.[1-3] Intimal hyperplasia, resulting in stenosis at the site of the venous anastomosis, usually leads to occlusion in nearly half of the patients.[4] Major disadvantages are bleeding from puncture holes, tendency of the graft to kink, and the stiffness of the material, which may imply technical difficulties. The repeated large needle punctures may finally result in graft disintegration, with formation of aneurysms.

Recently, a modification of the ePTFE graft has been introduced, with stretch properties leading to improved handling characteristics. The lengthwise compliance of the prosthesis may offer a better matching of the mechanical properties between the graft and native vessels. The conformability, increased resistance to kinking, and possibly ease of puncture and improved puncture hole healing of this graft might also result in a better performance with fewer complications.

In a prospective study, we compared the complications and patency rates of stretch ePTFE prostheses with standard ePTFE grafts implanted for hemodialysis vascular access.

Table 26-1. Patient Characteristics with Stretch and ePTFE A-V Grafts

	Stretch PTFE	ePTFE	P value
Mean age (years)	59 (31-73)	58 (15-74)	NS
Men/women	5/12	12/8	< 0.01
Mean number of previous fistulas	1.8 (0-6)	1.2 (0-4)	NS
Diabetes	43%	36%	NS
Cardiac disease	28%	43%	NS

Materials and Methods

Between April 1992 and September 1993, 37 chronic hemodialysis patients who needed secondary access procedures were randomized for implantation of either stretch ePTFE grafts (Stretch GORE-TEX, W.L. Gore & Associates, Flagstaff, Arizona) in 17 patients or standard ePTFE grafts (GORE-TEX) in 20 patients. The study group consisted of 17 men and 20 women with a mean age of 59 years (range: 15-74 years). In 31 patients, several previous A-V fistulas had failed before a PTFE graft was inserted, while six patients underwent primary implantation of a PTFE graft due to insufficient superficial veins in the forearm. The usual patient risk factors were observed: diabetes in 38%, cardiac disease in 35%, and cerebrovascular disease in 8% (table 26-I). All patients had preoperative Duplex scanning and/or phlebography to assess the arteries and superficial veins in the upper extremity. Stretch and ePTFE grafts, 6-mm in diameter and thick-walled, were used for implantation. The arterial anastomoses were placed at the brachial artery at the level of the elbow in all patients. Venous anastomoses were performed in an end-to-side fashion to the cephalic vein (10 patients), basilic vein (3 patients), cubital vein (12 patients) and deep vein (12 patients), all at the elbow region. There were no differences in outflow sites for venous anastomosis between the two types of grafts. Arterial and venous anastomoses were performed with 7-0 running polypropylene (Prolene) sutures. Completion angiography and perioperative Doppler studies with measurement of peak velocities and observation of turbulent flow were done during each procedure.

Patient follow-up ranged from 2 to 17 months (mean:10 months). Clinical evaluation of the functioning A-V graft was performed in the dialysis department. Blood flow and venous pressures on dialysis were regularly assessed. The time needed to stop bleeding from the puncture holes after the withdrawal of the needles was measured during each dialysis session. Duplex scans were performed two weeks postoperatively and at three-month intervals to assess graft patency and to detect stenoses. Significant stenoses (> 50% diameter reduction) were diagnosed according to previously outlined Duplex criteria.[5]

The elastic properties of the grafts and efferent vein were assessed with the use of vessel wall Doppler tracking (VWDT).[6] From the distension (in μm) and diameter (in mm), the following parameters were calculated: relative distension=$\Delta D/D*100\%$ and area increase=$\pi/2*D*\Delta D$. Relative distension (RD) gives the fractional diameter increase. Area increase (AI) represents the capacity of the vessel to store blood volume during cardiac cycle.

Table 26-2. Complications of Stretch and ePTFE A-V Fistulas

	Stretch PTFE (%)	ePTFE (%)	P value
Thrombosis	12	40	< 0.001
Puncture bleeding	-	13	NS
Aneurysm	-	5	NS
Venous hypertension	-	5	NS
Ischemia	6	5	NS
Infection	6	10	NS

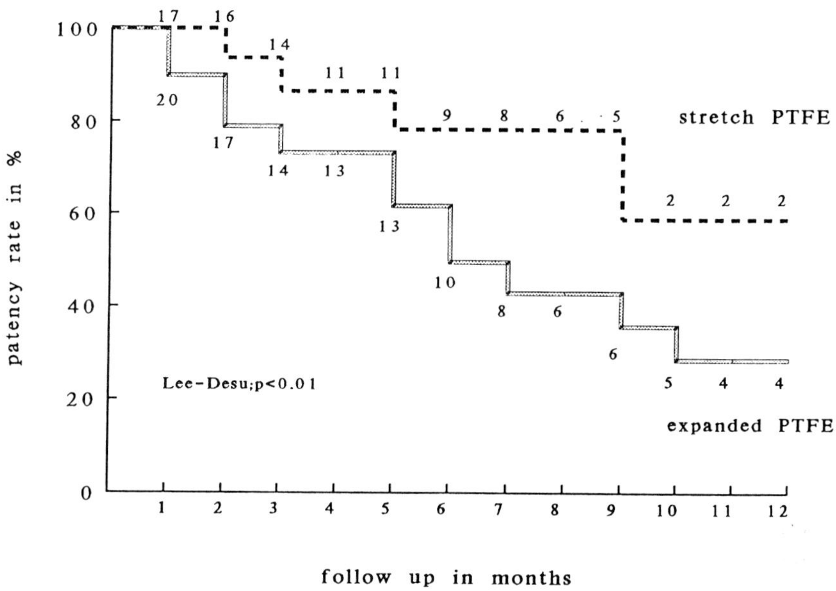

Figure 26-1. Cumulative primary patency rates of stretch PTFE and expanded PTFE A-V fistulas.

Statistical analysis of the differences in complications between the patient groups was performed by means of the nonparametric Mann-Whitney test. Primary and secondary graft patencies were calculated according to the life table method, and the Lee-Desu statistic was used for overall comparison of the two types of grafts.

Results

No deaths occurred within 30 days after the operative procedure. Two ePTFE grafts occluded within 24 hours of operation and successful thrombectomy was accomplished in both. Wound infection occurred in one stretch PTFE graft, leading to graft infection and finally necessitating graft explantation one month postoperatively. In the stretch group, two grafts occluded after two and five months. A successful thrombectomy with patch angioplasty at the venous anastomosis was performed in one patient, and in the other patient a new PTFE prosthetic A-V graft was created. One female patient developed severe ischemia of the ipsilateral hand, due to excessive

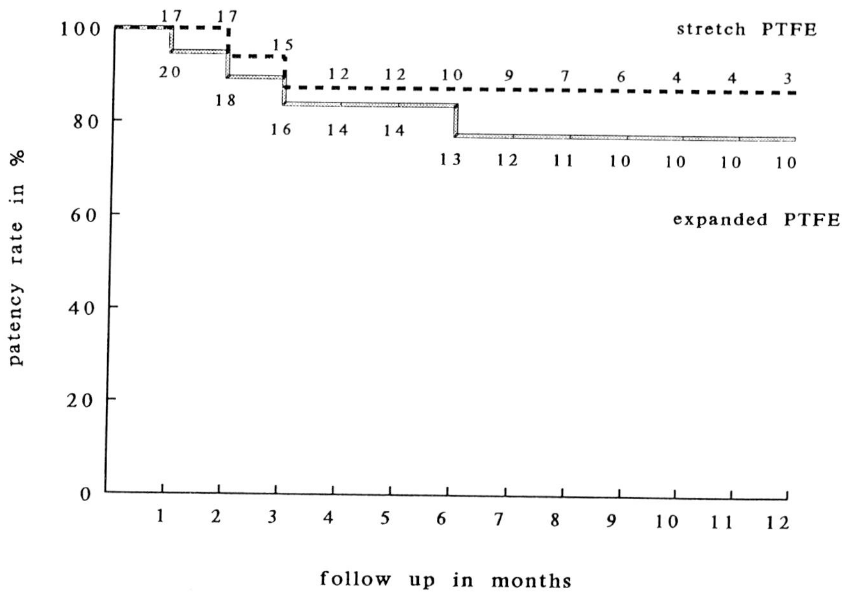

Figure 26-2. Cumulative secondary patency rates of stretch PTFE and expanded PTFE A-V fistulas.

Table 26-3. Number and Location of Stenoses in Stretch and ePTFE A-V Fistulas

	sPTFE	ePTFE
Total number of stenoses	10	24
Mean number/fistula	0.6	1.2
Location: arterial anastomosis	1	5
graft	-	5
venous anastomosis	6	9
efferent vein	3	5

volume flow in the A-V loop grafts. Flow was diminished by tapering the arterial anastomosis, and her complaints gradually disappeared (table 26-2). The primary and secondary cumulative graft patencies of stretch PTFE A-V grafts were 59% and 87% after one year, respectively (figures 26-1 and 26-2).

In the group of patients with ePTFE grafts, 12 thrombotic events occurred in eight grafts. A successful thrombectomy was achieved in five grafts, with additional PTFE interposition extended to the deep vein in the upper arm in four patients. Histological examination of excised stenotic lesions in all four patients showed occlusive intimal hyperplasia. New A-V grafts were created in three patients. Graft explantation was necessary in three patients, because of infection in two patients after one and 14 months postoperatively, and ischemia in one patient. Operative correction of puncture site bleeding and aneurysms was performed in four patients. One patient developed arm edema, due to venous hypertension caused by subclavian vein obstruction. This patient was treated by a jugular vein transposition (table 26-3). The primary and secondary patency rates of ePTFE grafts after one year were 29

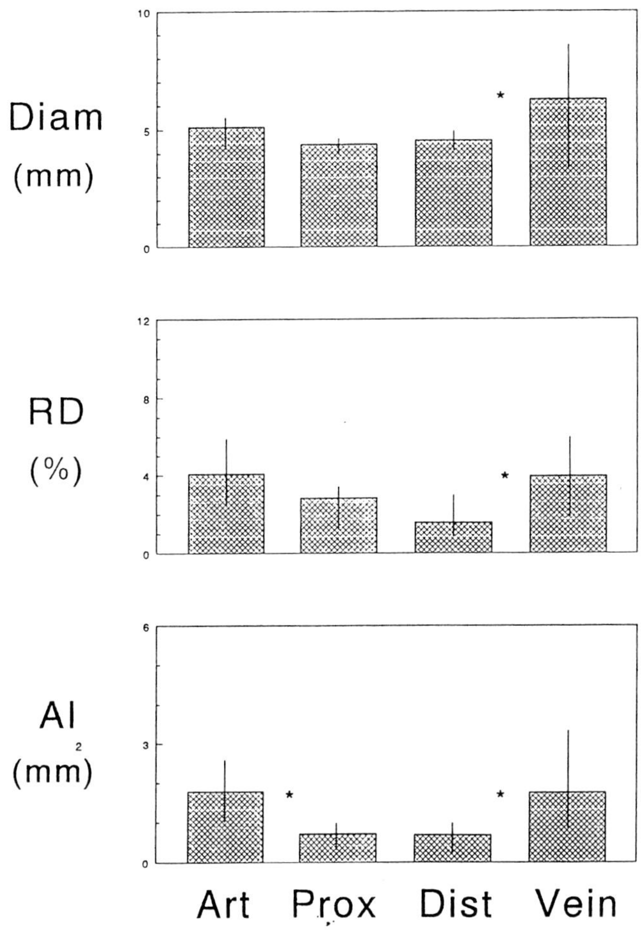

Figure 26-3. Stretch PTFE grafts. Median values and 25th and 75th percentile intervals of diameter (Diam), relative distension (RD), and area increase (AI) measured at the proximal (Prox), mid (Mid), and distal (Dist) segments of the grafts and the artery (Art) and vein segments (*p< 0.05).

and 77%, respectively (figures 26-1 and 26-2). During the follow-up period, seven patients (five in the ePTFE and two in the stretch group) died and three patients (all in the ePTFE group) received a kidney transplantation.

Early dialysis use (< two weeks) was permitted in 12 of the stretch PTFE prostheses (71%) and in eight ePTFE grafts (40%, $p < 0.05$). The stretch PTFE grafts were punctured after a mean postoperative period of 13 days (range: 2-30 days), while the ePTFE grafts could be punctured and used for dialysis after a mean period of 22 days (range: 4-34 days). No perigraft hematoma or infections occurred as a result of the early puncture. The mean time for bleeding to stop from the puncture sites was 16

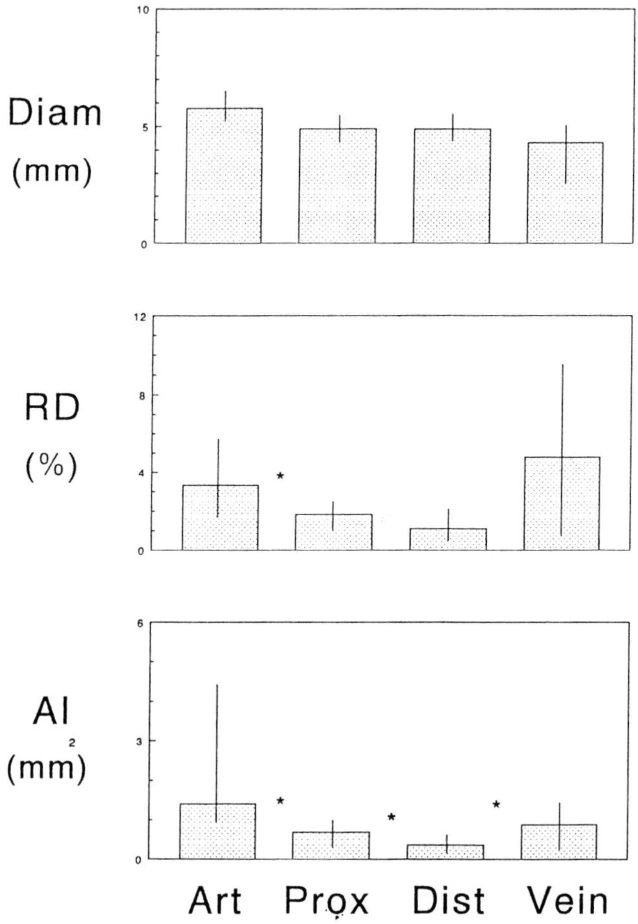

Figure 26-4. Expanded PTFE grafts. Median values and 25th and 75th percentile intervals of diameter (Diam), relative distension (RD) and area increase (AI) measured at the proximal (Prox), mid (Mid), and distal (Dist) segments of the grafts and the artery (Art) and vein segments (*p< 0.05).

minutes (range: 2-45 min) for the stretch prostheses and 24 minutes (range: 5-50 min) for the ePTFE grafts (p= NS).

Duplex scanning showed an increasing number of significant stenoses (> 50% diameter reduction) from two weeks to one year after graft implantation. The mean number of stenoses in the stretch group was 0.6 (range: 0-2) versus a mean of 1.2 stenoses (range: 0-3) in the ePTFE group (p< 0.01). These stenoses were located at the arterial anastomoses (15%), along the prosthesis (15%), at the venous anastomoses (45%), and in the efferent vein (24%). No difference in location of the stenoses was noted between both groups (table 26-3).

In the stretch PTFE prostheses, no differences in RD were observed around the arterial anastomoses and along the graft (figure 26-3). Relative distension increased around the venous anastomoses ($p < 0.05$). A decrease in AI was observed around the arterial anastomoses ($p < 0.05$), but an increase was found around the venous anastomoses ($p < 0.05$). Along the graft, no changes in AI were shown. A significant decrease in RD and AI from the arterial anastomoses into and along the graft were found in ePTFE (figure 26-4).

Discussion

Adequate vascular access remains the lifeline of end-stage renal disease (ESRD) patients treated by chronic intermittent hemodialysis. About 20-30% of these patients need secondary access procedures, of which the ePTFE A-V graft has been the most successful, with one-year patency rates of 60-80%.[3,4] Standard ePTFE prostheses have a high rate of thrombosis and puncture complications, usually necessitating multiple interventions. These complications are attributable to the properties of the material, with a high thrombogenicity and a low healing response on repeated punctures. Special features have been ascribed to the new stretch PTFE graft. Increased resistance to kinking and better matching of the prosthesis to the bevel of the arteriotomy may lead to less early postoperative thrombosis due to technical failures.

In this randomized study, we have not demonstrated any advantages of the stretch ePTFE prosthesis in the early postoperative period. No statistically significant differences were observed between the number of immediate postoperative complications in the two groups. However, during follow-up, a significantly greater number of occlusions occurred in the standard ePTFE grafts. Surgical exploration of these thrombosed grafts revealed arterial and/or venous anastomotic stenoses. Histological examination of the stenotic segments uniformly showed intimal hyperplasia. Primary patency rates were significantly better in the stretch group. Thrombosis occurred more often in the standard ePTFE grafts, and revision of these grafts was usually easily performed with prolongation of function for a considerable time, leading to similar secondary patencies of stretch and standard ePTFE grafts.

The unique lengthwise compliance of the stretch ePTFE may lead to better performance during and after puncture with large-bore needles. In the present study, we found no differences in the time needed to stop puncture site bleeding between the groups. However, because all surgical interventions for bleeding complications and aneurysm formation were done in the patients with standard ePTFE grafts, this might reflect a better capability to close puncture holes in the wall of stretch ePTFE grafts.

Long-term patency of PTFE grafts for vascular access is inferior to that of biologic materials.[7] This can be attributed to the occurrence of intimal hyperplasia in the anastomoses. Platelet deposition results in release of platelet-derived growth factor and subsequent migration of fibroblast and smooth muscle cells into the intima.[8] Several factors have been implicated in the development of intimal hyperplasia, including hemodynamic changes, low shear stress, and mismatch of mechanical properties between graft and native vessels.[9-11] Pärsson et al. found more thrombus-free surfaces in stretch ePTFE grafts as compared to standard ePTFE grafts.[12] The platelet deposition as measured by radioactive scanning was significantly lower in the stretch grafts, while in the distal region of the standard ePTFE graft, increased platelet activity was detected. A tendency to kink was noted in the midregion of the standard ePTFE prostheses, initiating turbulent flow and subsequently, areas of low shear stress, with a greater chance of platelet deposition. Histologic examination in occluded standard ePTFE grafts showed midgraft intimal hyperplasia, while in none of the explanted stretch grafts was intimal hyperplasia found.

The new stretch PTFE graft showed slightly better elastic properties as compared to the ePTFE grafts. In the stretch PTFE graft, the hemodynamic capacity was maintained along the graft, in contrast to the ePTFE prostheses, where a decrease in the hemodynamic capacity was observed. This indicates a better preservation of pulsatile energy of the stretch PTFE grafts. However, this did not result in a better match around the venous anastomoses. A higher AI was found in the venous outflow segments in the stretch PTFE group, indicating improved management of pulsatile flow at this point. This may contribute to a better hemodynamic environment of this flow segment, possibly leading to a decrease in the development of flow-induced hyperplastic lesions in the outflow segments of stretch PTFE A-V grafts.

In the present study, Duplex scanning showed a significantly greater number of stenoses in the standard ePTFE A-V grafts compared to the stretch ePTFE grafts. The distribution of these stenoses in the A-V grafts was similar in both groups. This difference in the number of stenoses can explain the improved primary patencies of the stretch graft. Less kinking and an improvement in elastic properties around the venous anastomoses may account for this feature.[13]

Our preliminary report shows that the longitudinal stretch properties of the new PTFE prosthesis may result in better primary patency rates compared to standard ePTFE A-V grafts. No differences in performance of the two grafts during and after dialysis puncture were noted. Further investigation into the mechanical behavior (i.e., kinking, compliance) of the stretch ePTFE prosthesis is needed. In addition, multicenter prospective studies need to be performed to demonstrate the better patency rates of the stretch prosthesis for hemodialysis access.

References

1. Raju S. PTFE grafts for hemodialysis access-techniques for insertion and management of complications. Ann Surg 1987; 206:666-673.
2. Rizzuti RP, Hale JC, Burkart TE. Extended patency of expanded polytetrafluoroethylene grafts for vascular access using optimal configuration and revisions. Surg Gynecol Obstet 1987; 166:23-27.
3. Tordoir JHM, Herman JMMPH, Kwan TS, Diderich PM. Long term follow up of the polytetrafluoroethylene (PTFE) prosthesis as an arteriovenous fistula for hemodialysis. Eur J Vasc Surg 1988; 2:3-7.
4. Palder SB, Kirkman RL, Whittemore AD, Hakim RM, Lazarus JM, Tilney NL. Vascular access for hemodialysis. Patency rates and results of revision. Ann Surg 1985; 202:235-239.
5. Tordoir JHM, de Bruin HG, Hoeneveld H, Eikelboom BC, Kitslaar PJEHM. Duplex ultrasound scanning in the assessment of arteriovenous fistulas created for hemodialysis access: comparison with digital subtraction angiography. J Vasc Surg 1989; 10:122-128.

6. Hofstra L, Ermers EJM, Langeveld APM, Hoeks APG, Kitslaar PJEHM. Vessel wall Doppler tracking: a new technique to assess vessel wall compliance. J Vasc Tech 1993; 17:65-68.
7. Veith FJ, Gupta SK, Ascer E. Six year prospective multicenter randomized comparison of autologous saphenous vein and expanded polytetrafluoroethylene grafts in infrainguinal arterial reconstructions. J Vasc Surg 1986; 3:104-114.
8. Swedberg SH, Brown BG, Sigley R, Wight TN, Gordon D, Nicholls SC. Intimal fibromuscular hyperplasia at the venous anastomosis of PTFE grafts in hemodialysis patients. Circulation 1989; 80:1726-1736.
9. Kohler TR, Kirkman TR, Kraiss LW, Zierler BK, Clowes AW. Increased blood flow inhibits neointimal hyperplasia and medial thickening in endotheliazed vascular grafts. Circ Res 1991; 69:1557-1565.
10. Abbott WM, Megerman J, Hasson JE, L' Italien G. Effect of compliance mismatch on vascular graft patency. J Vasc Surg 1987; 5:376-382.
11. Fillinger MF, Reintz ER, Schwartz RA, et al. Graft geometry and venous intimal-medial hyperplasia in arteriovenous loop grafts. J Vasc Surg 1990; 11:556-566.
12. Pärsson H, Jundzill W, Hallberg E, Thörne J, Norgren L. Acute thrombogenicity and 4 weeks healing properties of a new stretch-ePTFE graft. Eur J Vasc Surg 1993; 7:63-70.
13. Hofstra L, Bergmans D, Hoeks A, Kitslaar PJEHM, Tordoir JHM. Differences in mismatch of elastic properties in arterial and venous anastomoses of graft interposition for hemodialysis vascular access. J Am Soc Neprol (in press).

27

PTFE FOR A-V ACCESS: SIX YEARS OF EXPERIENCE WITH 310 REINFORCED AND STRETCH GRAFTS

Frantz J. Derenoncourt, M.D.

MAINTAINING VASCULAR ACCESS in chronic hemodialysis patients has been a challenge to vascular access surgeons. With improved medical therapy, patients with renal failure are surviving longer on hemodialysis. Assuring adequate sites for dialysis access remains a priority, and therefore improving on arteriovenous (A-V) graft survival is important. Expanded (nonstretch) polytetrafluoroethylene (PTFE) has proven to be second to the Brescia-Cimino fistula on long-term patency, easy accessibility, and complications.[1] In the present era of high-flux dialysis, many surgeons have used the loop forearm graft using the brachial-artery-to-antebrachial-vein as their primary graft.[2] The radial-artery-to-median-antecubital vein A-V graft has proved to be an excellent means of providing adequate arterial inflow, as previously reported.[3,4] The author's experience with 310 PTFE A-V grafts is reported. In an attempt to improve performance of the graft, the stretch PTFE replaced the standard PTFE two years ago, with gratifying results. Longer graft survival can be achieved as well as preservation of the brachial artery for later access.

Materials and Methods

From January 1988 to April 1994, 310 PTFE grafts were inserted in 210 patients. The expanded PTFE grafts were used from January 1988 to April 1992. In an effort to improve graft survival, the new stretch PTFE grafts were used from April 1992 to April 1994. All operations were performed by one surgeon. There were 119 male and 91 female patients. Ages ranged from 20 to 98 years (average: 62 years).

Table 27-1. Secondary Diagnosis

	No. patients	% of patients
Hypertension	159	76
Diabetes	58	27
Coronary artery disease	44	21
Peripheral vascular disease	29	14
Drug-related	5	2.4
Cardiac arrest	5	2.4
Kidney infections	4	2
Multiple myeloma	2	1
SLE	1	.5
Kidney obstruction	1	.5
Cancer	1	.5
Rhabdomyolysis	1	.5

Average female age was 66 and average male age was 58. There were 192 reinforced expanded PTFE grafts and 118 stretch grafts. Graft locations were as follows: left forearm radial to antecubital, 196 (63%); right forearm radial to antecubital, 55 (18%); left upper arm, 48 (15%); right upper arm, 9 (3%); left thigh, 1 (0.3%); right thigh, 1 (0.3%). Used as conduits were 6-mm diameter expanded reinforced PTFE or stretch grafts.

Hypertension was the primary cause of renal failure in 159 (76%) of the patients. Diabetes was present in 58 (27%) of the patients (table 27-1).

All primary operations were done with axillary nerve block. Thrombectomy and revisions were done under local anesthesia with mild sedation. Patients received 1 g of cephalothin I.V. prior to surgery and 4 doses of cephalothin postoperatively. Primary grafts were used 5-6 days after surgery. An indwelling catheter was inserted in the opposite subclavian vein for acute hemodialysis while the graft matured. Grafts that were thrombectomized or revised were used immediately after surgery prior to discharge on the day of surgery. Fistulograms were not done after thrombectomy and revisions. The occlusion test was adequate in predicting a good outcome.

All grafts were monitored in the dialysis units with recirculation studies. Elevated recirculation percentages above 15% were used as parameters to obtain fistulograms. Grafts with destroyed sections or venous outlet obstruction were electively revised. Only one patient in the series was ultimately placed on an indwelling central catheter because of several steal syndromes requiring takedown of multiple grafts. Two other patients needed to have grafts placed in the lower extremities. The remaining 207 patients had all their grafts in the upper extremities.

Results

Primary patency from graft insertion to clotting in the nonstretch grafts was 67% at six months, 55% at 12 months, 48% at 18 months, and was stabile at 25% up to 60 months (table 27-2). Stretch graft primary patency was 93% at 6 months and 79% at 18 months (table 27-3). Log rank analysis shows the difference between the grafts to be statistically significant, as outlined in figure 27-1 ($p = 0.0004$). Cumulative graft

Table 27-2. Primary Patency of Nonstretch PTFE from Graft Insertion to Clotting

Patency (months) Lower	Upper	No. at risk	Failed	Censored	Effective sample size	Survival	Survival standard error
0	6	165	46	48	141.0	1.0000	0.0000
6	12	71	9	11	65.5	0.6738	0.0395
12	18	51	8	11	45.5	0.5812	0.0445
18	24	32	5	7	28.5	0.4790	0.0492
24	30	20	1	10	15.0	0.3950	0.0530
30	36	9	1	1	8.5	0.3686	0.0556
36	42	7	0	2	6.0	0.3253	0.0638
42	48	5	1	1	4.5	0.3253	0.0638
48	54	3	0	0	3.0	0.2530	0.0808
54	60	3	0	0	3.0	0.2530	0.0808
60		3	1	2	2.0	0.2530	0.0808

Table 27-3. Primary Patency of Stretch PTFE from Graft Insertion to Clotting

Patency (months) Lower	Upper	No. at risk	Failed	Censored	Effective sample size	Survival	Survival standard error
0	6	90	5	41	69.5	1.0000	0.0000
6	12	44	5	23	32.5	0.9281	0.0310
12	18	16	0	13	9.5	0.7853	0.0643
18	24	3	1	2	2.0	0.7853	0.0643

survival in the nonstretch graft was 75% at 6 months, 68% at 12 months, 55% at 18 months, 39% at 36 months, and 34% at 60 months (table 27-4). Stretch PTFE grafts had cumulative patency rates of 96% at 6 months, 86% at 12 months, and 74% at 18 months (table 27-5). Life table analysis of the cumulative survival for nonstretch PTFE grafts compared to the stretch grafts (figure 27-2) highlights the significant improvement in survival of the stretch grafts (log rank $p = 0.0086$).

Complications were measured in terms of 100 graft-months of follow-up. Total graft follow-up was 9,231 months. Thrombosis was the most frequent complication, occurring at 2.93/100 graft-months. Infection occurred at 0.10, pseudoaneurysms and steal syndromes at 0.09, venous stenosis demonstrated by fistulograms at 0.72, and hematomas at 0.12. Total complication rate was 4.04/100 graft-months (table 27-6).

Discussion

Results presented in this retrospective study show that a statistically significant difference exists in primary patency and cumulative survival between nonstretch and stretch PTFE grafts. Long-term data up to 60 months show that the nonstretch PTFE graft primary patency survival (figure 27-1) is comparable to other reported data using life table analysis.[1,5] The statistically improved results with stretch grafts through 18-24 months compare favorably with the nonstretch expanded PTFE.

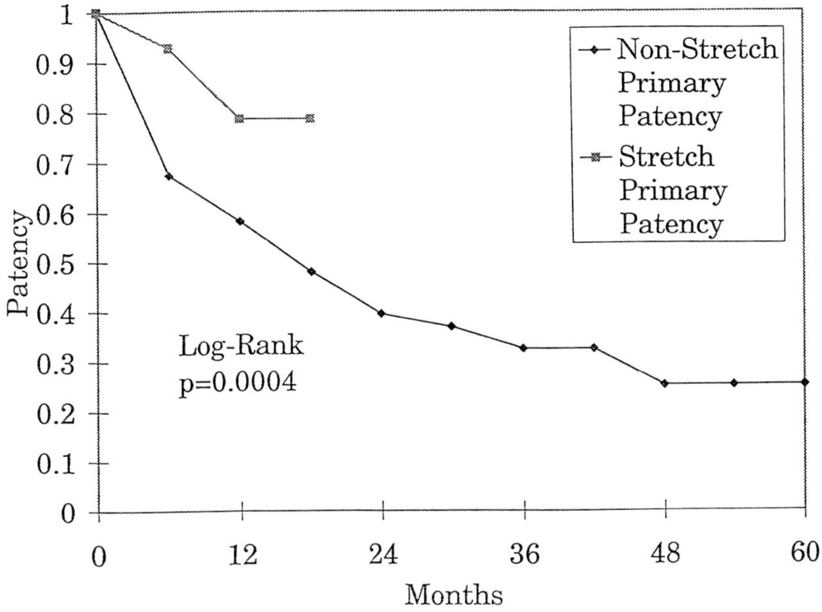

Figure 27-1. Primary patency of stretch versus nonstretch PTFE.

Table 27-4. Cumulative Patency: Life Table of Nonstretch PTFE

(Months) Lower	Upper	No. at risk	Failed	Censored	Effective sample size	Survival	Survival standard error
0	6	165	37	34	148.00	1.0000	0.0000
6	12	94	8	13	87.50	0.7500	0.2500
12	18	73	13	8	69.00	0.6814	0.3186
18	24	52	6	6	49.00	0.5530	0.4470
24	30	40	4	13	33.50	0.4853	0.5147
30	36	23	2	5	20.50	0.4274	0.5726
36	42	16	0	7	12.50	0.3857	0.6143
42	48	9	1	2	8.00	0.3857	0.6143
48	54	6	0	2	5.00	0.3375	0.6625
54	60	4	0	0	4.00	0.3375	0.6625
60		4	1	3	2.50	0.3375	0.6625

The use of recirculation studies in our patients proved to be a reliable screening test to pick up evolving venous stenosis before the grafts clotted. Fistulograms were done on these patients to define the area of stenosis. These grafts were revised with venous outflow patches when feasible or by extending the graft to a basilic vein or a cephalic vein across the elbow joint. It was possible to salvage most grafts with a simple patch of PTFE. Similar salvage techniques were used for nonstretch and stretch grafts.

The overall incidence of complications was 4.04/100 graft-months of follow-up. This is comparable to other reported series of PTFE grafts.[1] The rate of thrombosis of 2.93/100 graft-months is comparable to the rate of 2.96/100 graft-months reported in a summary of the published literature.[1] Our infection rate of 0.1/100 graft-months

Table 27-5. Cumulative Patency: Life Table of Stretch PTFE

(Months) Lower	Upper	No. at risk	Failed	Censored	Effective sample size	Survival	Survival standard error
0	6	90	3	37	71.50	1.0000	0.0000
6	12	50	4	23	38.50	0.9580	0.0237
12	18	23	2	16	15.00	0.8585	0.0517
18	24	5	2	3	3.50	0.7440	0.0877

Table 27-6. Complications per 100 Graft-Months of Follow-up (Total Graft-Months of Follow-up = 9,231)

Thrombosis		2.93
stretch	4.52	
nonstretch	2.64	
Infection		0.10
Pseudoaneurysm		0.09
Steal syndrome		0.09
Venous stenosis		0.72
Hematoma		0.12
Total		4.04

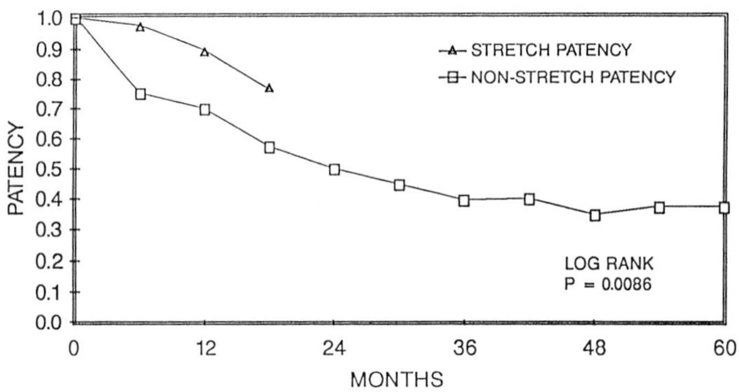

Figure 27-2. Life table curves: cumulative patency of stretch versus nonstretch PTFE.

compares very favorably to the overall average of 0.63/100 graft-months reported in the review referenced above. The rate of venous stenosis of 0.72/100 graft-months identified is higher than other reports. This is probably a direct result of our aggressive follow-up of grafts with recirculation studies as mentioned above.

It appears that stretch grafts have statistically significant improvement in primary patency and cumulative graft survival over nonstretch grafts. Longer follow-up of the stretch grafts will be necessary to show whether this modification of the PTFE graft has eliminated some of the problems that have plagued those of us who are forced to use PTFE for A-V access. It appears that this graft may be comparable to the Brescia-Cimino fistula in long-term survival.

References

1. Mehta S. Statistical summary of clinical results of vascular access procedures for hemodialysis. In: Sommer BG, Henry ML, eds. Vascular access for hemodialysis—II. Chicago: Precept Press, 1991; 145-157.
2. Rapaport A, Noon GP, McCollum CH. Polytetrafluoroethylene (PTFE) grafts for hemodialysis in chronic renal failure: Assessment of durability and function at three years. Aust NZ J Surg 1981; 51(6):562.
3. Pontari MA, McMillen MA. The straight radial antecubital PTFE angio-access graft in an era of high-flux dialysis. Am J Surg 1991; 161:450-453.
4. Raju S. PTFE grafts for hemodialysis vascular access. Ann Surg 1987; 206:666-673.
5. Rizzuti RD, Hale JC, Burkhart TE. Extended patency of expanded polytetrafluoroethylene grafts for vascular access using optimal configuration and revisions. Surg Gynecol Obstet 1988; 166:23-27.

28

EARLY EXPERIENCE WITH ePTFE DIALYSIS GRAFTS SODDED WITH LIPOSUCTION-DERIVED MICROVASCULAR ENDOTHELIAL CELLS

Scott S. Berman, M.D., Bruce E. Jarrell, M.D., Mary Anne Raymond, B.S., Leigh Kleinert, A.S., and Stuart K. Williams, Ph.D.

PROSTHETIC GRAFTS ARE PRESENTLY THE MOST COMMON vascular access created for hemodialysis. Despite excellent initial patency and successful dialysis, graft failure requiring intervention to restore patency occurs at a mean of nine months after placement. With more than 150,000 patients currently maintained on chronic hemodialysis, access-related complications remain the most common reason for hospitalization in this population.[1] The estimated annual cost to the health care system to maintain vascular access for hemodialysis is in excess of $500 million.

Failure of prosthetic dialysis access grafts can be divided into two time periods. Early thrombosis results from either technical errors at the time of placement or from an inherent thrombogenicity of the graft material. Late thrombosis usually follows the development of outflow stenosis in the venous anastomosis or outflow vein secondary to intimal hyperplasia.[2]

The technical considerations involved in creating a dialysis access graft are beyond the scope of this report, but include pre- and perioperative assessment of arterial inflow and venous outflow and the assurance of technically flawless construction of the arterial and venous anastomoses. Early graft thrombogenicity, however, results from the interaction of flowing blood with the base polymer of the graft and is enhanced by

This study is supported by a grant from Dialysis Clinics, Inc. The authors acknowledge the support of Drs. Victor M. Bernhard, Glenn C. Hunter, and W. Brad Carter in participating in the implant procedures.

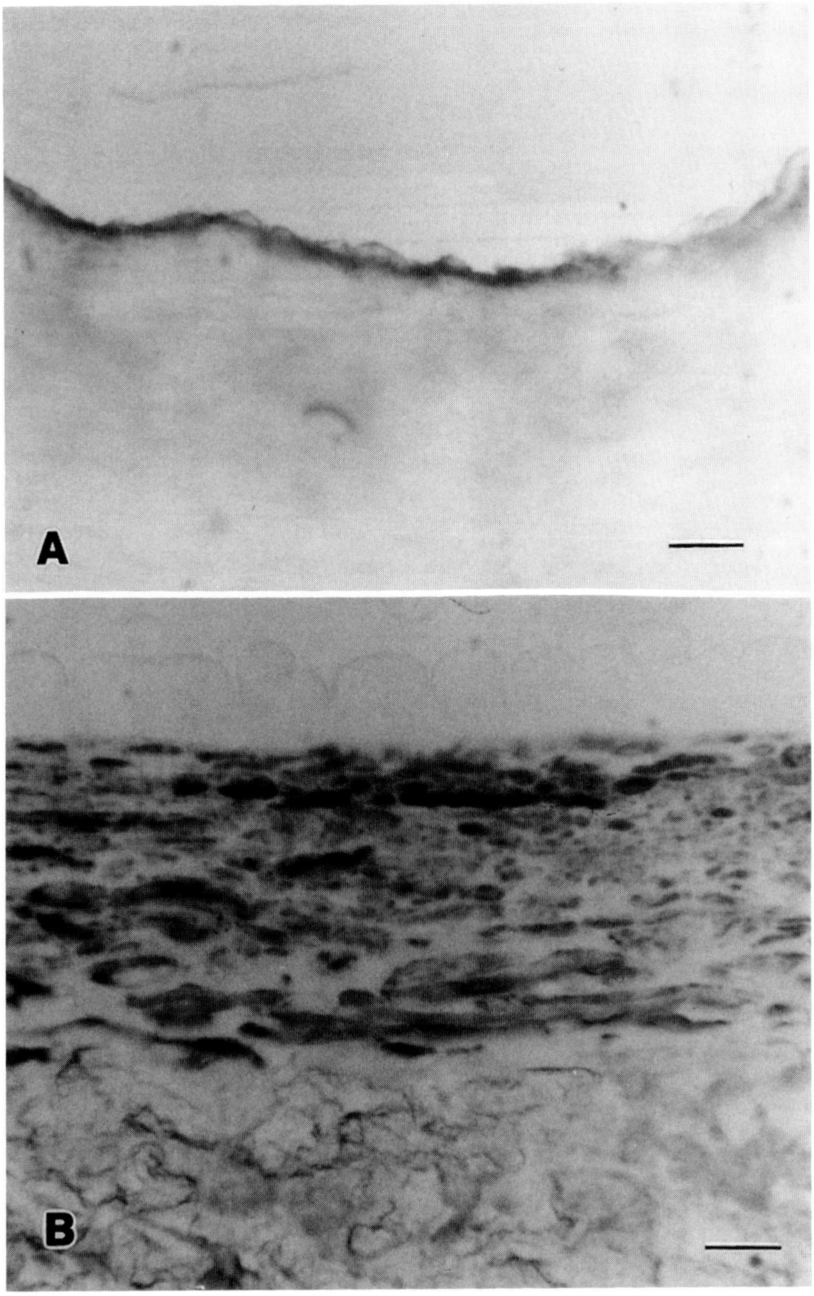

Figure 28-1. A—Immunosperoxidase staining of luminal surface positive for vWf (bar=14 microns). B—Thickened luminal lining staining positive with antibodies against α SMC actin (bar=14 microns).

Table 28-1. Inclusion and Exclusion Criteria for Sodded ePTFE Dialysis Access Trial

Inclusion criteria:	
	First-time access Previously failed access
Exclusion criteria:	
	Restricted inflow or outflow Active infection Lack of adequate subcutaneous fat Candidate for autogenous A-V fistula History of noncompliance Age < 18 or > 85 Life expectancy < 1 year

the inability in humans to spontaneously endothelialize the luminal surface.[3] Intimal hyperplasia, the underlying cause of most late graft thromboses, is a complex process that may involve hemodynamic and inflammatory factors centered around a response to injury. Hyperplasia frequently develops in proximity to the venous anastomosis, but may also occur at the arterial anastomosis or in the proximal outflow vein.[4] Regardless of the specific location in the rheologic circuit of the dialysis access, the end of this process is graft thrombosis. The mechanism of intimal hyperplasia is currently the focus of substantial research, as this process is a major factor not only in dialysis graft failure but also in thrombosis and failure of arterial bypass grafts and balloon angioplasty sites.[5] A primary relationship between thrombogenicity and intimal hyperplasia is hypothesized, but the mechanism remains ill-defined[6].

Our experience with endothelial cell (EC) sodding of vascular prosthetic grafts in the arterial circulation has been applied to arteriovenous (A-V) dialysis access grafts in an attempt to improve their long-term patency. *In vivo* and *in vitro* research conducted over the past decade has shown that coverage of the luminal surface of a prosthetic vascular graft with a confluent monolayer of ECs can prolong patency through modulation of both thrombogenicity and anastomotic intimal hyperplasia.[7-10] Our specific technique employs microvessel EC isolated from liposuction-derived adipose tissue and instilled under pressure (sodded) at confluent density into the interstices of expanded polytetrafluoroethylene (ePTFE). This method allows procurement of the ECs and graft preparation at the same time as graft implantation and is compatible with the operating room environment.[9]

Animal Experiments

In experiments using a canine model, paired sodded and control A-V grafts were created in the femoral position in a loop configuration. For the canine model, falciform ligament adipose tissue was used as the source for microvessel endothelial cells (MVEC). Grafts sodded with MVECs remained patent up to nine weeks. In contrast, all control grafts were clotted at the time of explant. Immunohistochemical analysis revealed von Willebrand factor (vWf) positive cells lining the experimental grafts from the arterial to the venous anastomosis. The cellular lining varied in thickness from a monolayer to regions that were several cell layers in thickness (figure 28-1). Where multiple layers were encountered, the surface cells stained positive for vWf, whereas the underlying cells stained positively for α smooth-muscle-cell (SMC) actin. The results of these *in vivo* experiments were used as the basis for proceeding with a study in human dialysis access patients.

Patients and Methods

The protocol for this randomized prospective study of 100 patients received approval from the Human Subjects Committee of the Institutional Review Boards at the University of Arizona Health Sciences Center and Kino Community Hospital, Tucson, Arizona. Patients in need of an A-V graft for hemodialysis access are eligible for inclusion in the study, as outlined in table 28-1 along with exclusion criteria. Eligible patients entered onto the study undergo a complete medical evaluation. Specific attention is paid to measuring blood pressure in all extremities; doing a complete hematologic, lipid, biochemical and coagulation profile; and performing a noninvasive vascular examination of potential access site extremities. The site of graft placement is left to the discretion of the surgeon based upon the preoperative evaluation, but most grafts to date have been in a loop configuration. Thus far, all patients have been treated under general anesthesia. All patients receive preoperative parenteral antibiotics (either cephazolin or vancomycin) before surgery. Just before surgery, patients randomized to receive an experimental graft are phlebotomized of 150 cc of blood to obtain serum for sodding the prosthesis.

The abdomen and the site for graft placement are prepped and draped. To obtain adipose tissue for MVEC isolation, liposuction of subcutaneous fat from the abdominal wall is performed with a liposuction cannula and specially designed 60-cc syringe. Approximately 50 g of fat (50 cc of aspirate) is required to adequately cover the luminal surface of the prosthetic graft at confluent cell density (1×10^5 cells/cm^2). This usually requires several passes of the cannula in different directions through the panniculus of the abdominal wall. All passes are made through a single 0.5 cm incision below or at the umbilicus. The fat is then washed and digested for 20 minutes in collagenase (4 mg/cc) containing 1% human serum albumin at 37°C with constant agitation. The resulting fat slurry is centrifuged at 100 *g* for seven minutes to pellet the vascular elements and separate them from the adipocytes and other components. Following a second wash, the MVECs are suspended in sodding media comprising M199 media (Gibco) and autologous patient serum 6:1, v:v). An aliquot of cell suspension is counted on a Coulter Counter to determine the cell concentration. On average, 1×10^6 MVECs are obtained from each gram of liposuction fat. Except for the collagenase digest, all cell isolation procedures are carried out in the operating room at room temperature (the collagenase digest is performed in a 37°C water bath).

Once liposuction has been completed, surgical exposure of the vessels for access creation is accomplished concurrent with the cell isolation and graft preparation procedures. Deposition of the MVEC on the luminal surface of the 6-mm ePTFE graft is performed using a pressure sodding technique. The cell suspension is diluted with enough sodding media to yield a cell density on the graft surface of twice confluence ($2x10^5$ cells/cm^2) and is injected into the graft. Additional sodding media is placed into a syringe and connected to the graft lumen along with an in-line pressure gauge. Four graft volumes of sodding media are then injected through the graft at 5 psi, thus completing the sodding procedure. The average time from liposuction to graft availability is 50 minutes.

The sodded graft is then implanted in the usual manner of other vascular prostheses. Care is taken to avoid kinking the sodded graft. Standard vascular surgery techniques are used to create the arterial and venous anastomoses using either 6-0 ePTFE or polypropylene suture in an end-to-side configuration. The venous anastomosis is completed, first using a venotomy at least 1.5 cm long. The outflow vein must have a minimum size of 3.5 mm. During the implantation procedure, the luminal surface is kept moist by dripping sodding media through the graft. Clamps are not applied to the graft itself; therefore, both the arterial and venous anastomoses are completed before flow is allowed through the graft. Both control and experimental graft recipients receive 2,500 U of I.V. heparin before vessel clamping. Once the graft is completed, intraoperative assessment is performed using palpation and interrogation with a hand-held Doppler.

Within 14 days of placement, all grafts are evaluated using a color flow Doppler duplex scanner (ATL Ultramark 9, Advanced Technology Labs, Bothell, Virginia). The arterial and venous anastomoses, as well as three evenly spaced areas in the midportion of the graft, are examined with color flow Doppler and B-mode imaging as well as Doppler determination of flow velocity. Following initiation of dialysis, usually more than two weeks postoperatively, each patient is monitored for venous pressure on a weekly basis. Additional graft monitoring includes calculation of recirculation percentage at a flow rate of 400 cc/min and color flow Doppler and duplex imaging every three months. Indications for further evaluation employing angiography include recirculation percentage of > 15%, venous pressure of > 150 mm Hg at a flow rate of 200-225 cc/min, or a detection of a stenosis of > 50% by noninvasive imaging either in the graft or at one of the anastomoses.

All patients are followed by the protocol outlined above. Study end points are listed in table 28-2. If a patient already enrolled in the study requires placement of a new graft, the second graft is of the same type (sodded or control) as the initial access. Follow-up of patients continues even after an end point is reached. Statistical analysis of access graft patency is reported using the life table and log rank methods. When appropriate, graft material is retrieved from study patients and subjected to evaluation using immunohistochemistry and electron microscopy.

Results

The results for the first 18 patients enrolled in the study have been compiled. Ten sodded grafts and eight control grafts have been placed in 12 females and 6 males. The control group comprises two males and six females who had placement of five upper-arm and three forearm loop grafts as first-time access in three patients and

Table 28-2. Sodded ePTFE Dialysis Access Graft Study End Points

Graft thrombosis
Need for intervention
Loss to follow-up > 60 days
Graft infection
Successful transplant
Initiation of CAPD
Refusal of dialysis
Death

Figure 2. Cumulative Patency of ePTFE Dialysis Access Grafts

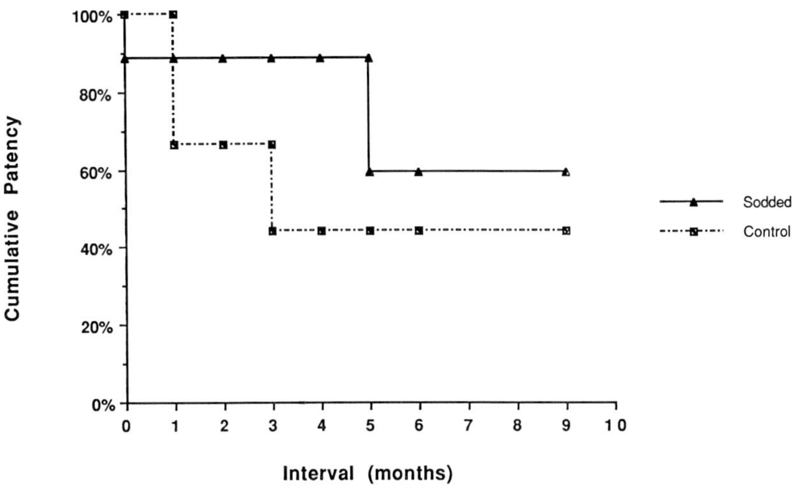

Figure 28-2. Cumulative patency of sodded ePTFE and control dialysis access grafts.

revisional access in five patients. The etiology of end-stage renal disease (ESRD) in the control group includes diabetes mellitus and hypertension in seven patients and lupus nephritis in one patient. No significant perioperative complications occurred in this group. In the sodded group, six females and four males had construction of five first-time and five revisional access grafts including one thigh, four upper-arm, and five forearm loop configurations. ESRD resulted from diabetes and hypertension in seven patients, polycystic kidney disease in one patient, lupus nephritis in one patient, and obstructive nephropathy in one patient. One patient developed a significant abdominal wall hematoma following liposuction that required transfusion of 2 U of packed red blood cells. Another patient had graft failure and thrombosis within the first week, requiring reoperation and replacement with a control graft. This patient, with lupus, was noted to have a thickened coagulum within her serum at the time of graft preparation.

Because of the small number of patients and the preliminary nature of this report, no attempt has been made to compare the groups in terms of demographic variables. Life table and log rank analysis of patency reveals no significant difference between the two groups at nine months follow-up; however, due to the small number of

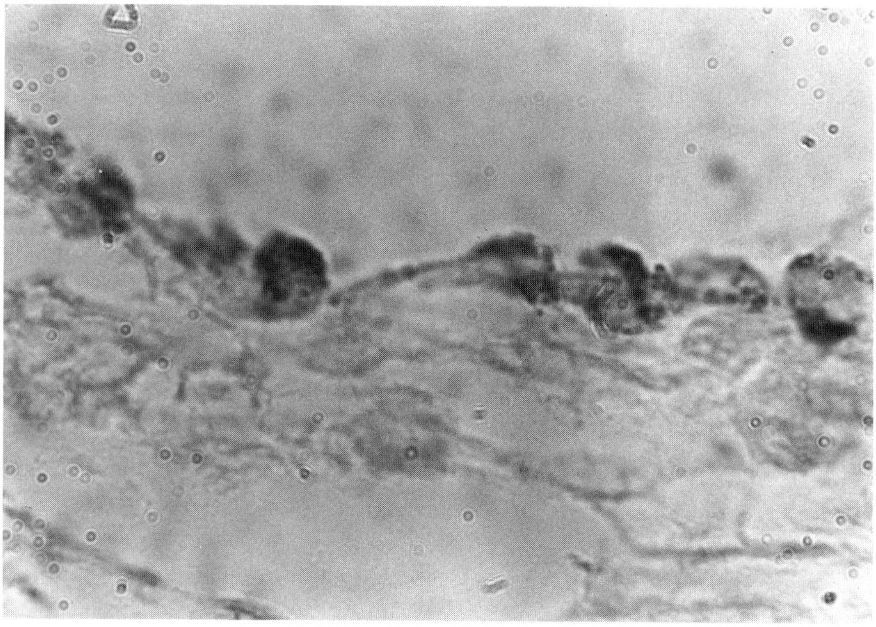

Figure 28-3. High-power view of human sodded dialysis access graft staining luminal cells positive for vWf (x1250).

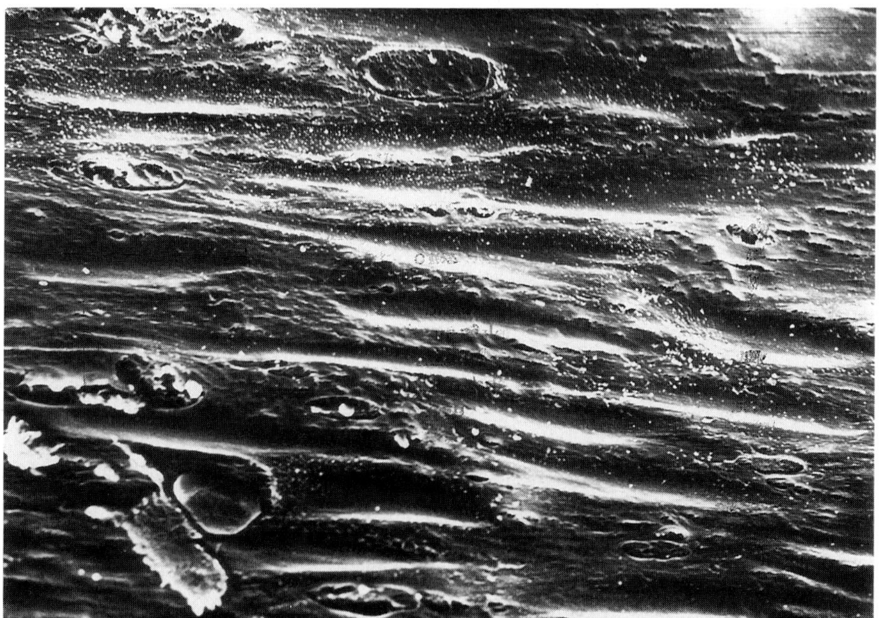

Figure 28-4. High-power scanning electron microscopy of luminal surface of human sodded dialysis access graft demonstrating ECs in a cobblestone configuration (x100).

patients in each group, the standard errors are quite large at the evaluated intervals (figure 28-2).

One patient died from sepsis unrelated to the access graft procedure a month and a half after placement. At the time the patient expired the sodded graft was patent and was immediately excised postmortem by permission of the patient's family. Immunohistochemistry performed on the graft demonstrates vWf-positive cells lining the surface throughout the length of the graft (figure 28-3). The amount and thickness of cells and matrix beneath the luminal layer varied but uniformly stained positive for α SMC actin. Scanning electron microscopy of the excised sodded graft displays a cellular lining comprising elongated cells in a cobblestone configuration characteristic of vascular ECs (figure 28-4).

Discussion

Maintaining vascular access for hemodialysis remains a major contributor to the morbidity and costs associated with ESRD.[1] Since their introduction in the mid 1970s, prosthetic grafts constructed of ePTFE are the most common forms of hemodialysis access.[11,12] However, despite their many advantages, including ease of placement, ready accessibility for dialysis, and ease of thrombectomy when clotted, little has been accomplished over the past two decades to prolong the primary patency of ePTFE and other prosthetic dialysis access grafts.

The fundamental process accounting for most access graft failures is intimal hyperplasia. This most commonly occurs in proximity to the venous anastomosis, but may also occur at the arterial anastomosis, in the proximal outflow vein, and at similar sites in autogenous A-V fistulas. Pursuit of the mechanism of intimal hyperplasia is the focus of much research in both access grafts and lower extremity arterial bypass grafts. Many theories have been postulated to explain the events that result in intimal hyperplasia. These include a response-to-injury theory, an immune-regulated theory, and a vessel-response-to-disturbed-hemodynamics theory. Fillinger and Kerns recently reviewed the available literature surrounding these processes and described many of the biologic factors that may play a role in the hyperplastic response.[4] It is not surprising that this exhaustive list of potential mediators includes many EC-derived elements.[13-15] The exact role that vascular endothelium plays is not clear; however, a goal of the present study is determining the functional significance of an intact EC layer within the lumen of a prosthetic dialysis access graft in regulating the evolution of intimal hyperplasia.

In an effort to improve patency, our experience with transplantation of MVECs onto the surface of experimental arterial grafts and canine A-V grafts has been expanded to a trial in human prosthetic dialysis access grafts. Our laboratory and others have shown that formation of an intact EC lining on a prosthetic graft may reduce thrombogenicity and prolong patency.[16-18] To accelerate this process, we have developed an O.R.-compatible method to isolate MVECs from liposuction-derived fat and place them on the lumen of a prosthetic graft at confluent density using a pressure sodding technique.[19] A significant criticism of this methodology has been the EC nature of the isolated cells and the origin of the cells lining the graft over time after EC sodding. The EC character of these cells has been verified using immunohistochemistry and electron microscopy.[20] Furthermore, using the membrane intercalating fluorescent dye PKH-26 (Xynaxis Cell Science Inc, Malver, Pennsylvania), sodded-liposuction-derived MVECs have been demonstrated to persist on the luminal surface for up to five weeks in a canine model.[21]

The hypothesis that sodding prosthetic A-V grafts with fat-derived MVECs will result in prolonged patency was tested in a canine model using 4-mm femoral ePTFE grafts.[22] In this paired graft study, all sodded grafts were patent at explant up to five weeks, whereas all control grafts were clotted. Immunohistochemical analysis and electron microscopy revealed a cellular lining on the luminal surface that demonstrated morphologic characteristics of ECs.

As noted, the present report consists of our results with the first 18 patients in a randomized, prospective trial of sodded ePTFE dialysis access grafts. The cumulative primary patency of the sodded grafts (63%) exceeds that obtained in the control group (44%) at nine months' follow-up. Unfortunately, the small number of patients in each group and resultant large standard errors yields no statistical significance in this comparison. What can be concluded from these preliminary data is that the method of sodding ePTFE dialysis access grafts with liposuction-derived MVECs is possible at the time of graft implantation without drastically prolonging the operative procedure. The method appears to be safe, as only one patient sustained significant complication due to the sodding technique. Although the number of patients in each group is small, the performance of the sodded grafts appears to be equivalent to standard ePTFE access grafts. The availability of limited tissue for detailed morphologic evaluation limits the conclusions that may be reached about survival of the MVEC lining after graft implantation and once dialysis has been initiated. However, the results of immunohistochemistry and scanning microscopy of the retrieved patent sodded graft suggests persistence of a cellular lining with EC characteristics up to 45 days after implantation and after the commencement of hemodialysis through the access.

Questions of prolonging patency and attenuating intimal hyperplasia by sodding the ePTFE grafts remain to be answered. Concomitant with the accrual of more patient experience is the expansion of our ability to access biologic factors that may play a role in regulating thrombogenicity and hyperplasia. Currently under investigation in both *in vitro* and *in vivo* experiments in our lab are morphologic studies using antibodies to growth factors, adhesion molecules, integrins, and cytokines in an effort to better elucidate the mechanism of intimal hyperplasia and interaction at the blood/polymer interface. Together with the ongoing clinical trial of sodded prosthetic access grafts, this effort represents a multidisciplinary approach to the significant health care issue of maintaining dialysis access.

References

1. Lazarus JM, Huang WH, Lew NL, Lowrie EG. Contribution of vascular access-related disease to morbidity of hemodialysis patients. In: ML Henry & RM Ferguson, eds. Vascular access for hemodialysis—III. Chicago: W.L. Gore & Associates, Inc., Precept Press, 1993;3-13.

2. Palder SB, Kirkman RL, Whittemore AD, et al. Vascular access for hemodialysis. Ann Surg 1986; 202:235-239.
3. Berger K, Sauvage LR, Rao AM, Wood SJ. Healing of arterial prostheses in man: Its incompleteness. Ann Surg 1972; 175:118-127.
4. Fillinger MF, Kerns DB, Bruch D, Reinitz ER, Schwartz RA. Does end-to-end anastomosis offer a functional advantage over end-to-side anastomosis in high output arteriovenous grafts? J Vasc Surg 1990; 12:676-690.
5. Clowes AW, Clowes MM, Fingerle J, Reidy MA. Kinetics of cellular proliferation after arterial injury. V. Role of acute distention in the induction of smooth muscle proliferation. Lab Invest 1989; 60:360-364.
6. Williams SK. Regulation of intimal hyperplasia: Do endothelial cells participate? Lab Invest 1991; 64:721-723.
7. Sharefkin JB, Latker C, Smith M, et al. Early normalization of platelet survival by endothelial seeding of Dacron arterial prostheses in dogs. Surgery 1982; 92:385-393.
8. Graham LM, Stanley JC, Burkel WE. Improved patency of endothelial-cell-seeded, long knitted Dacron and ePTFE vascular prostheses. ASAIO 1982; 8:65-73.
9. Jarrell BE, Williams SK, Stokes G, et al. Use of freshly isolated capillary endothelial cells for the immediate establishment of a monolayer on vascular grafts at surgery. Surgery 1986; 100:392-39.
10. Williams SK, Jarrell BE. Thrombosis on endothelializable prostheses. In: E Leonard, V Turitto, L Vroman, eds. Biomaterials research, Ann New York Acad Sci 1987; 516:145-157.
11. Baker LD, Johnson JM, Goldfarb D. Expanded polytetrafluoroethylene (PTFE) subcutaneous arteriovenous conduit: an improved vascular access for chronic hemodialysis. Trans Am Soc Artif Intern Organs 1976; 22:382-387.
12. Rizzuti RP, Burkart TE. Extended patency of expanded polytetrafluoroethylene grafts for vascular access using optimal configuration and revisions. Surg Gynecol Obstet 1988; 160:23-27.
13. Sumpio BE, Banes AJ, Levin LG, Johnson G. Mechanical stress stimulates aortic endothelial cells to proliferate. J Vasc Surg 1987; 6:252-256.
14. Fingerle J, AU YPT, Clowes AW, Reidy MA. Intimal lesion formation in rat carotid arteries after endothelial denudation in the absence of medial injury. Arteriosclerosis 1990; 10: 1082-1087.
15. Sharefkin JB, Diamond SL, Eskin SG, McIntire LV, Diffenbach CW. Fluid flow decreases preproendothelin mRNA levels and suppresses endothelin-1 peptide release in cultured human endothelial cell. J Vasc Surg 1991; 14:1-9.
16. Williams SK, Rose DG, Jarrell BE. Microvessel endothelial cell sodding of ePTFE vascular grafts: Improved patency and stability of the cellular lining. J Biomed Mat Res (in press).
17. Douville EC, Kempczinski RP, Birinyi LK, Ramalanjoana GR. Impact of endothelial cell seeding on long-term patency and subendothelial proliferation in a small-caliber highly porous polytetrafluoroethylene graft. J Vasc Surg 1987; 5:544-550.
18. Herring M, Gardner AL, Glover JA. A single-staged technique for seeding vascular grafts with autogenous endothelium. Surgery 1978; 84:498-504.
19. Williams SK, Jarrell BE, Rose DG, et al. Human microvessel endothelial cell isolation and vascular graft sodding in the operating room. Ann Vasc Surg 1989; 3:146-152.
20. Williams SK, Wang TF, Castrillo R, Jarrell BE. Human liposuction derived fat used for vascular graft sodding contains endothelial cells and not mesothelial cells as the major cell type. J Vasc Surg (in press).

21. Williams SK, Kleinert LB, Rose D, McKenney S. Origin of endothelial cells that line ePTFE vascular grafts sodded with cells from microvascularized fat. J Vasc Surg (in press).
22. Williams SK, Jarrell BE, Kleinert LB. Endothelial cell transplantation onto polymeric arteriovenous grafts evaluated using a canine model. J Invest Surg (in press).

29

CARBON-PTFE VERSUS STANDARD-PTFE A-V BRIDGE GRAFTS FOR CHRONIC HEMODIALYSIS

P. Bourquelot, M.D., J. Stolba, M.D., P. Cheret, M.D., F. Fournier, M.D., and A. Mouton, M.D.

IN VIEW OF THE FREQUENCY AND SEVERITY of the complications observed with the use of hemodialysis access arteriovenous (A-V) grafts, it seemed useful to evaluate a new polytetrafluoroethylene (PTFE) graft whose internal lumen is composed of a combination of PTFE and carbon, in comparison with a standard PTFE graft.

Materials and Methods

Between October 1, 1989, and July 1, 1991, 94 consecutive patients (39 males, 55 females) received 50 standard PTFE grafts (W.L. Gore & Associates, Flagstaff, Arizona) and 50 carbon-PTFE grafts (Impra, Tempe, Arizona) for chronic hemodialysis vascular access. (The U.S. Food and Drug Administration authorized the use of the carbon-PTFE graft.) Both of these grafts have a thin wall with an internal diameter of 6 mm. This was a randomized, prospective study. The mean age of the patients was 56 years (range: 9-89 years). Nine patients were insulin-dependent diabetics, and one of them had positive HIV serology. None of these patients had a superficial vein in the upper limb that could be used for the creation of an A-V fistula.

Almost all of the bridge grafts were performed linearly, either in the forearm (n = 69), arm (n = 29), or thigh (n = 2). Grafts in the forearm were performed under preventive hemostasis with a pneumatic tourniquet.[1] Perioperative prophylactic antistaphylococcal antibiotic therapy was administered in every case. Puncture of the graft was authorized from the tenth postoperative day forward.

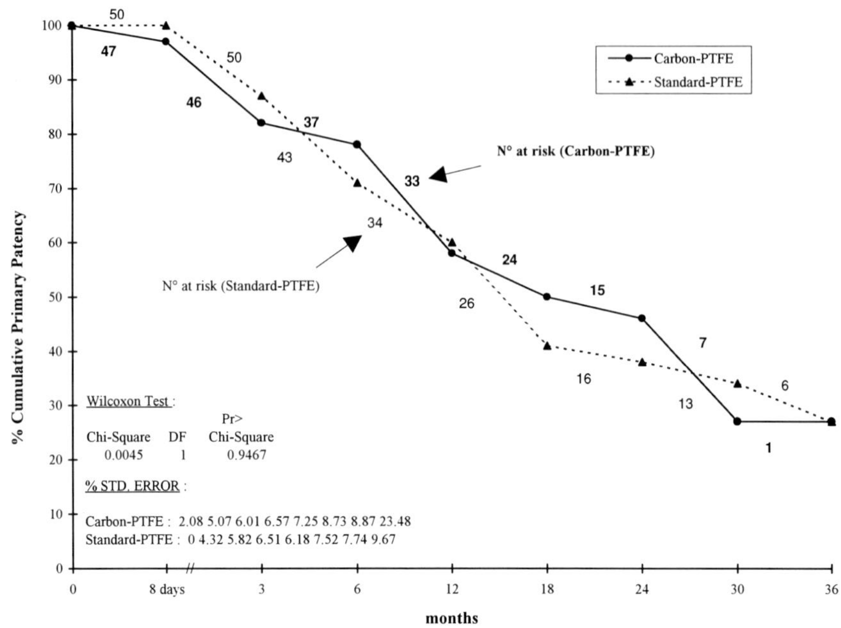

Figure 29-1. Primary patency of carbon-PTFE and standard-PTFE grafts: life table analysis.

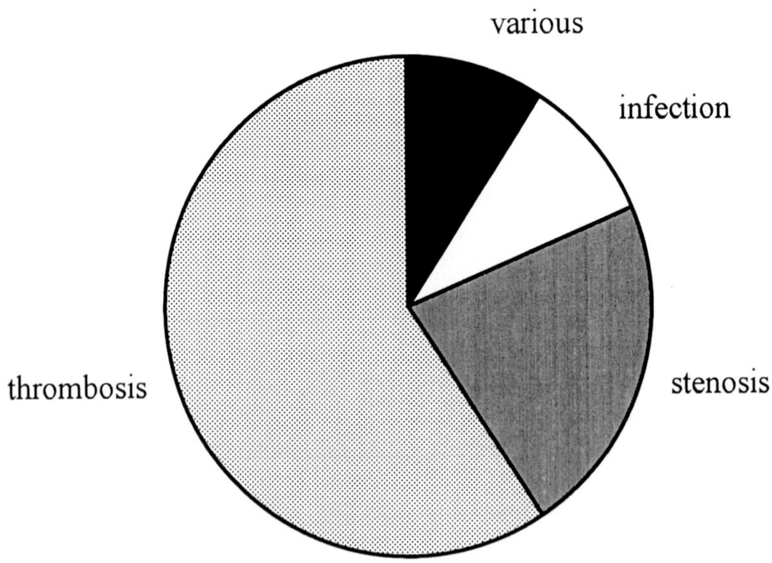

Figure 29-2. Primary complications observed in 97 grafts.

The evaluation criterion was the primary patency of the graft, and failure was defined as the development of the first complication. It should be noted that, in addition to classical complications such as thrombosis or infection, we also considered simple stenosis of the venous anastomosis to be a primary complication, whether it was detected by increased pressure in the graft or on routine angiographic or Doppler examination. All stenoses were considered to be hemodynamically significant and were treated. The primary objective of patient follow-up was, therefore, to assess the incidence of any type of complication, whether or not it was amenable to treatment.

Results

Three grafts, implanted in three patients who were immediately lost to follow-up, were excluded from the study. Thirty grafts were patent, with no complications, at the end of the study. Eight patients died, and five who underwent kidney transplantation had no complications. Comparison of the actuarial survival curves in terms of primary patency of the two groups of grafts did not demonstrate any significant difference (figure 29-1). Complications were observed in 24 cases of carbon-PTFE grafts and 30 cases of standard PTFE grafts. Distribution of the complications is shown in figure 29-2.

Early postoperative complications included one patient with an excessively deep subcutaneous tunnel, one with high flow rate and poor cardiac tolerance, one patient with limb acute ischemia, one with massive edema of the upper limb due to stenosis of a proximal vein, and one patient with periprosthetic seroma. These five patients were treated by ligation of the graft. Infection occurred in one patient early postoperatively (gram-negative infection) and four late infections at puncture sites. These were treated by excision of the graft. Eleven cases were treated by percutaneous transluminal angioplasty and one was treated by surgical angioplasty.[2]

Eighteen patients were treated locally. Fifteen successful radiological interventions using a combination of urokinase (UK)-aspiration-percutaneous endoluminal angioplasty were performed.[3] Three surgical manipulations were performed by grafting the venous anastomosis (one failure of UK, one in an intraoperative thrombosis, and one associated thrombosis of the brachial artery). Fourteen patients were treated by other teams. This included four successful surgical interventions and four surgical treatments followed by immediate or early failure, and six neglected thromboses.

Discussion

Carbon has been used in implantable biomaterials since 1960. Many papers have demonstrated its biocompatibility and lack of reactivity, even with blood products, particularly in the field of vascular prostheses.[4-7] These studies demonstrated a lower thrombogenicity of carbon, which is generally attributed to the negative charge on its surface. A negatively charged surface reacts less with blood cells, thereby reducing the thrombogenicity of the implant. The capacity of carbon to adsorb proteins is another factor responsible for this decreased thrombogenicity, especially when albumin is preferentially adsorbed.[4,7,8]

The carbon-PTFE graft used in this study is manufactured from active carbon powder complying with the purity standards of the United States Pharmacopeia. Carbon is an integral part of the internal wall of the graft. The general characteristics of this graft are similar to those of the usual standard PTFE graft.

For the purposes of statistical analysis, this study compared two types of grafts implanted, according to a randomized order, in 94 consecutive patients. The results were analyzed by the actuarial survival method. The onset of the first complication (primary patency) was studied, as studies based on secondary patency appear to be more representative of a certain degree of technical skill than of the intrinsic quality of the grafts used. The primary patency rates observed in this small patient sample are very similar to those reported by Mehta in his critical review of a large number of cases published in the literature. In his report, Mehta cited primary patency rates of 61% for one year, 37% for two years, and 22% for three years.[9] In the present study, these rates were 60% for one year, 38% for two years, and 28% for three years.

For a long time, it was thought that use of hemodialysis access grafts should be accompanied by an aggressive surgical approach to complications in order to preserve the patency of these grafts. This might even be at the cost of frequent surgical operations, which are unpleasant and sometimes dangerous for the patient. This attitude appears to be changing due to the influence of several factors: (1) the use of central venous catheters introduced via the internal jugular vein allowing temporary dialysis of the patient in the absence of an A-V vascular access; (2) prevention of thromboses by detection and treatment of stenosis of the venous anastomosis by percutaneous endoluminal angioplasty; and (3) percutaneous approach of thromboses treated by UK, with a high immediate success rate.[10] All of the postoperative complications and infectious complications in our series were treated surgically and not conservatively, while almost all of the stenoses of the venous anastomoses were treated conservatively and percutaneously. A slight (but not statistically significant), difference in the primary complication rate was observed between the two types of grafts. The major complication was stenosis of the venous anastomosis, causing thrombosis of the graft if left untreated. Together with the primary complications associated with this stenosis (simple stenosis and stenosis complicated by thrombosis), this lesion was responsible for 81% of the primary complications observed, affecting 40% of the carbon-PTFE grafts and 48% of the standard-PTFE grafts. This complication is probably related to the high flow rate and its associated turbulence rather than to the particular features of the different grafts.

Conclusion

This study of 100 chronic hemodialysis access grafts did not demonstrate a statistical superiority of the carbon-PTFE graft over the standard-PTFE graft in terms of primary patency, which was 28% at three years. However, an improvement associated with the use of carbon might be demonstrated on a longer follow-up and in a larger series of grafts. This study reconfirms that stenosis of the venous anastomosis is the main primary complication of A-V grafts, representing 81% of all complications, and demonstrates the major role of percutaneous endovascular techniques in the current management of vascular accesses.

References

1. Bourquelot P. Preventive haemostasis with an inflatable tourniquet for microsurgical distal arteriovenous fistulas for haemodialysis. Microsurgery 1993; 14:462-463.
2. Turmel-Rodrigues L, Pengloan J, Blanchier D, et al. Insufficient dialysis shunts: improved long-term patency rates with close hemodynamic monitoring, repeated percutaneous balloon angioplasty, and stent placement. Radiology 1993; 187:273-278.
3. Poulain F, Raynaud A, Bourquelot P, Knight C, Rovani X, Gaux JC. Local thrombolysis and thromboaspiration in the treatment of acutely thrombosed arteriovenous hemodialysis fistulas. Cardiovasc Interv Radiol 1991; 14:98-101.
4. Haubold AD, Shim HS, Bokros JC. Carbon in medical devices. In: DF Williams, ed. Biocompatibility of clinical implants material—vol. II. Boca Raton: CRC Press, 1990; 3-42.
5. Haubold AD, Norman JC. Ultra low temperature isotropically deposited carbon (biolyte): a promising new flexible interfacing biomaterial. Bull Tex Heart Inst Cardiovasc Dis 1992; 4:369-370.
6. Roon AJ, Moore WS, Golstone J, Campana G. Comparative surface thrombogenicity of implanted vascular grafts. J Surg Res 1977; 22:165-173.
7. Tschuchida H, Cameron BL, Marcus SC, Hye RJ. Indium 111-labeled platelet deposition on carbon-lined and high-porosity PTFE grafts. J Vasc Surg 1992; 16:643-650.
8. Clowes AW, Kirkman TR, Reidy MA. Mechanism of arterial grafts healing. Am J Pathol 1986; 123:220-230.
9. Mehta S. Statistical summary of clinical results of vascular access procedures for hemodialysis. In: BG Sommer, ML Henry, eds. Vascular access for hemodialysis—II. Chicago: W.L. Gore & Associates, Inc., and Precept Press, 1991; 145-157.
10. Roberts AC, Valji K, Bookstein JJ, Hye RJ. Pulse-spray pharmacomechanical thrombolysis for treatment of thrombosed dialysis access grafts. Am J Surg 1993; 166:221-226.

DISCUSSION

Moderator:

Ronald M. Ferguson, M.D., Ph.D.

Panelists:

Scott S. Berman, M.D.
P. Bourquelet, M.D.
John O. Colonna II, M.D.
Frantz J. Derenoncourt, M.D.
Jan H. M. Tordoir, M.D.

Discussant: Dr. Berman, my question is about your technique. Do you harvest arterial or venous endothelial cells, or is there no distinction? Are you seeing predominantly arterial or venous patterns with those cells?

Dr. Berman: These actually are capillary endothelial cells. We have shown all of the different cells in culture, arterial and venous. These are multiple types of endothelial cells, so I'm not really sure how yours compare. There are not a lot of data on the functionality of these cells once they are placed on a graft.

Discussant: We have found in the histologic examinations of stenotic lesions harvested from A-V fistulas that there is a lot denudation of the lining in the area of stenosis, in that only part of the stenosis is covered with endothelial cells. We think it is because of the high flow going by these cells. Do you think the seeded endothelial cells can resist these high shear rates in the graft?

Dr. Berman: Yes, we have shown that in animal studies, the cells persist as soon as flow is restored. Thirty minutes after the fact, the cells are still there. In our one human, endothelial cells are still there. Also, a few years ago a patient had a mesocaval sodded graft placed. It had to be revised, and at the time of revision there were still cells that had characteristics of endothelial cells. We have addressed this again in some more animal experiments where we fluorescently labeled the cells and sodded them. Up to five weeks after the cells are implanted on the lumen of the graft, they still display the fluorescent label, so we think that they persist and can hang on in the circulation. Part of the difficulty is getting them into the interstices of the graft.

Discussant: The early experience with the stretch graft reported by Dr. Dawidson was positive, and now we seem to have corroboration in the papers of Dr. Tordoir and Dr. Derenoncourt. The stretch graft seems to decrease the risk of complications, increase the primary patency rate, and decrease the early onset of graft stenosis. Dr. Tordoir, you mentioned those improvements but you did not mention the time period for follow-up.

Dr. Tordoir: The mean follow-up was 10 months. All patients were followed by serial duplex scannings from two weeks postoperatively to one year or more. We could see early on, even after two to six months, that there were stenotic lesions, especially in the expanded group. We don't know the reason for this high incidence of stenosis in this expanded group compared to the test group. Maybe the tests were made to exhibit better performance and compliance, as we have demonstrated, or maybe you can link it to the better meshing in the anastomosis and better configuration with less kinking. We don't know yet, but we are going to look at that in a prospective study.

Discussant: Dr. Berman, would you care to speculate how sodding of the PTFE might help in controlling the cause of failure, most of which is fibromuscular ingrowth at the venous end of these grafts?

Dr. Berman: If you look at the theories behind intimal hyperplasia, they revolve around inflammation, or there are some theories that propose angiogenesis. Some people believe that it is just clot that stimulates an inflammatory reaction, so our hope is that by putting down an endothelial cell surface on the graft, the endothelial cells are going to interact with the circulation so that the environment for hyperplasia is not initiated. Part of this involves better definitions of the entire mechanism. We are now at the point where there are so many different adhesion molecules involved and cell-cell interactions that those are the things that we are starting to investigate. We are interested as to what the endothelial cells that we put down do as far as causing platelets and leukocytes to stick and what's the role of that sticking in promoting clot and then hyperplasia. That's pretty much where our research is going and that is the theory that we are hoping to develop to explain how it would modulate hyperplasia.

INDEX